Children and Adolescents with Mental Health Problems

by

Wendy Sharman

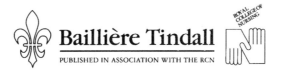

Baillière Tindall
PUBLISHED IN ASSOCIATION WITH THE RCN

London Philadelphia Toronto Sydney Tokyo

Baillière Tindall   24–28 Oval Road
London NW1 7DX

The Curtis Center
Independence Square West
Philadelphia, PA 19106–3399, USA

Harcourt Brace & Company
55 Horner Avenue
Toronto, Ontario, M8Z 4X6, Canada

Harcourt Brace & Company, Australia
30–52 Smidmore Street
Marrickville
NSW 2204, Australia

Harcourt Brace & Company, Japan
Ichibancho Central Building
22–1 Ichibancho
Chiyoda-ku, Tokyo 102, Japan

A catalogue record for this book is available from the British Library

ISBN 0-7020-1920-8

Typeset by Saxon Graphics Ltd., Derby
Printed and bound in Great Britain by Bath Press, Lower Bristol Road, Bath

CONTENTS

ACKNOWLEDGEMENTS

I would like to thank Stuart, and my parents, for their endless support, patience and encouragement.

It is impossible to acknowledge all those to whom I am indebted for ideas. However, I would like to express my appreciation to Christopher Bennett, William Crouch, Joanne Early, Nicole Harris, Peter Honig, Rachel Ibbs, Lisa Lewer, Andy Player and Samantha Swinglehurst whose work I have described in some of the case examples. I would also like to thank Anna Tate for revising and updating her guidelines for school visits, and Jeanne Magagna for reading the text and giving me her valued opinion and encouragement. Thanks also to Louise Burston who with the help of her son Nicholas Foundoukis provided many of the illustrations you will see.

Finally I would like to thank those children who have given me permission to include their drawings in this book.

PREFACE

I would like this book to be of practical use for nurses working with children and adolescents in a variety of settings. If we are to provide holistic health care, mental health problems must be recognised in all areas of nursing.

Working therapeutically with children and adolescents, requires great resourcefulness. The medical or psychiatric diagnosis may give the nurse some pointers for intervention, but often she or he will be left asking: 'But what should I do now?', 'How do I begin to relate to a child who is so withdrawn?', '…manage this aggressive behaviour?' and so on. I hope that this book will offer lots of practical suggestions for nursing intervention and encourage further creativity. Rather than be concerned with diagnoses, I have chosen to focus on the problems experienced by children and their families. Related problems have been grouped together for each chapter. However, the grouping is somewhat contrived and the reader will undoubtedly need to look at several chapters when considering a particular child. I hope that my cross-referencing will make this process easier.

Although nurses might often feel as though they are left on the front line to deal with problems as and when they arise, it is essential that they work as part of a multi-disciplinary team. Only then can the child, or adolescent, and their family, receive the broad spectrum of expertise that is necessary to provide holistic health care. Therefore, in each chapter, I have attempted to place nursing intervention within the context of a multi-disciplinary team approach. Although this book is intended primarily for nurses, other health professionals may find it useful.

For ease of reading, I have used the word child to mean child or adolescent, unless specifically referring to either. It should be clear from the text when I am writing exclusively about children, and I have made it clear when I am referring to adolescents only.

1 A HOLISTIC APPROACH

Mental health is an important component of the total well-being of a child. It cannot be considered in isolation, but must be seen in conjunction with physical health and in the context of the environment in which the child lives.

'Mental health' is described by *Mosby's Pocket Dictionary of Nursing, Medicine and Allied Professions*, as **'a relative state of mind in which a person...is able to cope with, and adjust to, the recurrent stress of everyday living' (Anderson and Anderson, 1995, p. 450). Mental health problems will therefore occur when this state of equilibrium is upset.** Most of us, if not all of us, will have experienced such a disturbance, when we feel unable to manage or deal with stress in our lives. Children are no exception; they cannot be protected from all potential stressors and indeed need some exposure, in order to learn how to cope with difficult or new situations and adapt accordingly. Starting a new school, the birth of a sibling, illness, hospitalisation, examinations, are just a few important stressors which come readily to mind. Subsequently, there will be times when children fail to cope with, or adjust to, such life events. The reader should not be led into believing that mental health problems are caused solely by outside stress, but that mental health problems are said to occur when the individual is failing to cope. Outside stressors may contribute to the aetiology, but a number of other factors, such as genetic predisposition, will also be important.

The *Mosby Pocket Dictionary* describes holistic medicine as **'a system of comprehensive or total patient care that considers the physical, emotional, social, economic and spiritual needs of the person, his or her response to illness, and the impact of illness on the person's ability to meet self-care needs' (p. 344).** This definition can be applied to paediatrics if developmental parameters and the significance of the family are recognised. A child's ability to care for him or herself will depend on their stage of development, as well as the impact of their illness. The family, on whom the child is still dependent, must play an integral part in the provision of care and will subsequently need support. By virtue of its title, this book may not appear to address the holistic care of children, as it clearly focuses on mental health. However, my intention is that it should be used within the context of a holistic approach, and in this first chapter I would like to explain how. There are six key issues that I would like the reader to consider, which highlight the importance of a holistic approach and how it can be promoted:

- ◆ Mental health problems should be the concern of all nurses.
- ◆ Mental health problems should be identified in addition to medical diagnoses being made.
- ◆ A multi-disciplinary approach to treatment is essential.
- ◆ A multi-cultural approach to treatment is paramount.
- ◆ Holistic nursing requires a wide range of interventions.
- ◆ Ethical issues must be considered in treatment.

MENTAL HEALTH PROBLEMS: THE CONCERN OF ALL NURSES

Holistic medicine recognises that health is a question of balance between mind, body and the environment. There is a state of homoeostasis, so that changes in one part of the system will effect a change elsewhere. Therefore, mind and body cannot be separated: there is an interrelationship and nurses from all backgrounds must ensure that the physical and psychological needs of the child are met.

Two main trains of thought regarding health and illness have predominated medicine, to a greater or lesser extent, throughout history. They date back to ancient Greece, when the Gods Hygeia and Aesculapius symbolised opposing views. The hygeian school of thought was dominant until and through the middle ages, and considered ill-health to be the result of an imbalance in the way one lived, which produced symptoms reflecting underlying distress and encouraged a change to a more healthy lifestyle. For example, influenza might be seen as resulting from exhaustion and the symptoms encourage rest. In complete contrast, the aesculapian theory took the line that ill-health resulted from specific identifiable causes, which resulted in specific symptoms and responded to a specific treatment. This approach became dominant at the time of the Renaissance and has come to represent orthodox medicine. Man or woman was seen as being made up of many parts, such as the digestive tract and neurological system, which required separate and specialist treatment (Chase, 1988). This reductionist approach (reducing the body into small separate units) proved to be very useful in advancing medical knowledge and treatment. However, its limitations are now being realised, and there has been a shift back towards the notion that, just as in nature and ecology, the different components of man and woman are in a state of balance, with one another and the environment. For example, it has been demonstrated empirically that our psychological state will influence our physical well-being and vice versa.

Grey (1993) reviewed the literature on the association of environmental stressors with the physical and psychological health of children. Examples cited include: the precipitation of leukaemia symptoms 2 years after a significant life event, the association of stress with the exacerbation of asthma and diabetic ketoacidosis, and with maladaptive behaviour, poor school performance and suicidal behaviour. Fritz et al (1987) highlighted the significance of psychological factors in childhood death from asthma. Depression, emotional precipitation of asthmatic attacks, an unsupportive family and a tendency to deny asthma symptoms were revealed in case examples where the child died. Perhaps more obvious is the psychological trauma caused by physical ill-health or disability. For example, Chapman (1993) talks about the misery felt by visually impaired children and young people; the difficulties it causes in everyday living and learning; and the negative way they feel others perceive them. The incidence of emotional and behavioural problems is reported as being significantly higher amongst those who are hearing impaired (Bond, 1993), and the self-esteem of those with epilepsy is likely to be battered by the general misunderstanding and stigmatisation of this disorder (Besag, 1993).

Research has therefore highlighted the significance of a holistic approach to treatment. For example, if the parents of a diabetic child are aware that stress can precipitate ketoacidosis, they may be able to prevent it, by ensuring that the need for extra emotional support is anticipated together with increasing the child's carbohydrate intake. Similarly, a child who is having frequent asthmatic attacks may benefit from psychological treatments, such as individual counselling or family therapy, as well as physical treatment, and indeed the need for drugs may be reduced.

If we consider the relationship between mind and body, and the significance that this has on effective health care, mental health must be seen as a concern for all nurses. However, despite the present talk of a holistic approach to nursing, mental health problems still tend to be placed firmly in the psychiatric arena by educationalists and clinicians. However, in reality, all nurses working with children – psychiatric and paediatric nurses, health visitors, school nurses and so on – must be able to identify mental health problems and intervene appropriately. This is not to say that all nurses will intervene to the same degree. Depending on their training and expertise, nurses will differ in the extent of their involvement. Some may refer to other specialists after their own assessment, whereas others may provide a more extensive assessment and therapy.

All nurses should be able to work therapeutically with children and their families, but some may have additional, specific skills, such as family therapy training. I would expect all nurses to acquire some skills in individual work, although nurses working in child psychiatry will obviously have greater experience. Milieu therapy, that is creating a therapeutic environment, is an important component of child psychiatric nursing, but has relevance for nurses working in other areas. Similarly, working with groups of children or parents is more commonly seen in psychiatry, but can be, and often is, used to great benefit elsewhere. All nurses working with children must be able to work with families, providing education and support. The individual, milieu and group work described in this book is therefore written with all nurses in mind, with the proviso that nurses use their own professional judgement, in conjunction with multi-disciplinary team consultation, to decide the extent of their involvement. Some of the work with families that is mentioned is also appropriate for nursing staff, but 'family therapy' requires a trained family therapist. Similarly, 'individual psychoanalytic psychotherapy', as opposed to 'individual work', requires specialist training. The team, and ultimately the consultant responsible for the treatment of the child, must decide which professional is most suitable to undertake a particular aspect of assessment and/or therapy. Effective communication between professionals will also prevent duplication of similar work with a particular child and/or family, which could have a detrimental effect on overall treatment.

Clinical supervision will enable the nurse to stretch and develop her/his repertoire of skills, as well as provide valuable objective criticism, which is so important when dealing with emotional issues. It appears that many paediatric nurses lack confidence in caring for children with mental health problems, often worrying that they might say something that could exacerbate the child's problem and feeling unable to cope with challenging behaviour, such as aggression (Sharman, 1993). Improvements in nursing education and training will be important if we are to achieve holistic care, but nurses should also take responsibility for their own professional development.

IDENTIFYING MENTAL HEALTH PROBLEMS

Identifying mental health problems enables infinite permutations to be considered, whereas a psychiatric diagnosis is limited by a finite list of signs and symptoms. This is not to say that medical diagnoses are unimportant; on the contrary, they facilitate the advancement of medical knowledge and treatment, and can provide the parents and child with a tangible disorder to deal with. However, holistic medicine requires us to recognise the uniqueness of the individual, something that a diagnosis cannot do. Multi-axial systems of diagnosis do go some way towards achieving a holistic description of the individual's condition. Two such systems exist: the tenth edition of the International Classification of Diseases (ICD-10) published by the World Health Organisation (1992) and the fourth edition of the *Diagnostic and Statistical Manual* (DSM IV) of the American Psychiatric Association (1994). A systematic formulation is arrived at using a set of axes. For example, ICD-10 has five axes: clinical psychiatric syndrome, specific delays in development, intellectual development, medical conditions and abnormal psychosocial situations. However, this approach to diagnosis still has limitations in terms of achieving a truly individual formulation and, in particular, the child is still given the label of a psychiatric syndrome, which will have a definitive list of signs and symptoms.

From a nursing point of view, and certainly from a holistic viewpoint, it is perhaps more important to identify the current problems faced by the child and their family, in order to provide care that is relevant to the present time and truly comprehensive. Where children have been referred for psychiatric treatment, only some of these problems are likely to fall under the description of their diagnosis, and where the primary reason for referral is a physical disorder, the child's medical diagnosis is unlikely to include any mental health problems.

I have therefore chosen to identify mental health problems rather than diagnoses and each chapter in the book identifies a group of related problems. However, it is important to remember that there is a relationship between these groups of problems and therefore no chapter can be considered in isolation. For example, a child who is aggressive may also be sad; another may have physical symptoms, show signs of sadness and fear, and later reveal problems related to sexuality. When the reader is considering an individual child, several chapters of the book will need to be reviewed. There is a considerable amount of cross-referencing by the author in order to help this process and to avoid undue repetition.

As previously mentioned, psychiatric diagnoses are important for evaluating and comparing treatment for like disorders and thus making progress in health care. It is therefore essential that nurses have some knowledge of psychiatric diagnoses, as the diagnosis will direct her or him to relevant research findings concerning positive intervention. Psychiatric diagnoses are therefore mentioned in this book, but are by no means comprehensive.

THE MULTI-DISCIPLINARY TEAM

All illnesses probably have a multi-factorial aetiology. Physical and psychological factors in the environment and those inherited are likely to play a part in causing ill-health. Similarly, ill-health will have physical and psychological sequelae, which will in turn have social implications. Therefore, a multi-disciplinary approach to treatment is essential in order to provide the broad spectrum of expertise required for holistic medicine.

The significance of the multi-disciplinary team is highlighted by the 'illness network' described by Lask and Fosson (1989), which represents the complex series of interactions between the child, his or her illness, the family and extra-familial factors (Figure 1.1).

The illness network, and indeed the concept of holism, is based on systems theory: each component of the network affects the others. For example, the type of illness, the treatment required and the constraints that either impose will influence the reaction of the child, family

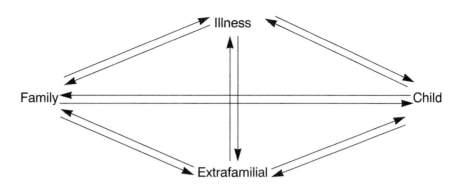

Figure 1.1 The illness network. Reproduced with permission from Lask and Fosson

and outside world. The child's temperament and level of understanding will influence their ability to cope with illness and the protective strategies that they use. Characteristics of the family, such as their communication style and ability to cope with stress, will influence their response to the illness. Relationships outside the family may offer support or be the cause of additional stress, which will in turn affect the course of the illness.

The psychosocial consequences of illness can be severely disabling and may even exacerbate the illness itself. On the whole, a child with a mild, acute and localised illness requiring simple, brief treatment will cope better than a child with a severe, chronic and generalised disease, who is having long, unpleasant and restricting treatment. However, many factors will come into play that may result in a child reacting adversely to the former. Children who do not adapt well to change will find illness more difficult, and those with lower intelligence will be less able to devise their own coping strategies. The attitude of a child and their family towards illness can influence their coping ability and directly affect the course of the disease. An over-acceptance of illness, manifested by preoccupation and extreme anxiety, may allow the illness to take over, and heightened emotional arousal may aggravate the illness itself. Conversely, denial of illness, characterised by a tendency to play down or even ignore the problem, may result in non-compliance with treatment. Illness will have emotional, financial and practical implications for the family, but family functioning will also have an effect on the illness. For example, families that encourage discussion of feelings are less likely to suffer from somatic symptoms than those that discourage, or bottle up, feelings. Lask (1988) identified family characteristics that lend to a better prognosis for the sick child. These include a good marriage, an optimal realistic attitude, satisfactory adaptation, stability, warmth, cohesion and satisfactory parental communication. The author suggests that a 'good partnership', where the couple is not married, would also be a significant positive family characteristic. Finally, the illness network reminds us that relationships outside the family will directly or indirectly influence the course of the illness. Grandparents, school friends and teachers, nursing and medical staff, and so on, can help to alleviate or aggravate disease. Miscommunications, inconsistencies, extremes of attitude or a lack of warmth and empathy are likely to have an adverse effect (Lask and Fosson, 1989).

Lask and Fosson cite two case examples which poignantly illustrate the illness network: one in which it works to the advantage of the child's health and one in which the converse applies:

Rowan, aged 9, had been admitted to hospital 22 times in three years because of unstable diabetes. His parents argued endlessly about how to manage his diet, and his mother became grossly over-involved, allowing him no independence whatsoever. The family doctor felt she could not help any further, and the paediatrician desperately tried to separate Rowan and his mother. The school refused to have him in class because of his frequent hypoglycaemic episodes. The family resented referral to a psychiatrist and refused to accept any of his suggestions. The paternal grandparents paid for a consultation from an international expert on diabetes, who recommended a change of treatment regime. This had no effect, and the paediatrician became increasingly exasperated with the parents' failure to comply. They transferred to another doctor, but by the age of 11 Rowan had been admitted to hospital on 13 more occasions.

Alex was 10 when he received an ileostomy for his intractable Crohn's disease. His parents, encouraged by medical and nursing staff, learned within three days how to change the ileostomy equipment, and taught him to do it for himself by the end of the first week. They helped him to return to school by devising with him a plan of what to say to other children, and how to cope in the showers and changing rooms. The school staff ensured that Alex was coping alright and nominated a teacher to whom he could go should there be any problems. Alex had no difficulties in settling back to a normal way of life, and remained in excellent health. At follow-up, aged 16 years, he was asked how he managed when he started dating. "Well when I told my first girl-friend, she gave me a funny look, and wouldn't see me again. With my next one, we were just cuddling, and she felt the bag and asked what it was, and I told her, and she said 'Oh' and we just carried on. It was great!"

The illness network highlights the importance of a holistic approach to treatment and the necessity of a multi-disciplinary model of care. Illness will touch every aspect of a child's life, and a wide variety of expertise will be required to address the numerous ramifications. This will not ensure a favourable outcome, but will go a long way to achieving one. It is also essential that professionals in different specialities work together. There is sometimes a tendency for professionals to become locked in their own view of illness and beliefs regarding appropriate treatment. In psychiatry, for example, behavioural therapy may take precedence over a psychodynamic approach to treatment, or vice versa. Some professionals do not believe that different psychotherapeutic approaches can work alongside each other. However, if we consider the complexities of illness, surely an eclectic approach is justifiable. A good example where specialities have failed to cooperate effectively is in the treatment of myalgic encephalitis (ME) or chronic fatigue syndrome, which has been the subject of much controversy in recent years. Feelings run high: some see it as a physical illness, caused by a virus, requiring medical treatment and rest, and others view it as a psychiatric disorder, depression, requiring a psychological approach. The reality is that the cause is unknown. However, it is likely that a number of factors, both physical and psychological, contribute to its aetiology. Simplistically, perhaps stress and exhaustion enables a virus to be contracted, which leads to further physical exhaustion and feelings of depression. The reality is no doubt more complicated, but a holistic approach to the treatment of chronic fatigue syndrome should involve both physical and psychological therapies. Benierakis (1995) highlights the importance of each individual in a multi-disciplinary team and suggests that, if the team is supportive rather than critically destructive towards its members, professional advancement will be enhanced. 'A well functioning team with a strong sense of shared responsibility can have a synergistic effect, i.e., the team can produce significantly more and better work than its individual members working as solo practitioners' (p. 348).

Although this book focuses on nursing intervention, it also highlights the intervention of other professionals in the multi-disciplinary team. It is important that nursing assessment and intervention is seen in the context of a multi-disciplinary team approach. Reference is also made in the text to liaison between specialities. In some hospitals, communication between disciplines and specialities has been improved through the organisation of 'psychosocial meetings'. These ideally include a paediatrician, nurse, child psychiatrist, psychologist, psychotherapist, play specialist, teacher, social worker and other appropriate personnel, such as physiotherapist or dietician. Their function is to discuss the physical, emotional and social needs of the children under their care and to initiate appropriate intervention.

A MULTI-CULTURAL APPROACH

'Culture consists of the shared values, norms, tradition, customs, arts, history, folklore and institutions of a group of people' (Wun Jung Kim, 1995, p.126). Our culture influences our ideas about illness and treatment; it may even affect the symptoms that we experience and our response to medical or nursing care. Therefore, it is not surprising that holistic medicine requires that we are culturally responsive and, because we live in a multi-cultural society (Figures 1.2 and 1.3), it is essential that we acquire an understanding of, and respect for, cultures that are different from our own.

Unfortunately cultural sensitivity is a neglected area in health care and requires considerable attention if truly holistic medicine is to be achieved. Health-care provision essentially reflects

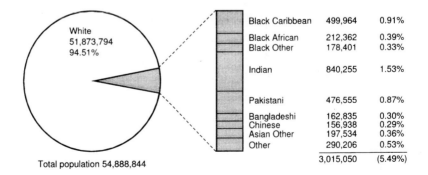

Figure 1.2 Ethnic breakdown of the population of Great Britain, according to 1991 Census figures.

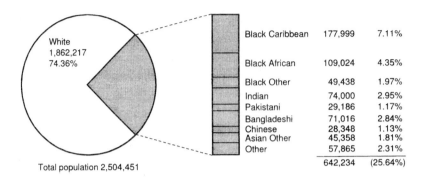

Figure 1.3 Ethnic breakdown of the population of inner London, according to 1991 Census figures.

the dominant culture in which it exists (Vargas and Berlin, 1991), and the preferences and beliefs of ethnic minority groups tend to be given token consideration. Some of the areas in which this is clearly demonstrated include:

◆ *Physical environment* Furniture, colour schemes, paintings, and so on, tend to reflect the tastes and preferences of the dominant culture. An environment that should convey concern and sensitivity may actually evoke unease in ethnic minority children and their families.

◆ *Staff group* There is a tendency for health professionals to recruit from the same culture group as their own,. i.e. the dominant culture. It is probably easier to work with individuals who have a similar educational background, have similar ideas about issues such as child rearing, and where there are no language difficulties to be overcome. However, this not only conveys a subtle message of non-acceptance to children and their families, but can actually be an obstacle to effective health care. A one-culture staff group will lack the resources to deal with the problems faced by minority groups entering the health service.

◆ *Policies and procedures* The typical family structure, beliefs and values, including ideas about child rearing, gender roles and inter-generational relationships, are reflected in health policies and procedures. For example, legally we require a child's parents to consent to their treatment, even though in some cultures, such as that of native the Americans, the approval of an extended family member may be necessary.

Hospitals generally have procedures for managing patients' belongings. On an inpatient child psychiatric unit there may be individually allocated lockers. However, although ownership has become an important aspect of Western culture, in many others the concept of sharing is valued. Vargas and Berlin (1991) cite a case example where this cultural difference was initially overlooked. A 7-year-old Pueblo Indian boy continuously took toys belonging to other children without permission. Staff became angry and frustrated when he 'refused' to mind his behaviour. When the 'problem' was addressed, it became apparent that his upbringing had stressed the need to share.

◆ *Diagnosis* Conceptualisation of normal and abnormal behaviours, and attitudes towards illness, will vary in different culture groups. For example, in Western culture, the development of independence and self-reliance is considered important, whereas in many other cultures, such as African American, the idea of group interdependence and cooperation is valued (Lorrie Yoos et al, 1995). This can lead to the diagnosis of 'problem' behaviour, which is in fact normal within the culture that it exists in. However, similarly, care must be taken not to mistake psychopathology for a cultural difference. For example, the mutual cooperation of some culture groups must be distinguished from an unhealthy enmeshment.

Symptoms may also be affected by culture and so lead to misdiagnosis. In the Chinese culture, self-control and composure are idealised and the expression of emotion is frowned upon. In addition, there is a strong fear of the stigmatisation of mental illness, which is thought to be caused by punishment from the Gods, a failure in guidance and discipline from the family leader, or a hereditary weakness. Weddings might even be cancelled if mental illness is discovered in future in-laws. Consequently, somatic symptoms are likely to mask mental illness and may therefore be overlooked. In the psychiatric clinic at Taiwan University Hospital, 70% of patients initially complained of physical symptoms (Kuo and Kavanagh, 1994).

◆ *Treatment* Our expectations of a child's, and their family's behaviour, is likely to be determined by our own upbringing, which is culturally influenced. This can lead to misunderstanding and inappropriate treatment when working with those from a different culture to our own. For example, native American children are taught that looking directly at the face of an adult, especially when being disciplined, is a sign of disrespect. Conversely, a child in mainstream American culture is taught the complete opposite (Vargas and Berlin, 1991). It is easy to imagine how misunderstanding could arise on an inpatient unit and result in inappropriate and harmful reprimanding. Similarly, teaching a Chinese child to talk openly about their feelings, will lay them open to criticism from their own community.

Our culture will influence our ideas about treatment. For example, the Chinese tend to prefer medical and cognitive approaches to treat mental health problems than psychotherapeutic approaches. If a treatment modality is forced upon a child and their family, which is at odds with their cultural belief, it stands to reason that it is likely to be unsuccessful.

'Cultural competence' is not only reasonable and humane, but can also influence treatment success. It is defined as 'a set of knowledge-based and interpersonal skills that allow individuals to understand, appreciate and work with individuals of cultures from other than their own' (Wun Jung Kim, 1995, p.126). Gerrish and co-workers (1996) highlighted the inadequacy of nurse training in England, in relation to promoting cultural competence. Only 25% of programmes made meeting the health needs of ethnic minority communities an explicit learning outcome. Wun Jung Kim (1995) proposes a curriculum for American trainee child and adolescent psychiatric residencies, which is aimed at improving cultural competence. It includes improving their basic knowledge base in topics such as the cultural diversity of the United States; ethnic characteristics of families and ethnic attitudes towards mental health; enhancing clinical skills, such as interviewing children and families from different ethnic groups, using interpreters and formulating treatment plans that are culturally appropriate; and addressing attitudes, such as the trainee's own prejudices.

Efforts should be made to create a multi-cultural environment, which respects the values and beliefs of those from all different backgrounds. For example, although a certain framework of policies and procedures will be necessary, where these are at odds with a particular culture, time must be taken to explain why they are in place. Nurses must continuously address their own cultural biases and prejudices. Most of us have prejudices against other races because we have been conditioned by early experiences in our family and the community in which we live. Our prejudice may be unconscious and our discrimination subtle. Migration brings with it many stresses, including racial discrimination, and a multi-cultural staff group may be intuitively more able to deal with subsequent hostile and challenging behaviour than a single-culture staff group. Unless you have experienced discrimination or been emotionally close to someone who has, it is difficult to fully comprehend the effect that it can have.

It is beyond the scope of this book to address fully the cultural issues that will arise in caring for children, and the author is concerned that the reader does not adopt culturally stereotypical ideas, based on the research mentioned in this chapter. For example, it would be wrong to assume that all non-Westerners have a tendency to somatise. It is essential to remember that there will be considerable diversity in beliefs within ethnic groups as well as across them. There are also many factors, in addition to culture, that influence our behaviour.

The nursing and multi-disciplinary interventions in this book are typically based on Western research, but I have tried to mention some important cultural phenomena, and implore the reader always to question whether the approach suggested is culturally appropriate for the child and family with whom they are working. Further reading and liaison with ethnic minority support groups and services is essential.

SOME USEFUL ADDRESSES

The Department of Health, in conjunction with the British Broadcasting Corporation, has published a directory of services for mental health, which includes a number of organisations that can provide advice to professionals and/or culturally sensitive therapy to those from ethnic minority groups. This booklet is available from the Department of Health, PO Box 410, Wetherby LS23 7LN. Services listed include:

Afro-Caribbean Mental Health Association
35–37 Electric Avenue
London SW9 8JP
Tel: 0171-737 3603

NAFSIYAT (Intercultural therapy centre)
278 Seven Sisters Road
London N4 2HY
Tel: 0171-263 4130 (24 hours)

Asian Family Counselling Services
74 The Avenue
London W13 8LB
Tel: 0181-997 5749

Jewish Association for the Mentally Ill
707 High Road
London N12 0BT
Tel: 0181-343 1111

A WIDE RANGE OF INTERVENTIONS

As well as requiring the wide range of expertise of a multi-disciplinary team, holistic medicine depends on the nurse using a variety of approaches to health care. Nurses need to expand their repertoire of skills and consider 'alternative', or complementary, therapies, such as aromatherapy, relaxation therapy and massage. As Newbeck and Rowe (1986) has pointed out, it is unfortunate that the term 'alternative' is often attached to these more unusual treatments, as this implies that they are used instead of orthodox approaches. Holistic medicine does not exclude any treatment possibility or recognise one aspect of treatment as being more important than another. Therefore, the term 'complementary' is perhaps more appropriate, implying mutuality. As well as learning new skills and undertaking appropriate training, nurses can also widen their expertise in mental health care by drawing on their own creativity and imagination. I hope that this book will stimulate your own inventiveness.

Nurses working in non-psychiatric areas need to develop some of the skills more usually associated with psychiatric nursing, if holistic care is to be achieved and the mental health of all children given important consideration. I appreciate that many of the techniques suggested in the text will be difficult for some nurses to implement, for example those working on a busy paediatric ward. However, every effort must be made, as holistic medicine depends upon it. Some ideas on how the nurse can promote mental health care in non-psychiatric areas include:

◆ *Being involved in the design of wards, health centres and school health-care facilities* On a ward, separate rooms may be useful for children with emotional or behavioural problems, as well as for those who are critically ill or infectious. Space to play and run around is essential, as is a quiet place to meet families or children individually, where no interruptions can be guaranteed. Today's health centres are usually well designed for private consultation, but often do not have sufficient resources for children. A child-oriented room with a variety of toys, puppets, drawing materials, and so on, is essential for effective individual work. Similarly, schools may have a 'sick room', but there is often no space for counselling.

✦ *Promoting the multi-disciplinary team* Nurses arc in an ideal position to coordinate the multi-disciplinary team. Setting up psychosocial meetings and encouraging liaison with psychiatric colleagues should both be feasible.

✦ *Attending courses on mental health care and complementary therapies* Nurses must strive constantly to increase their range of mental health skills as well as other abilities.

✦ *Ensuring that mental health care is given equal consideration to physical well-being* So often, mental health care is considered to either be 'a luxury item', one that receives consideration if time or resources allow, or 'a last resort', if all other treatments fail. A truly holistic approach requires that the 'whole' person is considered right from the start. Obviously there will be priorities of care, but this should not mean that mental health is not discussed from the outset.

ETHICAL ISSUES

'Special ethical problems in child and adolescent psychiatry relate to the nature of the child as a developing being, with changing morals, cognitions and emotions, and as a dependent being, reliant on adults – whether parents or professionals' (Green and Stewart, 1987, p. 5). It is essential that nurses always put the interest of the child and family first; recognising their rights as fellow human beings and continually questioning the ethics of professional practice.

The nurse will be faced by many ethical issues during the course of his/her career. The author wishes to highlight two fundamental issues in child mental health: the child's right to consent to, or refuse, treatment, and health professionals' responsibility in planning treatment.

A holistic approach to treatment must recognise the developing personality of the child and growing ability to make informed decisions. The Children Act 1989 recognises that children have 'rights' concerning the way in which they are treated and that parents have a responsibility to ensure that they receive appropriate care (White et al, 1990). The judgement in the case of Gillick vs. West Norfolk and Wisbech Health Authoriy and DHSS (1985) has been important in shaping current law in Britain. The Gillick judgement made three points:

✦ Parental powers are for the protection of the child.

✦ Parental powers dwindle as the child matures (Lord Scarman said, 'Parental rights yield to the child's right to make his own decisions when he reaches sufficient understanding and intelligence to be capable of making up his own mind on the matter requiring decision').

✦ Parental powers depend on the understanding of the individual child, not on any fixed age' (Black et al, 1991, p. 82).

The Gillick principle is pertinent when considering a child's ability to refuse or consent to treatment. A number of factors must be borne in mind when attempting to establish whether a child is capable of making such decisions:

✦ *The child's stage of cognitive development* Piaget describes cognitive development as an essentially biological process, the child progressing through identifiable age-related stages. Below the age of about 7 years, Piaget describes the child as basically egocentric and unlikely to consider the views of others. Their ideas tend to be based on immediate concrete perception and therefore will probably be inconsistent over time. After the age of 7, although still thinking concretely, the child begins to recognise the relationships between external perceptions, and by the age of 9 or 10 the child has grasped the concept of cause and effect. By now the child is also less egocentric and becoming aware of the opinions of others. At the age of 12 or so, the adolescent is able to be more reflective in thought and to understand more abstract concepts. Piaget recognised that environmental factors could facilitate this cognitive development, but also that emotional and physical stress could cause developmental regression.

◆ *The child's physical and emotional state* In a case described by Honig and Bentovim (1996), the High Court overruled an adolescent's refusal of treatment for anorexia nervosa on the basis that self-induced starvation had impaired her cognitive capacity. Lord Donaldson said, '…it is a feature of anorexia nervosa that it is capable of destroying the ability to make an informed choice. It creates a compulsion to refuse treatment or only to accept treatment which is likely to be ineffective. This attitude is part and parcel of the disease and the more advanced the illness, the more compelling it may become' (p. 290).

◆ *Whether the child has special needs* A child's ability to make a considered decision may be affected by learning difficulties. Each child must be assessed individually with respect to their specific difficulties.

◆ *Cultural differences* Assessment must consider the child's and cultural background. For example, a child whose background has encouraged the expression of opinions and development of autonomy may find it easier to convey their wishes than a child who has been brought up to respect the opinions of elders, and where dependence is seen as a positive and integral part of family life.

Health professionals are faced with the decision of whether to respect the wishes of the child, to be instructed by the parents or to seek directions from the Court. In Britain, two separate legal routes may be taken; one uses the Children Act 1989 and the other the Mental Health Act 1983. The former legislation has the advantage of being designed specifically to represent the wishes and needs of children. It is also less likely to have long-term adverse repercussions, such as affecting employment prospects and personal insurance (Honig and Bentovim, 1996). Whether legal action is taken or not, the wishes of children must be ascertained and given serious consideration in any decison-making regarding their care.

Another important area for health professionals to consider, in relation to ethical issues, is their choice of treatment approach. It is much easier to see the ethical problems attached to theories and therapies that you do not support, than to those that you do support (Green and Stewart, 1987). In reality, each mode of therapy poses ethical dilemmas. For example, individual therapy may succeed in helping a young person to develop a sense of self, but in doing so may alienate that young person from their family, especially if the values and attitudes of the therapist are fundamentally different from those of the parents. Similarly, family therapy may result in an improvement in the identifed child, but in the process siblings may be adversely affected or the parental marriage may suffer. Sometimes there is a danger that practitioners of different therapies become so personally identified with their theoretical position that any possible ethical problems become invisible to them.

A holistic approach to treatment, which necessitates communication between practitioners with different professional backgrounds and recognises the child as a multi-faceted individual, is hopefully more likely to address such ethical dilemmas. However, nurses must continually question the ethics of their approach for each individual child. For example, for some children it may be considered helpful to facilitate their expression of anger, but for others containment and facilitating self-control may be thought to be paramount. Similarly, it may be considered in the child's best interest to change their method of coping with stress, which might involve obstructing obsessional behaviour. The additional stress caused by such action must be considered in the context of the total well-being of the child. Although such issues are also relevant in adult mental health nursing, they are perhaps particularly pointed when working with children, owing to their dependence on adults and relatively impressionable nature (Green and Stewart, 1987).

REFERENCES

American Psychiatric Association (1994) *Diagnostic and Statistical Manual of Mental Disorders*, 4th edn (DSM IV). Washington, DC: American Psychiatric Association.

Anderson KN and Anderson LE (eds) (1995) *Mosby's Pocket Dictionary of Nursing, Medicine and Professions Allied to Medicine*, UK edn. London: Mosby.

Benierakis CE (1995) The function of the multidisciplinary team in child psychiatry – clinical and educational aspects. *Canadian Journal of Psychiatry* **40(6)**: 349–353.

Besag F (1993) Coping with unhappy children who have epilepsy. In Varma V (ed.) *Coping with Unhappy Children*, pp 72–79. London: Cassell.

Black D, Wolkind S and Harris Hendriks J (1991) Children and the law. In *Child Psychiatry and the Law*, pp 81–82. London: Gaskell.

Bond D (1993) Mental health in children who are hearing impaired. In Varma V (ed.) *Coping with Unhappy Children*, pp 31–51. London: Cassell.

Chapman E (1993) Coping with unhappy children who are visually impaired. In Varma V (ed.) *Coping with Unhappy Children*, pp 17–30. London: Cassell

Chase HD (1988) Holistic medicine – What is it and what are its clinical implications? *Maternal and Child Health* **13(10)**: 292–296.

Fritz GK, Rubinstein S and Lewiston NJ (1987) Psychological factors in fatal childhood asthma. *American Journal of Orthopsychiatry* **57(2)**: 253–257.

Gerrish K, Husband C and MacKenzie J (1996) *Nursing for a Multi-ethnic Society*. London: Open University Press.

Gillick vs. West Norfolk and Wisbech Area Health Authority and the DHSS (1985) Vol. 3, WLR: 830.

Green J and Stewart A (1987) Ethical issues in child and adolescent psychiatry. *Journal of Medical Ethics* **13**: 5–11.

Grey M (1993) Stressors and children's health. *Journal of Pediatric Nursing* **8(2)**: 85–91.

Honig P and Bentovim M (1996) Treating children with eating disorders – ethical and legal issues. *Clinical Child Psychology and Psychiatry* **1(2)**: 287–294.

Kuo C-L and Kavanagh K (1994) Chinese perspectives on culture and mental health. *Issues in Mental Health Nursing* **15**: 551–567.

Lask B (1988) The highly talented child. *Archives of Disease in Childhood* **63**: 118–119.

Lask B and Fosson A (1989) *Childhood Illness: The Psychosomatic Approach*. Chichester, UK: John Wiley.

Lorrie Yoos H, Kitzman H, Olds DL and Overacker I (1995) Child rearing beliefs in the African–American community: implications for culturally competent pediatric care. *Journal of Pediatric Nursing* **10(6)**: 343–353.

Newbeck I and Rowe D (1986) Going the whole way. *Nursing Times* **82(8)**: 24–25.

Sharman WJ (1993) A bar to holistic care? Effect of patients with mental illness on nurses in paediatric settings. *Professional Nurse* **8(6)**: 384–389.

Vargas LA and Berlin IN (1991) Culturally responsive care of inpatient children and adolescents. In Hendren RL and Berlin IN (eds) *Psychiatric Inpatient Care of Children and Adolescents – A Multicultural Approach*, pp 14–33. New York: John Wiley.

White R, Carr P and Lowe N (1990) *A Guide to the Children Act 1989*. London: Butterworth.

World Health Organisation (1992) *The ICD-10 Classification of Mental and Behavioural Disorders – Clinical Descriptions and Diagnostic Guidelines*. Geneva: WHO.

Wun Jung Kim (1995) A training guideline of cultural competence for child and adolescent psychiatric residencies. *Child Psychiatry and Human Development* **26(2)**: 125–136.

2 SAD AND SELF-HARMING

INTRODUCTION

Occasional feelings of sadness are a normal part of every child's life. However, parents or professionals may identify a problem that requires specialist help when the extent of unhappiness is such that the child's quality of life and general functioning is significantly impaired. Relationships within or outside the family may break down or school achievement may deteriorate. There is considerable controversy surrounding the concept of depression in childhood, many being doubtful that it can occur prepubertally. However, a traditional diagnosis of depression depends largely on the young person's ability to verbalise feelings and does not consider important developmental criteria. Infants and prepubertal children can be diagnosed as suffering from depression, if developmental parameters are recognised (Trad, 1987). When working with children, it is important to identify not only the signs of full-blown clinical depression, using adult diagnostic criteria, but also depressive-like phenomena using a developmental model. Nurses working in the community or in general paediatrics may be foremost in identifying depression in children and initiating appropriate help.

Diagnosis of depression, using the *Diagnostic and Statistical Manual of Mental Disorders* (fourth edition), **depends on the presence of at least five of nine symptoms, of which a dysphoric mood and/or the loss of interest or pleasure in everyday activities must be apparent. Other symptoms include weight loss or gain, insomnia or hypersomnia, psychomotor agitation or retardation, poor concentration, lethargy, feelings of worthlessness and recurrent thoughts of death** (American Psychiatric Association, 1994). The ICD-10 (tenth edition of the World Health Organisation's international classification of diseases) classification of mental and behavioural diseases recognises similar signs and symptoms. Nikelly (1988) suggests that there is a danger of missing depression in non-Western patients because the criteria for diagnosis essentially reflect Western values of behaviour. In societies where self-containment is fostered, such as China, patients suffering from depression are likely to present with physical symptoms and not to disclose feelings of despondency. Similarly, it is neccesary to look for other signs of depression in prepubertal children, who may be developmentally unable to verbalise feelings. Infants and toddlers may be apathetic, irritable, refuse to feed and spend much of their time crying or rocking. Failure to thrive and developmental delay may ensue. Similarly, older children may first present with physical symptoms, such as head or stomach aches. Poor concentration and social withdrawal may be noticed at school and an inability to cope with minor frustrations leading to temper outbursts.

There are likely to be many contributing factors to the aetiology of depression, unless there is a clear precipitating event, such as the death of a significant person. However, even if the trigger for depression is straightforward, the coping strategies used by the individual will be influenced by genetic and other environmental factors. It is important to assess the context in which depression arises, as various factors will influence its development, nature of presentation and maintenance:

- ✦ Genetic predisposition
- ✦ Neuroendocrine changes

◆ Viral infection before the development of signs of depression

◆ Acute or chronic psychosocial stressors

◆ Temperament characteristics

◆ Culture

(See *Assessment* below for further explanation.)

Given the controversy surrounding the existence of depression in infants and young children, there do not seem to be any significant studies to indicate the prevalence. Rutter et al (1970), in the Isle of Wight study, found that 10% of 10–11 year olds showed signs of unhappiness and misery, and 1.4% showed signs of full-blown depression. The prevalence increased to 4% amongst 14–15 year olds (Rutter et al 1976).

A significant relationship exists between depression and suicidal behaviour in children, although depression is not a necessary antecedent to self-destructive behaviour. Feelings of hopelessness, which are associated with depression, are also associated with suicide. Suicidal behaviour is rare before the age of 12 years, although suicidal ideas, threats or attempts are relatively common. Children from any social background are at risk of self-harm. **'Suicidal behaviour in children is any self-destructive behaviour that has the intent to hurt oneself seriously or to cause death'** (Pfeffer, 1986, p. 21). In 1990, the suicide rate for 15–19 year olds in England and Wales was 57 boys and 14 girls per million. No suicides were recorded in children aged under 10 years and for 10–14 year olds a rate of 1.5 boys and 1.0 girls per million was registered between 1981 and 1990 (McClure, 1994).

ASSESSMENT

The assessment of a child who is sad and self-harming will overlap considerably with any nursing or multi-disciplinary intervention plan. Assessment will include establishing the extent of unhappiness and starting to unravel the possible reasons behind such misery. Both these processes will be an important part of ongoing treatment. Therefore, if possible, the professionals involved in assessment should continue with treatment. If this is not feasible or appropriate, the assessment process should be kept to a minimum, so that the child and family do not form a therapeutic attachment with professionals who will promptly stop working with them. The multi-disciplinary team must plan the assessment process, to ensure that it is well coordinated, and, in non-psychiatric areas, colleagues in mental health should be consulted. Nursing staff and, indeed, other professionals should not work in isolation. A multi-disciplinary approach, with psychiatric liaison where appropriate, ensures a holistic approach and will enable the child and family's distress to be contained more successfully. The assessment process itself may trigger emotional and behavioural responses which the team must be able to hold.

INDIVIDUAL ASSESSMENT

The aim of the individual nursing assessment will depend on whether you are likely to continue working with the child. If the child is likely to be referred on to other professionals for treatment, then the assessment should aim to establish the extent of the child's unhappiness, possible pre-cursors and the level of risk for self-harm. Therefore, it may be necessary to select only part of the following individual assessment work.

'Getting to know children' and 'beginning a relationship'

It is important to find somewhere comfortable and free from distraction to meet with the young person. Having introduced yourself, it may be useful to ask the child why they think you are meeting them. What the child thinks that others have noticed about their behaviour or mood may be a starting point for the conversation. Some children will welcome the opportunity to talk, whereas others may find this too difficult. The nurse should not push the child to reveal their innermost thoughts or feelings, but must go at the young person's pace. Sensitivity and creativity are essential. Many children find it easier to communicate through play and drawing. The following are just some examples of how to start getting to know a young person and begin a therapeutic relationship:

◆ *Play a non-threatening game* – one that does not inquire into the child's world.

◆ *Use fun questionnaires* Use ready-made questionnaires or create your own, to start getting to know the child (see, for example, Figure 2.1).

◆ *Getting to know games* There are specific games available for getting to know children; for example, 'All about me' (Hemmings, 1991) is a non-competitive board game which aims to provide a non-threatening medium through which the child can start to talk about themselves.

◆ *Draw a family tree* Help the child to draw a family tree and then talk about the family. Ask who is most like each other, which family members are closest to each other, what does the child think that each person in the family makes of their unhappiness and so on. The family tree could also include other significant people in the child's life (Figure 2.2).

◆ *Make a 'button picture'* The child chooses individual buttons, from a large collection in a tray, to represent different family members and/or friends, and sticks them on to a sheet of paper. The nurse can ask the child to explain why particular buttons have been chosen or simply comment on the characteristics of the buttons and talk about where the buttons have been placed in relation to each other on the paper. The buttons may have become a useful metaphor to describe the characteristics of family members and their relationships to each other (see Plate 1 which appears in the unfolioed section between p56 and 57).

◆ *Paint or draw a picture* Ask the child whether they would like to paint a picture. What to paint could be left open to the child or you could pick a theme, such as their family doing something, the child at school, any person, their favourite hero, something that irritates them or they find boring or something that they enjoy doing (see Chapter 10 for indicators of possible abuse – *Assessment, Facilitating disclosure of abuse*).

◆ *Design a personal or family coat of arms* Ask the child to create a coat of arms with special symbols incorporated to represent important characteristics, interests, activities and so on.

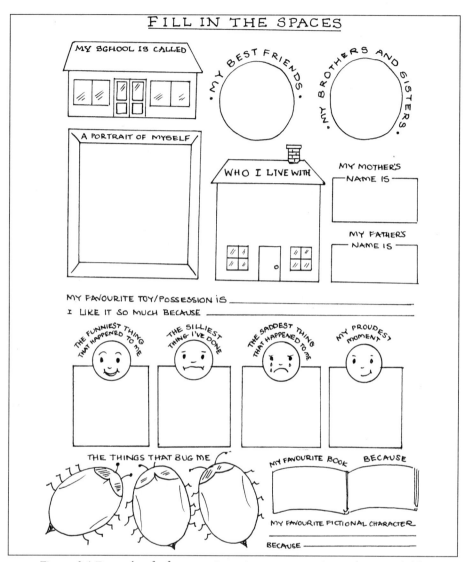

Figure 2.1 Example of a fun questionnaire to start getting to know a child.

◆ *Use a doll's house*. An older child could be asked to show a typical scene at home (who is where and what they are doing), whereas a younger child would probably enjoy playing freely. Simply stating what is seen may encourage further discussion or at least give the child an opportunity to correct any misconceptions the nurse has made. It is important not to attempt to analyse what is observed; the child will show you what they want you to see in their own time.

◆ *Create a world in sand* In 1929, Margaret Lowenfeld developed a sand tray technique through which children could express and demonstrate symbolically their inner world (Lowenfeld, 1939). This tool continues to be of great value today. A blue plastic tray, about 40 cm by 30 cm and 8 cm deep is placed on a table at waist height for the child. If possible two or three types of sand (coarse, medium and fine) are provided, together with a jug of

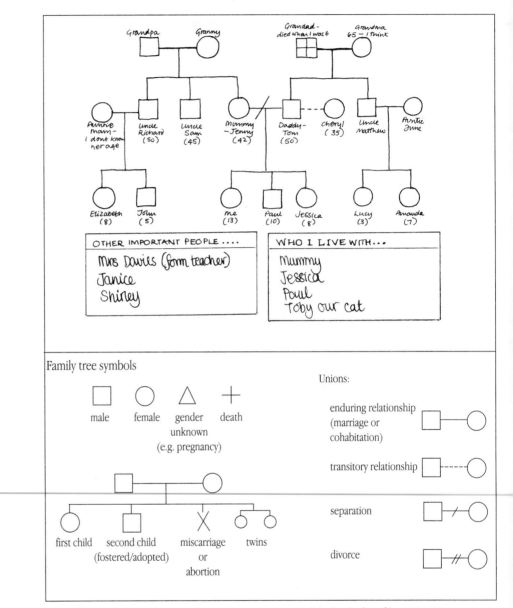

Figure 2.2 Family tree drawn by a teenager with the help of her Key Nurse.

water to wet the sand and allow it to be moulded. A collection of five or six trays containing different small figures and objects are available for the child to add to their sand world. For example, individual trays could contain realistic people, fantasy characters, jungle animals, domestic animals, buildings, fences, road signs, and so on. The child is asked to make whatever they like in the sand, using any of the tray items. The nurse comments on what is observed and asks questions to clarify what they see; the child may not be using objects realistically and there may be a good reason why, for example, a tree is being placed upside down. The first time this technique is used there may be only a very superficial demonstration of the child's inner world, and so it is usually helpful to have a series of sessions. The sand world can be kept in a safe place until next time or a drawing made to record the first session and the child given a fresh tray at the following session (Lowenfeld, 1939, 1950) (Figure 2.3).

◆ *Use puppets* Some children may find it easier to communicate through puppets. A good choice of glove puppets will enable the child to identify with their chosen character or animal. The nurse should also choose a puppet and then the conversation or story can begin. The child may find it easier to talk about themselves in this once-removed position.

◆ *Using telephones or computers* Toy telephones or real telephones can be used to have a conversation. It may feel less threatening for the young person to talk at some distance,

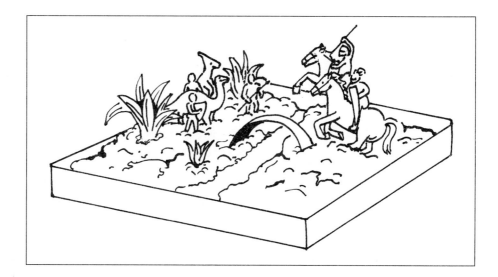

Figure 2.3 Lowenfeld sand tray technique. Lucy, aged 10, was admitted to the psychiatric unit with anorexia nervosa. In an individual session, she made her world in sand. Lucy wet the sand and divided it into two 'lands'; one she called the 'good land' and the other the 'bad land'. A bridge connected the two lands. Soldiers on the good land were having to defend their territory from the invading 'bad soldiers'. Lucy commented that the good soldiers were poor and their commander was absent, so they had to fight without their leader. The bad soldiers were rich and rode horses. Lucy's father had recently been made redundant from a high status position in an international company. The family was on the brink of having to sell their house. The battle in Lucy's world also represented her inner conflict: the healthy versus the unhealthy part of her. The anorexia (the unhealthy part of her) had brought outside help to the family (perhaps represented by the helpful dinosaurs) and prevented her sitting a school entrance exam, thus affording some relief from her fear of failure. Therefore, the healthy part of Lucy was struggling to win. Perhaps the 'absent commander' symbolised Lucy's father who was currently suffering from depression.

be that literal distance or in role play. Similarly, computers provide a mode of communication with which the young person is likely to be familiar.

◆   *Talk about a 'special' object* The child is asked to bring something to the session which has great importance for them, such as a doll, particular article of clothing, some artifact, anything that has significance. In the session the child is asked to talk about their object and its special meaning.

◆   *What if my…could talk* Ask the child to guess what their special object (see exercise above) would say if it could talk. Alternatively, if the family has a pet animal, what stories could it tell?

◆   *Draw a road* Hanes (1995) describes the use of road drawings to elicit spontaneous imagery that represents the origins, life history, past experiences and future expectations of the artist. His work is essentially with adults, but road drawings can be used equally as well with children. They are familiar and simple to draw, and so can reduce the child's anxiety about feeling a need to be artistic. Your instructions to the child could go something like this: 'I would like you to draw a road' – pause – 'Think of all the different types of roads…fast roads…slow roads…bendy roads…straight roads… What type of material is your road made of? What sort of condition is your road in? How many lanes are there? Is there more than one road? Are there any junctions? Are there any road signs? What is surrounding the road? Does it go through a built-up area or countryside? Where is your road heading?' (Figure 2.4).

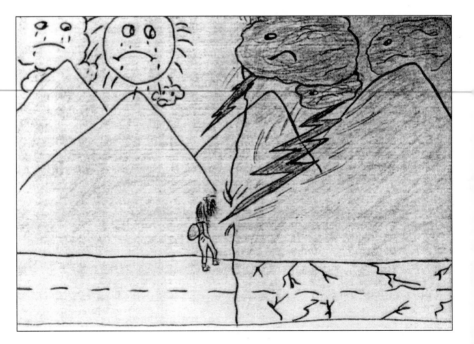

Figure 2.4 Road drawing. Reproduced from Hanes (1995) Utilising road drawings as a therapeutic metaphor in art therapy. American Journal of Art Therapy 34, 19–23, with permission.

Assessing the extent of the child's unhappiness and their risk of self-harming

The nurse must look for signs of clinical depression or depressive-like phenomena, such as somatic symptoms, and establish whether the child has injured or attempted to injure themselves, or is contemplating doing so.

Areas to cover and examples of questions to ask to identify depression or depressive-like phenomena include:

◆ *Affect and feelings of worth*

How often do you feel sad?

Do you ever feel bored and, if so, how often? (Children often describe themselves as bored rather than sad.)

How often would you say you cry?

Do you often get angry or irritable?

How are you getting on with your friends?

Do you ever fight with other people?

Who do you feel cares about you?

Do you blame yourself if things go wrong?

Do you ever feel like hurting yourself?

◆ *Physical symptoms*

Do you have difficulty sleeping?

Do you ever feel tired during the day?

How are you eating at the moment?

How well can you concentrate in lessons at school?

Do you get any aches or pains, such as stomach or head aches?

◆ *Current life situation and potential triggers of unhappiness.*

How are things going at school?

Is it a new school or have you been there a while?

Do you worry about doing well in school?

Do you have a special friend?

How are things at home?

Are your family well?

Is there anyone else who is feeling sad?

Who are you closest to at home?

Are there many fights at home?

If so, who is involved?

Depression increases the risk of self-harm, including suicide. Any self-harm or suicidal ideas must be taken seriously and the situation assessed regularly. If there are signs of depression and/or self-destructive ideas, a psychiatric opinion should be sought. If there is an acute suicidal risk, immediate measures will need to be taken to ensure the child's safety, which may include admission to hospital. Consciously or unconsciously, suicidal children have a wish for someone to care for them (Pfeffer, 1986). By taking them seriously, the nurse can actually reduce these suicidal impulses as a sense of hopefulness is generated in the child.

Examples of areas to cover and questions to ask in evaluating suicidal risk (taken from Pfeffer, 1986, p. 187) include:

◆ *Suicidal fantasies or actions*

>Have you ever thought of hurting yourself?

>Have you ever threatened or attempted to hurt yourself?

◆ *Concepts of what would happen*

>What did you think would happen if you tried to hurt or kill yourself?

>Did you think you would die?

◆ *Circumstances at the time of the child's suicidal behaviour*

>What was happening at the time you thought of killing yourself or tried to kill yourself?

>Was anyone else with you or near you when you thought of killing yourself?

◆ *Previous experiences with suicidal behaviour*

>Have you ever thought about killing yourself or tried to kill yourself before?

>Do you know anyone who has either thought about, attempted or committed suicide?

>How did this person carry out their suicidal ideas or action?

◆ *Motivations for suicidal behaviours*

>Why do you want to kill yourself?

>Did you wish someone would rescue you before you tried to hurt yourself?

>Did you feel rejected by someone?

>Did you hear voices telling you to kill yourself?

◆ *Experiences and concepts of death*

>What happens when people die?

>Can they come back again?

>Do you know anyone who has died?

Observation of a child's play might reveal suicidal thoughts. Typical play characteristics of suicidal children include:

>◆ Games involving loss and retrieval (e.g. repeatedly throwing toys out of windows, jumping from heights, attempting to fly).

>◆ The repetition of dangerous or reckless behaviours.

✦ The abuse or misuse of play things (e.g. aggressively breaking toys).

✦ Play that involves acting out omnipotent fantasies; for example, the child acts as a superhero in sadistic or dangerous play. Play is so intense that someone may end up being hurt.

✦ It is more difficult to interrupt suicidal children during play than non-suicidal children, because they are less in touch with reality.

✦ Drawings may illustrate a general theme of violence and destruction or specific suicidal tendencies (Figure 2.5).

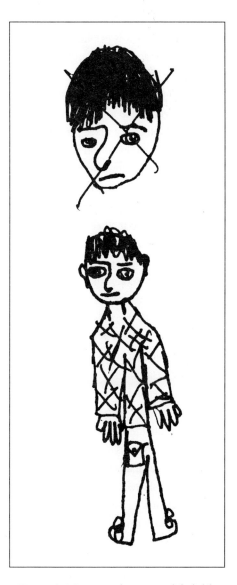

Figure 2.5 Drawing by a suicidal child.

MEDICAL ASSESSMENT

If the child is suffering from physical symptoms and/or presents with developmental delay, it is imperative to exclude any organic cause. This may be achieved by means of a simple medical examination or may require more extensive investigation. A medical history may reveal that the signs of depression began following a viral infection. Measles and mononucleosis are particularly associated with triggering mild depression. If there are concerns about the child's mental state, a child psychiatrist should be requested to contribute to the assessment and be involved in discussion regarding physical investigations (see Chapter 5 – *Medical assessment*).

INDIVIDUAL ASSESSMENT BY A PSYCHOANALYTICAL PSYCHOTHERAPIST

If possible, it is helpful to have a psychotherapist's assessment. There are a number of psychoanalytical theories that link early separation and loss with depression later in childhood and adult life.

Melanie Klein hypothesized that all children go through a developmental stage when they are vulnerable to depressive symptoms. At about 6 months of age the infant starts to recognise the mother as a whole person separate from him or herself, who can be 'good' and 'bad', present and absent, loved and hated. The infant sees that the mother has her own separate life and discovers their absolute dependence on her and jealousy of other people. At the same time the infant's ego becomes whole and separate, and the infant recognizes that their good and bad feelings about the mother are their own. The child's main anxiety is that their own bad feelings towards the mother will destroy her – the very person they love and are dependent on. The infant is left with feelings of guilt and helplessness, characteristic depressive experiences. In favourable circumstances, the mother's continued return after absence, and constant love and attention, modify the child's sense of their own destructive omnipotence and the infant is more able to separate fantasy from reality. However, losses in later life may re-awaken these depressive feelings (Segal, 1973).

Bowlby (1980) identified depressive reactions in infants aged between 6 months and 4 years following separation from their mother. He identified three stages of mourning: protest, despair and detachment. During the protest phase, the child attempts to prevent the separation by means of anger and having temper tantrums. This anger is directed towards those who the child holds responsible. Such signs of protest are often seen in suicidal children, who may be attempting to restitute the loss of an emotionally important nurturing person. During the phase of despair, the child continues to long for the return of the mother, but experiences feelings of helplessness and becomes apathetic. The phase of detachment, which follows, represents a stage of recovery when the child reduces their hope of the mother returning and starts to form new relationships. Fostering new attachments for suicidal children can help to reduce self-destructive impulses (Pfeffer, 1986). Bowlby suggests that an early experience of loss, for which there was no successful mourning process, may be re-activated later in childhood or adult life, resulting in depression.

Although it is important to consider the influence of past experiences on a current state of depression, it is essential to try to understand the child's present psyche. It may be that the young person is experiencing feelings of extreme anger towards a significant person, but is so terrified by the intensity of such feelings and frightened of the damage that could be caused if they were unleashed, that the anger and loathing are turned inwards. The result is that the child feels depressed, but cannot connect these feelings with anger. Schechter (1957) views childhood suicide as an expression of murderous feelings towards one who is loved. Physical harm is directed towards this internalised representation rather than the actual person. The process occurs at an unconscious level, as the child would experience tremendous feelings of guilt and anxiety if aware of their murderous inclinations towards a loved one. Ackerly (1967), who links childhood suicide with psychosexual development, talks about a punitive superego and the child's fear of losing control over aggressive sexual impulses toward the parents.

There is considerable controversy surrounding the importance of early loss and its link with depression. A number of studies have looked at the significance of parental death, separation or divorce in the development of depression later in life; some have identified a link and some have not (e.g. Reinherz et al, 1989; Goodyer and Altham, 1991; Paykel, 1982). However, in line with psychoanalytical theories, what seems to be more important is a lack of early nurturing and insecure attachment (e.g. Bifulco et al, 1987). Nevertheless, the psychotherapist will want to focus on what is happening in the child's mind now and link this with significant past experiences.

FAMILY ASSESSMENT

Important information can be obtained from talking with the child's parents, although a more thorough picture will be achieved by one or two family therapy meetings. Whichever approach is chosen or most practical, certain areas should be covered in discussion:

Parents' understanding of the child's unhappiness

It is important to establish the history of the child's unhappiness and the parents' understanding of its origin. There may be a concern about physical illness, if depression seemed to be triggered by a viral infection and/or the child currently complains of symptoms. If physical symptoms mask feelings of sadness, the parents may be unaware that their child is depressed. The parents may feel to blame if they acknowledge that their child has a mental health problem, whereas a physical illness can be more easily explained. It is important to be sensitive and to explain to parents that there may be many contributing factors. A holistic approach to management, which includes investigating and treating physical and psychological symptomatology, is not only appropriate but may also ease the parents into addressing their child's depression. Family culture will influence the child's presentation of depression and the family attitudes towards mental illness (see *Introduction* above and Chapter 1 – *A multi-cultural approach*).

Family history of depressive or other mental illness

Depression in parents or relatives may be significant in the development of the child's depression. Research suggests that there is a genetic component to depression (e.g. McGuffin and Katz,

1986; Kendler et al, 1992); that mental illness in one or other parent is likely to produce environmental conditions that contribute to the development of depression, such as a lowered responsiveness to the child or hostility and marital discord (e.g. Rutter and Quinton, 1984; Cox et al, 1987; Schwartz et al, 1990) and that identification with a depressed parent, which is a natural part of development, may result in the child internalising the parent's depression.

Child's temperament

Temperamental characteristics seem to predispose or protect a child from depression (Harrington, 1993). Children who have a propensity to withdraw and are less able to adapt to change may cope less well with crises and be more prone to develop depression. Conversely, adaptable children will find it easier to cope with change and therefore perhaps have an inbuilt protection against depression.

Child's school attendance and peer relationships

A child's school attendance and/or performance is likely to be adversely affected by depression. The young person may be staying off school with somatic symptoms such as stomach aches, or teachers may be reporting lethargy or aggressive outbursts to parents. Peer relationships may noticeably deteriorate, with the child preferring to be alone rather than go out with friends.

A family assessment may reveal family processes that foster the child's depression or suicidal tendencies. For example, Sabbath (1969) believes that a child may commit suicide if they feel they are expendable. The relationship toward the child is likely to be an ambivalent one from birth and, when the child rebels with behavioural disturbances, the rejecting family atmosphere intensifies. The only way to win the parents' affections may be through death. Orbach (1988) talks about 'the unresolvable problem' in relation to childhood suicide, where the only way out is death. For example, when there is extreme hostility between parents but such feelings are denied, their aggression may be directed toward the child, who becomes a scapegoat. Any attempt to escape this predicament will result in further attacks by the parents in order to maintain family equilibrium; the problem is unresolvable except through death.

SCHOOL AND HOME VISIT

A school and home visit by the nurse may shed more light on the child's sadness (see *Family assessment* above). It is important to meet the people at school who are significant for the individual child, for example the head teacher, class teacher and school nurse. On a home visit it is useful to ask the whole family to be present, in order to gain some insight into family dynamics at home. If the child has shown a propensity to self-harm, it is necessary to establish the level of safety in the home environment and the parents' ability to reduce the risk of self-harming. For example, the nurse should establish what drugs are available to the child at home. In 1996, the British government called for a reduction in the number of paracetamol tablets sold in one packet, as impulsive overdose attempts depend on the ready availability of drugs. (See Appendices A and B – *Home visits* and *School visits.*)

NURSING/MULTI-DISCIPLINARY INTERVENTION

During assessment a decision must be made regarding the necessity of an admission to a child/adolescent psychiatric unit. If there are serious concerns regarding the child's mental state and/or a desire not to live has been expressed, the child should be admitted for safety and intensive therapy.

MAINTAINING THE CHILD'S SAFETY

Safety of the ward environment must be ensured

The basic structure of the ward must be as safe as possible; for example, windows should not open so wide that a child could climb out. Any items that could easily be used to cause self-harm, such as scissors and knives or drugs or other chemicals, must be out of the young person's reach.

Writing a contract with the young person who is self-harming

It can be helpful with some older children or adolescents to draw up a contract, which clearly states that they must not harm themselves. Sanctions are identified for any breaks in the contract. The nurse needs to identify something that the young person would not want to miss, such as joining in a particular group activity. This period away from the group must be for a specified length of time and might include some individual work (see below) with a nurse. Sanctions must always be appropriate for the individual child, in order to ensure that they are meaningful and do not reinforce the very behaviour that is meant to be discouraged (for some children, being away from the group and having individual time with a nurse would be experienced as a reward and would therefore reinforce self-destructive behaviour). Contracts may be particularly helpful for young people who cut themselves, but are not suicidal. A child who is intent on killing her/himself or who is severely depressed is unlikely to respond to a contract. For other children, it may not be right on ethical grounds to sanction self-harming behaviour. Such an approach must be discussed in the multi-disciplinary team and with the parents.

Level of child supervision

A decision must be made regarding the level of supervision that is required to ensure the child's safety. If the young person is actively suicidal, **constant supervision** will be essential, meaning that the child is kept in sight and reach of a designated nurse at all times. Nursing staff must rotate in order to prevent fatigue and a lapse in concentration. When parents or other members of the multi-disciplinary team are with the child, it must be made clear who is taking responsibility for supervision. If the child is expressing a wish to self-harm, but is not considered to be actively suicidal, a decision may be made to ensure **close**, but not constant, **supervision**. This will mean that the nurse checks on the child at regular intervals, for example every 15 minutes. Having someone constantly in the same room as the young person can lead to an unhealthly dependence on company and a fear of being left alone. This should be borne in mind when establishing the level.

> Gavin, aged 14, was admitted to the inpatient unit after attempting suicide. A decision was made to supervise him constantly. It soon became apparent that Gavin yearned for attention and emotional nurturing, having had a perverse strict upbringing. Once Gavin stopped attempting to hurt himself, nursing staff began to withdraw their constant supervision and replace it with close observation, only to find that Gavin resumed attempts to self-harm. Gavin had learnt that demonstrating a wish to hurt himself gained the attention he needed.

Physical restraint

The Children Act 1989 states that physical restraint is appropriate if a child is attempting to harm themselves or others (White et al, 1990). It is important that all nurses learn how to restrain safely, in order to prevent injury to the child or themselves. The author suggests some important principles to adopt in relation to restraint and describes two methods of restraint, but insists that a more comprehensive knowledge base and practical training must be undertaken by the nurse.

The number of nursing staff involved in the restraint should be kept to the minimum required to ensure safety for all. The procedure will be more easily coordinated with fewer staff, which is likely to reduce the risk of physical injury and perhaps reduce any psychological trauma caused to the child by the restraint process. The degree of force used must be kept to the minimal amount required. The child must be held firmly enough for them to feel safe and secure, but not so tight as to cause discomfort. It is important not to apply pressure to the joints or to force them out of their natural alignment. The method of restraint used and the manner in which it is executed must ensure that the child's rights and dignity are safeguarded. Inappropriate, potentially sexual contact must be avoided and staff should ensure the child is not inappropriately exposed during the restraint. For example, staff should only restrain a child on the floor as a last resort, avoid contact with breasts or genital areas and replace clothing which becomes misplaced during the restraint.

One nurse should always coordinate the restraint and talk to the child, in order to achieve a safe hold swiftly and reduce the fear that this experience will undoubtedly engender in the child. The nurse must always weigh up the risk of not restraining with the psychological impact of doing so. Other children should be removed from the scene and the situation explained to them. It will be very distressing for onlookers, and their needs must not be overlooked by nursing staff. Staff who are not directly involved in the restraint should periodically check that those who are involved do not need assistance or relief. A new adult entering the scene may help to diffuse the aggression and/or offering the child tranquillising medication that has been prescribed for them, may act immediately as a face-saver for the child as well as eventually calming them. Releasing the hold should be done gradually, one part of the body being released at a time as the child calms down. It is essential to talk to the child in a calm and reassuring voice, and explain to them what is happening to them at each stage of the restraint.

After the episode of restraint, the child must be given an opportunity to talk about it, offered a drink, and if appropriate, helped to change into fresh clothes. The nurses involved in the restraint should also meet to evaluate the restraint process and share feelings. It is always distressing to hold a child against their will and additional or more complicated feelings may also give the nurse some insight into how the child was feeling. Where a child has been sexually abused, the counter-transference experienced by the nurse may include sexual and/or abusive feelings. When other children have witnessed the restraint, such as on an inpatient psychiatric unit, it may be useful to call a meeting with all the children, to allow them the opportunity to talk about what they saw and/or heard and the feelings that it evoked in them. The nurse coordinating the restraint must record the incident in the child's notes and in an audit book, which will enable staff to monitor their use of restraint.

A number of different restraining techniques have been devised and several training courses are available. Nurses must decide which method best suits their area of work. It is beyond the scope of this book to fully cover this aspect of care, and training must in any case include demonstration and practice. However, in order to illustrate some of the key points of good practice, the author will describe three 'Price' (Protecting rights in a care environment) techniques. 'Price' techniques were developed by Nicholson in response to difficulties experienced by staff and injuries incurred by children in residential child care (Nicholson, 1997). (See figures 2.6, 2.7 and 2.8)

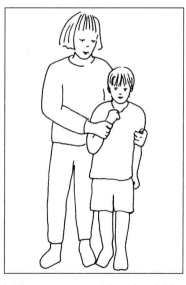

Figure 2.6   Embrace hold. The nurse approaches the child on one side, slightly behind him. Her leading arm encircles the child's back and collects his upper arm. The child's other arm is held flexed and close to his side. A close adjacent body position is maintained between the adult and child to secure the hold.

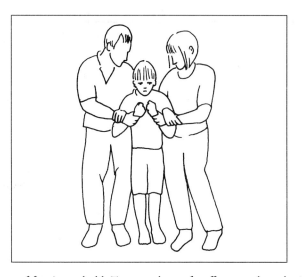

Figure 2.7 'Figure of four' arm hold. Two members of staff approach each side of the child from behind. Each nurse takes hold of the child's arm nearest to them. The nurse's inner hand passes between the child's body and arm, at the same time the nurse's outer hand grasps the outside of the child's forearm above the wrist joint, the nurse's hand palm-up. The nurse's inner hand passes over the child's forearm and grasps his or her own outer forearm. The nurse's inner hip is pushed towards the child's to achieve close body contact, which helps secure the hold.

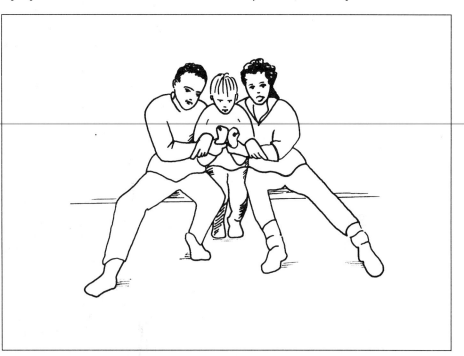

Figure 2.8 Sitting using the 'figure of four' arm hold. Having initially taken hold of the child using a figure of four arm hold, the child is taken to sit down as greater containment is needed. The child is bent forward to secure the hold, as well as the adults continuing to push in towards the child with their hips. It is important not to talk directly into the child's face; this will make the child feel too claustrophobic and provoke further struggles to break free.

Inpatient units should have a policy for the use of restraint, training provision for staff and a system of audit. There is always a danger that incidents of restraint can escalate in number, either for individual children or more generally, if nurses start to rely on this method of containing undesirable behaviour. Most children will be reassured that they have not been allowed to hurt themselves; however, it is important that they do not learn to rely on others to intervene but, instead, learn self-restraint. The use of restraint to prevent a child from self-harming must be discussed with parents before admission and parents themselves need to be taught how to restrain their child safely.

Locking the unit door

If a child is threatening to abscond from the ward, it may be necessary temporarily to lock the main door, rather than constantly having to restrain the child. The Children Act 1989 states that, if a child is likely to come to harm from absconding, restricting their liberty in this way is permissible (White et al, 1990). However, unless the ward is a 'secure unit', Court approval should be sought if the door is locked for more than 72 hours in 28 days. A system of audit is therefore essential. All parents of children on the ward must be notified that the door is locked and it should be made clear that other children on the ward can move as freely as usual. The length of time that the unit is locked should be kept to a minimum.

INDIVIDUAL WORK

It is essential that the child feels accepted by the nurse undertaking individual work and that a genuine wish to listen and try to understand is conveyed to the child. Building a therapeutic relationship will be an essential component of individual work (see *Assessment – Getting to know children* above).

Helping the child to recognise and express their own thoughts and feelings

A child who is depressed is likely to feel numb, being disconnected from their own thoughts and feelings. One of the aims of individual therapy will be to help the child to recognise and express what they are thinking and feeling. A number of techniques can be used by the nurse, such as:

◆ A 'feelings' thermometer could be used to enable the child visually to convey the extent of unhappiness (Figure 2.9).

◆ A series of drawings of different facial expressions could be presented to the child, who is asked to point to the one that represents most closely how they are feeling. Visual methods are particularly useful when working with very withdrawn children (Figure 2.10).

◆ Asking the young person to keep a diary, which can be discussed at the end of the day.

◆ Reflecting on what the child tells you and/or hypothesising on how you think the

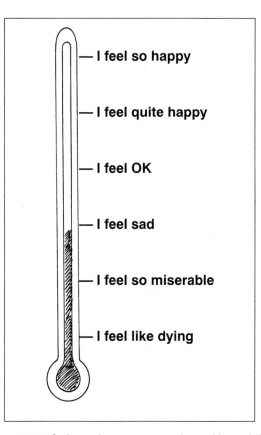

Figure 2.9 A feelings thermometer coloured by a child.

child might be feeling given their observable behaviour. For a child who is mute, this may be all that you can do. It is important to stress to the child that you may be wrong in your guessing. The nurse can encourage the child to indicate verbally or non-verbally whether he/she is accurate.

> Leanne, aged 13, sat hunched up with her hair covering her face. She had been mute for several weeks. It later became apparent that she had been sexually abused. Initially her only means of communication was to affirm or discount nurses' suggestions regarding how she was feeling. She achieved this by moving one finger to affirm their conjecture.

Children who are self-harming need to be encouraged to vent the destructive feelings that they are directing towards themselves. This may be achieved through 'angry times' (see Chapter 3 – *Targeting the behaviour problem*) and/or during individual sessions.

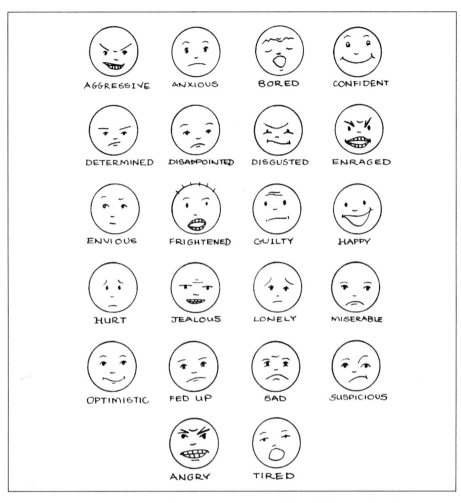

Figure 2.10 Drawings of facial expressions to help children indicate how they are feeling.

Fiona, aged 14 years, had been sexually abused by a stranger near her home. She had run out of the house at night, after arguing with her parents, and felt to blame for the assault. She was admitted to the psychiatric unit with a diagnosis of anorexia nervosa and self-harming behaviour. Fiona had taken one overdose and cut her arms repeatedly. Eventually she was able to disclose her abusive experience and begin to express her anger through drawing (see Plate 2 which appears in the unfolioed section between p56 and 57) and 'angry times'.

Separating the positive and negative self

For the suicidal child, it may be helpful to talk with them about having two sides: a negative side that is self-hating and wants to die and a positive side, albeit small, that wants to live. By splitting off these two sides, the nurse can encourage nurturing of the positive side. When the child is talking negatively, the nurse can comment, 'That's your self-hatred talking. I'd like to talk with your positive side' (Orbach, 1988). This idea could be developed further using visual demonstration, for example:

◆   Balancing scales could be used to assess how heavy or strong each side is. Counters represent positive and negative thoughts, feelings and ideas, and each counter is clearly identifiable by the application of a sticky label. As counters are labelled, they are placed into the positive or negative bowls of the scales. For example, a wish to return to school would go into the positive bowl, whereas a feeling that 'I'm horrible' would go into the negative one. This exercise may help the child to identify the part of them that wants to live, and could be repeated at intervals to demonstrate improvement.

◆   Drawings could be made to represent the positive and negative sides. The child might draw a monster for the negative side and 'Superman' for the positive. These analogies can then be used in discussion with the child and in further individual work, always with the aim of helping 'Superman' to win (see Chapter 5 – *Individual work* on using imagery to fight against the symptom).

Cognitive–behavioural work

Lewinsohn et al (1990) demonstrated the efficacy of cognitive–behavioural treatment for depressed adolescents. A modified version of the 'coping with depression course' for adults was used which addresses the problematic areas for depressed individuals: discomfort and anxiety, irrational and negative thoughts, poor social skills and a low rate of pleasant activities. The course ran for 7 weeks, with 2-hour sessions twice weekly. Skills training included teaching relaxation techniques, increasing pleasant events, controlling irrational and negative thoughts, and improving social skills, in particular conflict resolution.

Relaxation techniques

As anxiety is often associated with depression, teaching a child skills in relaxation may improve their sense of well-being and reduce their feelings of helplessness by giving them some self-control (see Chapter 4 – *Relaxation*).

Reframing

Because of feelings of paranoia, a depressed individual may misintepret a banal and harmless situation. Reframing aims to help the child see things more objectively and to think rationally. The child must learn to connect their thoughts to subsequent mood and behaviour. A diary could be kept to record each time they feel sad. It is useful to divide the pages into three columns (Figure 2.11) to help the child identify irrational thoughts which may be confounding their feelings of sadness and to recognise how their own behaviour can influence what happens around them, which may also reinforce their depression. In the example given in Figure 2.11, the situation can be reframed in a number of ways: the other children were unaware of the child's presence because of their own excitement, or they were aware of the child but thought he/she showed no interest in joining in.

TUESDAY 5 MAY		
HOW I WAS FEELING AND WHAT I WAS THINKING ABOUT	WHAT WAS HAPPENING	WHAT I WAS DOING
I was feeling sad, thinking that nobody cared about me or wanted to play with me	The other children in the unit were planning to play a board game together. They were noisy— all trying to choose the game. They didn't ask me if I wanted to play	I was sitting on my own looking out of the window

Figure 2.11 Page of a teenager's diary aimed at helping her or him to recognise irrational thoughts and identify patterns of their own behaviour which may contribute to their sadness.

Problem-solving

Another cognitive–behavioural approach involves problem-solving. The young person identifies a problem, such as the example above: being left out of games by peers. Together, the child and nurse generate solutions to the problem, such as the child asking to join in, initiating games or showing interest when games are suggested. After brainstorming a number of solutions, the child picks one to try. The next time a similar situation arises, the child implements the solution and then evaluates its effectiveness in a subsequent individual session. Role-playing in the individual session may help to boost the child's confidence in putting the plan into action.

Developing coping strategies

Helping the child to develop coping strategies is an important adjunct to reframing and problem-solving. It is important that the young person does not feel a failure if they are unable to reframe or problem-solve effectively. Coping strategies might include:

♦ *Avoiding potential difficulties* Using the example above, the child could choose to spend time on their own or with one other child, when group games are going on.

◆ *Seeking support from others* The child could seek support from nursing staff after the group game has started and they feel excluded.

◆ *Making a decision to try harder next time* Problem-solving may have been unsuccessful this time, but it is important that the child does not feel a failure and, instead, must decide to try harder on the next occasion.

◆ *Controlling self-destructive behaviour* Help the child to find someone to talk to rather than hurt him/herself.

◆ *Using relaxation techniques* (see Chapter 4 – *Relaxation*).

Improving self-esteem

Helping to improve a child's self-esteem is a relevant part of individual work for each chapter in this book and therefore, despite overlapping with other areas of individual work, such as cognitive approaches, it warrants special attention. The nurse may create her/his own exercises, but some possibilities are as follows:

◆ *Bedtime review of accomplishments* The child writes a diary with the help of the nurse, who helps the young person to identify their achievements of the day.

◆ *Life book* With the help of the nurse and parents, the child creates a 'life book'. This is a record of the child's life in the form of writing, pictures, documents, memorabilia and so on, and aims to give the young person a sense of who they are. Life books are particularly useful for children who do not live with their birth families. They not only facilitate discussion about the past and present, but can also be used to help the child think about their future and how to move forwards (Ryan and Walker, 1985).

◆ *Draw a map* Another exercise to help build a sense of self is for the child to draw a map to represent their life to date. The road, river or railway starts in one corner of the picture and ends in another. Different buildings, trees, and so on, represent different people or events.

◆ *Write an advertisement* With the help of the nurse and/or another child, the identified child writes an advertisement for her/himself. This could be kept in a special file for self-esteem work.

◆ *Interviewing others* With the help of the nurse, the child writes a short questionnaire to find out what others think of her/him. One question might be, 'What do you think my strengths are?' Together, the child and nurse approach different children, staff and family members.

◆ *Body outline* The nurse draws around the child on a life-size piece of paper and together they write in the child's strengths, such as big brown eyes on the face, neat handwriting on the right hand, and kind heart on the chest. The young person can then stick the final work on their bedroom wall to act as a reminder of their good points.

◆ *Teach others* Having discovered a particular skill that the child has, the nurse prepares the child to teach others. This may take place on a one to one basis with the additional support of the nurse or, if the child feels confident enough, group teaching sessions could be arranged. Skills might include cooking a particular recipe, calligraphy, make-up, plaiting hair, and so on.

MILIEU THERAPY

A daily timetable comprised of purposeful activities with other children and/or nursing staff together with some 'free time' alone provides the young person with limited time for depressive ruminations but some space to be alone and in touch with their feelings. If the child is requiring constant supervision, observing them from a distance or through an open door to their bedroom can allow the child some freedom from intrusion.

An important part of milieu therapy for the child who is extremely unhappy and possibly suicidal is for nursing staff to respond to cues of sadness by commenting to the child on what they observe. Simply stating, 'You look really sad' indicates to the child that you are aware of how they feel or at least trying to understand. A suicidal child will be less inclined to take any drastic actions to show how bad they feel, if adults caring for them are clearly making efforts to hear and understand their distress.

GROUP WORK

Group activities and therapy can play an important part in building the child's self-esteem and self-reliance. The views of other children may hold more weight than those of adults. It is also likely that some of them will be experiencing similar worries and can demonstrate a different level of empathy as peers, which is not possible in the professional nurse–child relationship. Examples of group activities to boost self-esteem and self-reliance include:

◆ *Advertising your partner* Children are divided into pairs. Each child writes an advertisement for themselves with the help of their partner. Group facilitators will need to circulate to offer assistance. Returning to the group, children introduce their partners using the advertisement. The presentation may include a poster, exhibits, such as samples of art work or music that the child likes, acting, and so on. Although a depressed child is unlikely to be able to recognise any strengths in themselves, another child will, with or without the help of staff. Similarly, the depressed child will probably be able to see the strengths of others.

◆ *Practising giving and receiving compliments and criticism* This involves the use of role play and perhaps videotaping for group discussion.

◆ *Assertiveness training* Titles of sessions might include: 'coping with bullying', 'making yourself heard' and 'asking for help'. Nursing staff could role-play situations that demonstrate assertiveness, aggressiveness and passivity, which are then discussed in the group. The children should be encouraged to identify the features of an interaction that characterise assertiveness and then practise for themselves situations in which they would like to be more assertive, using role play.

◆ *Problem-solving exercises* Peers are used to help individual children find solutions (see *Individual work above*). Role play could be used to test out different solutions.

◆ *Creating the circumstances that will attract positive reinforcement from peers and other staff* Establish what activities the child is good at, perhaps from parents, and provide opportunities for these, so that the child can receive positive reinforcement from their peers and staff.

Fine and colleagues (1991) demonstrated the immediate effectiveness of a therapeutic support group for treating depressed adolescents. In this group, adolescents were encouraged to share common concerns, discuss ways of dealing with difficult situations and offer mutual support. The therapeutic support group was compared with a social skills training group, where the adolescents learnt problem-solving skills, how to recognise feelings in themselves and others, assertiveness, giving and receiving positive and negative feedback, and conversational skills. The therapeutic support group was found to be more immediately effective in reducing depression. However, at 9-month follow-up, adolescents assigned to the social skills training group caught up and showed a similar level of improvement. Perhaps this early discrepancy in effectiveness suggests that adolescents experiencing a more severe mood disturbance are not ready to utilise social skills training. However, at a later stage in treatment, social skills training can be effective.

FAMILY THERAPY

Brief cognitive–behavioural work

Rotheram-Borus and co-workers (1994) describe a brief standardised cognitive–behavioural treatment for adolescent suicide attempters and their families. A series of activities are aimed at helping the family to problem-solve and change the family's understanding of their problems, to one of troublesome or difficult situations rather than of a troublesome individual, the adolescent. At the beginning of each session, the family therapist gives each member of the family some tokens, perhaps counters. The therapist instructs the family to hand a token to another person whenever they have a positive feeling towards that person or want to express their agreement. This approach encourages positive interactions. The family is asked to make a hierarchy of problems and each family member gives a thermometer reading for each problem. A problem of medium proportion ('warm' on the thermometer) is selected to work on, in order to increase the likelihood of success. The family is taught how to analyse the problem situation and positively reframe underlying causes to the conflict. For example, a recurring argument between a mother and daughter over when the teenager should return home at night could be seen as an example of a mean controlling mother and disrespectful teenager or, more positively, a concerned caring mother and a teenager trying to struggle with her own issues of autonomy. Having a greater understanding of what lies behind a problem situation, the family then brainstorm possible solutions and select one to role play. This family therapy approach aims to challenge the family's beliefs and raise self-esteem and coping abilities.

Identifying the function of the child's unhappiness

Problems within the family may be hidden to the outside world, but become located in one particular child, who is presented as the 'problem child'. Strong denial of difficulties is likely to lead to such scapegoating. The child's problem or unhappiness becomes a living representative of the family's problem. Covert hostilities are more likely to lead to self-destructive tendencies rather than outward aggression. Orbach (1988), who believes that children attempt suicide when confronted with an unsolvable problem, suggests that the therapist constantly ask her/himself, 'Why does this child feel that there is no other way out?'. Meetings with different combinations of family members may be important to address problems hinging around particular family relationships. Parents may need to have some sessions together to address marital difficulties. However, in other situations the whole family's presence may be important, for example if there has been a death in the family for which there has been no bereavement. Therapy aims to give the family permission to express feelings openly, which in turn should allow the defusion of destructive covert fury.

INDIVIDUAL PSYCHOANALYTICAL AND INTERPERSONAL PSYCHOTHERAPY

Psychotherapy may enable the child to have a better understanding of their feelings and a greater sense of self. For example, the therapist may help the child to recognise feelings of anger which are being turned inwards causing self-hatred and self-harming behaviour. Giving the child permission to have 'negative' feelings may help to reduce their feelings of guilt and self-loathing, and facilitate the open expression of such emotion.

It appears that interpersonal psychotherapy (IPT) can be an effective form of treatment for depressed adolescents (Mufson et al, 1994). This is a brief treatment that focuses specifically on addressing current interpersonal problems. Depending on the treatment resources available and the individual needs of the teenager, this form of individual therapy may be chosen in preference to psychoanalytical psychotherapy. Training in IPT is relatively short and straightforward, and so members of the multi-disciplinary team, other than those trained in psychoanalytical psychotherapy, could undertake this form of treatment.

MEDICATION

For severely depressed children and adolescents, medication may be prescribed. Tricyclic antidepressants, such as imipramine and amitriptyline, may be considered for 'slowed up' and agitated children, respectively. The dose for either drug should be in the range of 2–5 mg kg^{-1} day^{-1}. Puig and Weston (1983) demonstrated a 100% response rate when plasma levels were maintained at 155 ng ml^{-1}. Low plasma levels resulted in a rate of response of only 33%. The dose of imipramine or amitriptyline must be slowly increased to the therapeutic level and the child monitored for side-effects. These include a dry mouth, sedation (particularly amitriptyline), postural hypotension, tachycardia, blurred vision, tremors, sweating, rashes, nausea, constipation, appetite disturbance, behavioural disturbances and cardiac arrhythmias. Electrocardiography should be arranged by medical staff if high doses are prescribed, and nursing staff should monitor the child's pulse, lying and standing blood pressure, and observe for other side-effects. Improvement in the child's mood should be seen in 10 days and, if there is no improvement after 3 weeks, the medication should be stopped. If the drug is effective, it should be stopped after about 2 months. The drug must be slowly reduced at the end of treatment to minimise the likelihood of withdrawal effects, which include gastrointestinal complaints, drowsiness, decreased appetite, tearfulness, apathy or withdrawal, headaches, agitation and insomnia.

Selective serotonin re-uptake inhibitors, such as fluoxetine, have become more popular for the treatment of depression, because of reduced cardiotoxicity. However, insomnia, agitation, headaches and restlessness may occur and, of particular concern, self-injurious behaviour has been reported (King et al, 1991). Gastrointestinal complaints, including nausea, vomiting, abdominal pain, constipation and diarrhoea are fairly common side-effects. Effective dosage seems to be in the range of 0.33–0.73 mg kg^{-1} day^{-1}.

FOLLOW-UP

Pfeffer et al (1994) looked at the risk of recurrent suicidal episodes in prepubertal and young adolescents following discharge from psychiatric inpatient treatment. Those with a history of suicidal ideation or suicide attempt had a significant risk of attempting suicide within 6 months of discharge and a heightened risk for the first 2 years. This study highlights the need for careful and thorough discharge planning. Community nurses can play an important part in the provision of long-term care and treatment.

CONCLUSION

Developmentally, children are less likely to verbalise feelings of sadness. Instead, they may be withdrawn, irritable or develop somatic symptoms. Therefore, nurses will need to draw on all their creative and non-verbal skills to build a therapeutic relationship and facilitate change.

The most fundamental aspect of nursing children who are self-harming is to do everything possible to ensure their safety. However, it is important to remember that professionals and parents can only do their best, and a child who is intent on killing themself is likely to succeed.

Relevant areas of work include: helping the child to recognise, accept and openly express his/her own feelings, rather than turn negative thoughts inwards; helping to raise self-esteem; facilitating the development of coping strategies; and teaching problem-solving skills. It is likely that a number of factors will contribute to a child's sadness and/or self-harming behaviour. In working with the family it will be important to identify whether the child's mood and behaviour serve a family function and, where a child is suicidal, to establish why the child feels that death is the only solution.

REFERENCES

Ackerly WC (1967) Latency-age children who threaten or attempt to kill themselves. *Journal of the American Academy of Child Psychiatry* **6**: 242–261.

American Psychiatric Association (1994) *Diagnostic and Statisical Manual of Mental Disorders*, 4th edn (DSM IV). Washington, DC: American Psychiatric Association.

Bifulco A, Brown GW and Harris TO (1987) Childhood loss of parent, lack of adequate parental care and adult depression: a replication. *Journal of Affective Disorders* **12**: 115–118.

Bowlby J (1980) *Attachment and Loss. Vol. 3: Loss: Sadness and Depression*. New York: Basic Books.

Cox AD, Puckering C, Pound A and Mills M (1987) The impact of maternal depression in young children. *Journal of Child Psychology and Psychiatry* **28**: 917–928.

Fine S, Forth A, Gilbert M and Haley G (1991) Group therapy for adolescent depressive disorder: a comparison of social skills and therapeutic support. *Journal of the American Academy of Child and Adolescent Psychiatry* **30(1)**: 79– 85.

Goodyer IM and Altham PME (1991) Lifetime exit events and recent social and family adversities in anxious and depressed school-age children and adolescents – I and II. *Journal of Affective Disorders* **21**: 219–238.

Hanes MJ (1995) Utilizing road drawings as a therapeutic metaphor in art therapy. *American Journal of Art Therapy* **34(1)**: 19–23.

Harrington R (1993) Predisposing and precipitating factors. In *Depressive Disorder in Childhood and Adolescence,* pp 97–124. Chichester, UK: John Wiley.

Hemmings P (1991) *All about me*. Ilford, Essex: Barnados.

Kendler KS, Neale MC, Kessler RC, Heath AC and Evans LJ (1992) A population-based twin study of major depression in women: the impact of varying definitions of illness. *Archives of General Psychiatry* **49**: 257–266.

King RA, Riddle MA, Chappell PB et al (1991) Emergence of self-destructive phenomena in children and adolescents during fluoxetine treatment. *Journal of the American Academy of Child and Adolescent Psychiatry* **30(2)**: 179–186.

Lewinsohn PM, Clarke GN, Hops H and Andrews J (1990) Cognitive–behavioural treatment for depressed adolescents. *Behavior Therapy* **21**: 385–401.

Lowenfeld M (1939) The world pictures of children. *British Journal of Medical Psychology* **18**: 65–101.

Lowenfeld M (1950) The nature and use of the Lowenfeld world technique in work with children and adults. *Journal of Psychology* **30**: 325–331.

McClure GMG (1994) Suicide in children and adolescents in England and Wales 1960–1990. *British Journal of Psychiatry* **165**: 510–514.

McGuffin P and Katz R (1986) Nature, nurture and affective disorder. In Deakin JFW (ed.) *The Biology of Depression*, pp 26–52. London: Royal College of Psychiatrists.

Mufson L, Moreau D, Weissman MM, Wickramaratne P, Martin J and Samoilov A (1994) Modification of interpersonal psychotherapy with depressed adolescents (IPT-A): phase I and II studies. *Journal of the American Academy of Child and Adolescent Psychiatry* **33(5)**: 695–705.

Nicholson B (1997) Price techniques. *Professional Social Work* **March**: 8.

Nikelly AG (1988) Does DSM-III-R diagnose depression in non-Western patients? *International Journal of Social Psychiatry* **34(4)**: 316–320.

Orbach I (1988) *Children Who Don't Want to Live*. London: Jossey-Bass.

Paykel ES (1982) Life events and early development. In Paykel ES (ed.) *Handbook of Affective Disorders*, pp 146–161. Edinburgh: Churchill Livingstone.

Pfeffer C R (1986) *The Suicidal Child*. New York: The Guilford Press.

Pfeffer CR, Hurt SW, Kakuma T, Peskin JR, Siefker CA and Nagabhairava S (1994) Suicidal children grow up: episodes and effects of treatment during follow-up. *Journal of the American Academy of Child and Adolescent Psychiatry* **33(2)**: 225–230.

Puig J and Weston B (1983) The diagnosis and treatment of major depressive disorder in childhood. *Annual Review of Medicine* **34**: 231–245.

Reinherz HZ, Stewart-Berghauer G, Pakiz B, Frost AK, Moeykens BA and Holmes WM (1989) The relationship of early risk and current mediators to depressive symptomatology in adolescence. *Journal of the American Academy of Child Psychiatry* **28**: 942–947.

Rotheram-Borus MJ, Piacentini J, Miller S, Graal F and

Castro-Blanco D (1994) Brief cognitive–behavioural treatment for adolescent suicide attempters and their families. *Journal of the American Academy of Child and Adolescent Psychiatry* **33(4)**: 508–517.

Rutter M and Quinton D (1984) Parental psychiatric disorder: effects on children. *Psychological Medicine* **14**: 853–880.

Rutter M, Tizard J and Whitmore K (eds.) (1970) Education, Health and Behaviour. London: Longman.

Rutter M, Graham P, Chadwick OFD and Yule W (1976) Adolescent turmoil: fact or fiction. *Journal of Child Psychology and Psychiatry* **17**: 35–56.

Ryan T and Walker R (1985) *Making Life Story Books*. London: British Agencies for Adoption and Fostering.

Sabbath JC (1969) The suicide adolescent – the expendable child. *Journal of the American Academy of Child Psychiatry* **38**: 211–220.

Schechter DM (1957) Explaining child suicide. In Orbach I. (ed.) (1988) *Children Who Don't Want to Live*. London: Jossey-Bass.

Schwartz CE, Dorer DJ, Beardslee WR, Lavori PW and Keller MB (1990) Maternal expressed emotion and parental affective disorder: risk for childhood depressive, substance abuse or conduct disorder. *Journal of Psychiatry Research* **24**: 231–250.

Segal H (1973) The depressive position. In *Introduction to the Work of Melanie Klein*, pp 67–81. London: Hogarth Press.

Trad PV (1987) *Infant and Childhood Depression*, New York. John Wiley.

White R, Carr P and Lowe N (1990) *A Guide to the Children Act 1989*. London: Butterworth.

3   RESTLESS, DISTRACTED OPPOSITIONAL AND AGGRESSIVE

INTRODUCTION

This chapter considers some of the most challenging problems for the nurse. The child who is restless, distracted, oppositional and perhaps aggressive. Working with these children requires great patience, perseverance and understanding. It is essential that professionals work in a team where there is space for discussion and mutual support. Strong feelings and emphatic disagreements regarding treatment are likely to occur and should be predicted. Perhaps then it is possible to look at the 'split' in the team more objectively and for constructive decisions be made on behalf of the child and those caring for him/her. Otherwise it is so easy to 'give up' on these children and for them to be moved from one school or treatment centre to another. Such a poor outcome serves only to lower the child's self-esteem further, and to lower the self-confidence of parents and professionals involved.

Challenging behaviour is a part of healthy development and necessary for children to acquire important social skills. All children must explore and experiment in order to learn. Infants strive to discover the limits of their parent's authority and, given appropriate boundaries and role models, develop self-control and assertiveness. Children naturally seek new experiences and, provided with guidance and supervision, learn about safety and develop prudent inhibitions. The ability to concentrate and problem-solve are skills that develop throughout pre-school and school years. Toddlers can focus their attention, but the ability to sustain concentration and problem-solve takes time to acquire. When children deviate from these developmental norms a number of problems, such as learning difficulties, family dysfunction, peer rejection and low self-esteem, are likely to ensue. Unchecked, these problems are likely to perpetuate into adult life.

There has been much controversy surrounding the diagnosis, aetiology and treatment of attention deficits and overactivity in children. Diagnostic terminology has also changed over recent years, adding to the confusion. The term 'hyperactive' is sometimes used very loosely but generally implies overactivity with inattentiveness and impulsivity. The *Diagnostic and Statistical Manual of Mental Disorders* (American Psychiatric Association, 1994) identifies three subgroups for 'attention deficit–hyperactivity disorder' (ADHD) which distinguish between children in whom inattentiveness, hyperactivity and impulsivity are equally prevalent, inattentiveness is the dominant feature and where hyperactivity and impulsivity prevail. A diagnosis of ADHD requires that symptoms first appeared before the age of 7 years, have persisted for at least 6 months and are outside the developmental norms for the age of the child. In addition, there must be clear life impairment in areas such as school, family and peer group.

A 'conduct disorder' is characterised by a persistent pattern of antisocial behaviour. The child may be aggressive towards people and/or animals, deliberately destroy property, be deceitful or steal, be truant from school or violate other rules (American Psychiatric Association, 1994). Aggressiveness and defiance are often associated with hyperactivity, and vice versa. Therefore, there are some similarities between a diagnosis of ADHD and a conduct disorder.

Whatever the medical diagnosis, the aetiology and/or maintenance of such behavioural problems is likely to be multi-factorial. Possible contributing factors include:

◆ Genetic predisposition

◆ Neurological dysfunction or damage

◆ Biochemical factors

◆ Perinatal factors (e.g. maternal substance abuse during pregnancy and low birth weight)

◆ Temperament

◆ Physical environment (e.g. lead poisoning)

◆ Dietary factors (e.g. food additives)

◆ Psychological stressors (e.g. physical illness or disability, maternal depression, marital conflict between parents)

◆ Ineffective parenting

ASSESSMENT

A thorough and comprehensive assessment is necessary to clarify the behavioural problem and make an appropriate referral. Nurses working in the community are in an ideal position to identify children for whom a psychiatric referral would be beneficial. Given that the problems dealt with in this chapter are likely to continue, and indeed worsen into adult life, effective primary health-care screening is paramount. Many parents will have some concerns about their child's behaviour and some will benefit from simple advice, perhaps from a health visitor, whereas others will require specialist psychiatric help. Ambiguous statements regarding a child's behaviour will need to be clarified and an understanding of the context in which it occurs gleaned. Assessment will need to be approached from a number of different angles to gain a reasonably clear picture of the problem and make useful suggestions regarding appropriate intervention.

Once a behavioural problem has been picked up by parents or professionals, a decision must be made concerning the most appropriate place to undertake a thorough assessment and, following this, where the child and family should recieve help. This may all take place in the community or the child may be admitted to a child/adolescent psychiatric unit.

Factors indicating that admission will be necessary include:

◆ The child is in danger of hurting him/herself or others.

◆ The parents or school cannot cope with the child's behaviour.

◆ A 24-hour assessment by specialist nursing staff in a relatively neutral and therapeutic environment is necessary to clarify the issues.

FAMILY ASSESSMENT

The family assessment and observation of parent–child interaction (see below) will overlap to a certain extent and may actually be incorporated into a few family meetings involving the same professional(s). Ideally, a family therapist should be involved. Meeting the whole family enables the therapist to start building a picture of the environment in which the behaviour problem arose and its impact on the family. Certain information regarding the problem and reason for referral must first be established:

◆ *The nature of the problematic behaviour* A clear, precise and non-ambiguous description of the behaviour, including its frequency, should be obtained. For example: 'If I say he can't do something like getting out a certain video, Keith hits or kicks me and then runs off. Sometimes he'll run off for several hours. It's not unusual for him to run off all day or evening and not return until midnight or 1 o'clock in the morning. This is now happening two or three times a week.' A vague and ambiguous description might be: 'Keith's a nightmare if he doesn't get his own way'.

◆ *The context in which it occurs* This should include a description of when, where and with whom the behaviour occurs and the type of situation that might provoke it. For example: 'It happens at home and in school, but more at home. It only happens with me (mother) at home – never with Simon (step-father). At school he's kicked his teacher badly. As I said before, it's when Keith's told that he can't do something, although I have also noticed it's worse if he's recently seen his dad'.

◆ *When the parents first noticed that the child's behaviour was problematic* Have there always been difficulties or are they more recent, and if so, are the parents aware of any significant trigger? Keith had always been 'a handful' according to his mother: boisterous, accident prone and argumentative.

◆ *The consequences of the child's behaviour* How do the parents and school manage the child's behaviour? For example: 'Simon goes looking for him and gives him a right telling off.' 'What do you mean by a right telling off?'(therapist). 'He's grounded for a week. The school were sending him home for a few days, which didn't help because I can't cope and now they've suspended him indefinitely.'

◆ *How the parents would like the child to behave* What are the parents' expectations of the child? Asked directly, Keith's parents are likely to feel patronised and answer: 'We want him to stop being aggressive, running off and to do as he's told!' However, it would be helpful to know what the rules are regarding behaviour at home and what limits are set concerning going out alone.

◆ *What help the parents want* Keith's parents wanted him to return to the same school (he had been expelled from two previous schools), but for him to receive help. They were uncertain about the benefit of admission to the inpatient psychiatric unit.

Establishing the history of the family and significant events, together with more general information concerning the child's personality and temperament will form an important part of the family assessment. Children who have not had a stable, secure and consistent family are likely to have difficulties in acquiring socially desirable behaviour. Wolkind and Rutter (1973) found that deviant behaviour in later childhood was associated with being 'in care' in early childhood. Wolff (1985) discussed the influences of marital discord, violence within the family, the absence of a father figure, large sibship and maternal depression on aggressive behaviour in children. A child's temperament will affect parenting style, which in turn may provoke aggressive behaviour. For example, a child's awkwardness may evoke greater criticism from parents, which in turn contributes to the aetiology of aggressive behaviour.

Mary described her own childhood as complicated, with her mother having several partners. She had married at 18 when she became pregnant with Keith. Keith's father (David) had left Mary when Keith was 2 and had susequently been in prison. His contact with Keith was inconsistent and unreliable. Keith said he had a great time with his dad and would like to see more of him. Mary had divorced David and re-married when Keith was 4. Keith was said to get on well with his step-father but fought constantly with his younger half-brother, James. Mary had an uneventful pregnancy and straightforward birth. Keith was very 'clingy' as a young child and Mary had great difficulties leaving him at nursery school. However, as he became older, he had become more adventurous and outgoing. He made friends easily, but the relationships did not last, as other boys and girls got fed up with him always wanting his own way and breaking their things. Keith was described as being a lively 11-year-old boy who was bright but had difficulties in school. Mary said he was good at what he liked doing, but he didn't like school work.

This is a brief summary of the information obtained from Keith's family and gives an idea of the sort of information that is helpful, but is by no means comprehensive. Constructing a family tree is a useful tool for facilitating a discussion on family history, relationships and personalities.

OBSERVATION OF PARENT–CHILD INTERACTION

Observation of the parent–child interaction will give useful information regarding parenting style. Research (Gent, 1992, p. 32) indicates that 'parents of problem children differ from other parents in their interactions by:

- ◆ Being more punitive
- ◆ Issuing more commands
- ◆ Providing more attention after unacceptable behaviour
- ◆ Being less likely to perceive oppositional behaviour as such
- ◆ Being more involved in extended coercive hostile interchanges
- ◆ Giving vague commands
- ◆ Being generally less effective in stopping their child's non-compliant behaviour'

Specific observation of the parent–child interaction may be organised by means of a video link or one-way mirror, or may be part of an inpatient assessment or home visit. In an observation session using a video link or one-way mirror, the parents and child would be set a task, perhaps to play a game, and observations would be recorded. On an inpatient unit, nurses can observe the parents and child in a variety of situations, such as mealtimes, free play, going into school, bed-time and so on. A home visit by nursing staff provides an opportunity to meet the family in their own environment and may give important clues concerning the nature of home life (see Appendix A – *Home visit*). A one-off observation of the parent–child interaction will give a false representation of reality, but a comprehensive assessment providing various different opportunities to see the parents and child together will help to form a more accurate picture.

OBSERVATION OF CHILD IN PEER GROUP AND WITH OTHER ADULTS

An inpatient admission to a psychiatric unit will allow nursing staff to observe the child's inter-action with peers and other adults in the absence of their parents. Questions to be answered include:

✦ Does the child relate easily with peers or is he/she reserved, awkward or aggressive?

✦ Does the child show warmth and empathy towards other children or is he/she egocentric?

✦ Can the child share with others?

✦ Is the child highly competitive?

✦ How does the child handle loosing in a game or not achieving as well as others in school?

✦ Is the child unusually familiar, reserved or aggressive with adults?

✦ Does the child respond to limit-setting by other adults?

An inpatient assessment will reveal whether the child's behavioural problem is all pervasive or specific. Most children entering a new situation, such as a new school or an inpatient unit, will have a 'honeymoon' period, when the problem behaviour disappears temporarily. An inpatient assessment must be long enough to allow the problem behaviour to materialise. LaBarbera and Dozier (1985) assessed the changes in intensity of behavioural problems in 28 children admitted to a child psychiatry inpatient unit and found that uncontrolled aggression, misbehaviour and dependency became more vivid after 60 days of admission than after 14 days.

SCHOOL VISIT

A school visit provides an opportunity for nursing staff to experience the atmosphere of the child's school as well as to learn about its philosophy and to meet significant teachers. It is important to establish how the child behaves and functions in class, his/her behaviour in the playground, the parents' involvement in the school and whether the staff consider the school to be appropriate for the child (see Appendix B – *School visit*).

OBSERVATION CHARTS AND DIARIES

It is often very helpful if parents, or nursing staff on an inpatient unit, observe and record every incident of the problem behaviour using an ABC chart or diary (see Chapter 4 – *Assessment, Baseline recording*) in order to identify the triggers and evaluate adult responses. The frequency of problem behaviour may not be as high as first suggested, or the parents be fully aware of how they react to their child (perhaps aggravating the problem), until a written record has been made. Inconsistency between parents, excessive criticism or covert rewards for inappropriate behaviour may come to the fore (see Figure 3.1).

MEDICAL OR PSYCHIATRIC ASSESSMENT

The medical history should include the parents' memories of their own childhood, as a familial pattern in behaviour may be discovered. There is a high risk for ADHD among children of parents with childhood onset of the disorder (Biederman et al, 1995).

Any problems in pregnancy, birth and the early postnatal period may also be significant. Antenatal difficulties, low birth-weight, diseases of infancy and early neurological injury have

ANTECEDENTS	BEHAVIOUR	CONSEQUENCES
Keith had spent morning waiting for his father to pick him up. David didn't turn up. James had painted a picture which he said he wanted to give to Simon.	Keith tore up James' picture. James was holding it up to show Keith. Keith took it from him laughing and joked around with it. I told him not to be so nasty. He tore it up.	When he wouldn't give it back to James, I told him not to be so nasty. After he tore it, I said he was really spiteful and he couldn't go out with Simon tomorrow.
James and Simon went out for the day. Keith was grounded.	He kicked out at me when I had to stop him trying to leave with Simon and James. Then he ran off.	Simon and James stayed back. Simon went after Keith. We were all really angry with Keith for ruining the day.
Keith and James were arguing over something – I can't remember what.	A fight started	I told them to pack it in at once. I said when they stopped we'd go out. To my surprise they stopped after a minute or so and we went out.

Figure 3.1 Example of an ABC chart completed by a parent

been related to ADHD (Cantwell and Hanna, 1989; McCormick et al, 1990) and it seems likely that substance abuse during pregnancy may induce disinhibition, learning difficulties and behavioural problems (Brown et al, 1993).

There is no impressive evidence that dietary factors cause hyperactivity. Possibly, there is a minimal effect on the behaviour of a small number of young children. Food additives and sugar eaten with protein or carbohydrate alone have been implicated in provoking hyperactivity and deviant behaviour (Pollock, 1991; Werbach, 1992; Rowe and Rowe, 1994). Interestingly, sugar eaten as part of a balanced diet may actually improve intellectual functioning and reduce activity levels. Severe elimination diets can lead to malnutrition and occasionally the syndrome of Munchausen by proxy (see Chapter 5) may present as dietary intolerance. Although the role of diet in the aetiology of hyperactivity is highly controversial, exposure to lead in the environment is associated with overactivity, attention deficit, impulsivity, disruptive behaviour, disinhibition and learning difficulties. Early signs of lead poisoning include reduced appetite, prolonged diarrhoea, irritability, behavioural problems, gastrointestinal colic, vomiting and slow developmental progress (Hallaway, 1993). If there are concerns that the child has been exposed to toxic levels of lead, blood levels should be estimated.

The child should have a neurological examination and appropriate tests to identify the presence of damage or dysfunction. Less than 5% of children with ADHD have demonstrable brain damage, although 'neurological soft signs' such as abnormal reflexes or tremors will often be detected. The significance of these is controversial (Cantwell and Baker, 1987). Rivara et al (1994) demonstrated that traumatic brain injury was associated with a decline in academic functioning but not with a change in behaviour. Nevertheless, antisocial behaviour is more common among children with brain damage and so the presence of pathology should be excluded.

PSYCHOMETRIC TESTING

Given that a child with behavioural problems is likely to have learning difficulties, evaluation of intellectual potential will be important for future school planning. Psychometric testing, performed by a clinical psychologist, should be looked at alongside reports from the child's school and, if the child has been admitted for assessment, from the unit teacher. Simple administration of psychometric instruments may not fully reveal the child's strengths and difficulties, but will be valuable in conjunction with reports from the child's school together with an assessment by an inpatient unit teacher.

INDIVIDUAL ASSESSMENT BY A PSYCHOANALYTICAL PSYCHOTHERAPIST

Unconsciously a child's problematic behaviour may symbolize unresolved conflicts, typically emanating from earlier caregiver–child interactions. It has been suggested that a failure of bonding can lead to insecurity which is then acted out in the child's behaviour. A child must learn that he/she can survive separation from his/her primary caregiver and this is achieved through consistent care and positive nurturing experiences (Winnicott 1960; Balbernie, 1974; Bowlby, 1977).

The aim of a child psychotherapist's assessment is to identify unresolved conflicts which, although they may originate from early infancy, must be understood in their present form so that treatment addresses the current struggles that are occurring.

NURSING/MULTI-DISCIPLINARY INTERVENTION

Admission to an inpatient psychiatric unit for treatment may be considered necessary (see *Assessment* above). The essential difference between inpatient and outpatient treatment is that the inpatient setting provides milieu therapy. However, many of the elements of milieu therapy are also important for home and school life, and treatment in the community may include training parents and teachers in creating a therapeutic environment for the child.

MILIEU THERAPY

Safety

Safety is always an important consideration in childcare, but is paramount when the young person is restless, impulsive or aggressive. The nurse must ensure that the risk of harm or damage is at a minimum for the child, others and the material surroundings. The physical environment should be made as safe as possible without loosing a sense of normality. It is impossible to create a totally safe environment, and it is worth remembering this. However, important precautions that should be implemented include:

◆ *Ensuring the basic structure of the environment is safe* There should be no accessible heights from which to fall. Windows should have safety catches so that they open only a short distance and stairs should have gates for young children.

◆ *Objects that can easily cause damage should be kept out of the child's reach* Sharp implements, like scissors or knives, or potentially hot objects, such as a kettle, should not be accessible. This does not necessarily mean that the child should not have access to these things, but supervision must be provided. This is a good example of how the child's environment should reflect a degree of normality; if children are cutting paper in school, it would be unfair to exclude one child from the activity unless absolutely necessary.

◆ *Assessing the need for supervision* A child may require 'close' or 'constant' supervision to ensure their safety or the safety of others (see Chapter 2 – *Maintaining the child's safety, Level of child supervision*).

◆ *Assessing the need for physical restraint or holding* The Department of Health's (1993) guidelines for permissible forms of control in children's homes state that staff may take 'any action immediately necessary to prevent injury to any person, or serious damage to property'. In Chapter 2, the use of physical restraint is described in relation to the child attempting to hurt themself (see *Maintaining the child's safety, Physical restraint*). The same method of restraint may be used to prevent a child from hurting others or seriously damaging property, if alternative measures are unlikely to arrest the behaviour, such as neutralising the provocative situation by removing the target of the child's aggression. Sometimes the child may need simply to be physically guided away from a situation. The author refers to the latter as 'holding' as opposed to 'restraint'. Holding should only ever require one member of staff. The reader should be alerted to the fact that some literature will refer to 'therapeutic holding', but is actually describing restraint by several adults. Barlow's (1989) description of 'therapeutic holding' is one such example. In this article, it is suggested that restraint itself can reduce the incidence of aggression in children, by providing containment. However, in the author's experience, using frequent physical restraint can become punitive and, ironically, reinforce the aggressive behaviour. For some children the physical contact of restraint rewards their antisocial behaviour, but for many who have been abused it reinforces their belief that they deserve to be dominated and hurt. Even when restraint is used safely, the fact that the child is pushing against those restraining means that he or she is likely to experience some pain and may be bruised as a result. Children who are physically aggressive must be taught alternative ways of expressing their feelings (see below – *Targeting the behavioural problem*) and if they are 'seeking' restraint the underlying reason should be tackled. A child who seeks physical contact can be given hugs when they are not aggressive and the child who feels that they deserve to be hurt must be taught otherwise.

◆ *Locking the door of the treatment centre* If the child is likely to abscond and cause harm to themselves or others, it may be advisable to lock the inpatient unit door rather than use frequent restraint (see Chapter 2 – *Maintaining the child's safety, Locking the unit door*).

Structure and individual attention

Children who are restless, distracted, oppositional and aggressive need structure to help them to feel safe, to gain self-control and to facilitate them in achieving realistic goals, which in turn will improve their self-esteem. All children will be used to a timetable at school and to a certain amount of structure and routine at home, but some will actually benefit from more detailed and constant structure. A child who can settle in one activity for only a short space of time will benefit from a timetable that divides the day into short and achievable activities. Children who need a great deal of structure will also benefit from a high level of individual supervision. Some children cannot cope with long periods of unsupervised, unstructured time; they do not have the capacity to play on their own or with others without someone to facilitate and provide guidelines. Children with conduct disorders will feel more contained and secure if the day has routine and is predictable. 'Angry times' may even be included, when the child is encouraged to release pent-up feelings of anger (see *Individual work* below).

> David, aged 9, could not play with other children but could play for hours with his train set, which he became totally absorbed in to the exclusion of anyone or anything else. In the mornings his mother found it impossible to get him ready for school. When she insisted that he leave his train set to get washed and dressed, David became oppositional and aggressive. Once in school, he was restless and rushed through his work. If David was set a task that he found difficult, he became agitated and distracted. If the teacher was unable to attend to him, David became disruptive and, when reprimanded, became aggressive. He was admitted to an inpatient psychiatric unit for assessment and was diagnosed with Asperger's syndrome. David responded well to individual attention and a highly structured day. A behaviour therapy programme was established to teach him how to wash, dress and undress himself, which divided the task into small achievable goals (see *Targeting the behavioural* problem below) and during the day he was given special times to play with his train set together with times when he was helped to join other children in activities (see Plate 3 which appears in the unfolioed section between p56 and 57).

It is a good idea if timetables are drawn up with the child, so that they feel included in planning their own day and the child has his/her own copy, which could be stuck on the bedroom wall or kept more discreetly in a diary. Nursing staff should refer to the timetable throughout the day to reinforce the structure. It is also imperative that staff adhere to the timetable. Where possible (shifts permitting), nursing staff providing individual supervision/attention should be named.

Positive reinforcement

Creating a positive therapeutic environment where children's potential is realised and achievements are recognised is not only important for their well-being, but also essential if certain behaviours are to change (see *Targeting the behavioural problem* below).

Boundaries and limit-setting

All children need to learn how to behave appropriately and what is socially acceptable and unacceptable. Establishing boundaries is an essential part of teaching children to respect others and develop self-control. Adults must be clear, concise and consistent when setting limits to behaviour. Ambiguous, over-elaborate or inconsistent limit-setting is confusing for the child and ineffective. It is important that children understand why certain rules must apply and that they know the consequences of breaking them. Sanctions must be appropriate for the individual child. Missing a trip to the park may be a deterrant for one child but not for another. Sanctions should occur as soon as possible after the child has misbehaved and, once a penalty has occurred, the subject of the child's misbehaviour forgotten. Parents may have smacked their child in order to teach discipline and, although this is not illegal in the home, it should be discouraged, as it gives the child a confusing message concerning physical aggression, and limit-setting can be achieved without resorting to these means.

Observation and feedback

An important part of milieu therapy on an inpatient psychiatric unit is providing constructive feedback to the young person and parents. Showing empathy with the child may be the first step in changing their behaviour, and providing the parents with alternative ways of understanding the child's behaviour will be important if they are to change their management of the problem.

Keith (described above) was diagnosed with attention deficit disorder and found it impossible to sit at the meal table waiting for other children to finish eating. Nursing staff acknowledged that they could see that it was frustrating for him to wait but suggested that perhaps a system could be worked out to overcome the problem (see *Targeting the behavioural problem* below). Keith's parents saw his behaviour at mealtimes as being naughty and attention seeking until they appreciated that he had a short attention span and that restlessless was typical of someone with ADHD.

TARGETING THE BEHAVIOURAL PROBLEM

Changing a child's behaviour is far more likely to be successful if one problem is dealt with at a time. If several problems are tackled simultaneously, the child is likely to become confused and demoralised. It is also essential to keep in mind, and provide opportunities for, activities that the child is good at. In this way the child's self-esteem is enhanced, which will in turn facilitate a behaviour programme tackling a problem in another area and help to maintain a positive attitude towards the child in both parents and professionals alike. Westmacott and Cameron (1981) described a useful written exercise to identify the child's positive points, problems, priority problem and goal for change (Figure 3.2). They suggested that the exercise should include all those who have direct contact with the child – parents, teachers, the child him/herself and siblings – together with a 'neutral' person to facilitate discussion. The multidisciplinary team must decide whether such an exercise is carried out in a family session, a meeting with teachers and the parents, or with parents alone. A family therapist or key nurse may be the most suitable person to facilitate.

Once the priority problem has been identified, a behaviour programme can be drawn up. Essentially, in order to change behaviour conditions must be right for the desired behaviour to occur so that it can be positively reinforced; the problem behaviour must elicit no rewards and perhaps be positively discouraged.

Keith (described above) could not sit at the meal table for more than 4 or 5 minutes once he was no longer eating. Whilst waiting for other children to finish he would become agitated and destructive; perhaps pouring salt or tomato sauce on to the table. When reprimanded, Keith was verbally aggressive and became more disruptive. A management plan was established which allowed Keith to leave the table before he reached this point and so create the conditions for him to achieve a problem-free mealtime. When he felt that he could no longer cope with sitting at the table, Keith would ask to go to his room. If Keith managed to stem his aggressive behaviour by going to his room and behaved appropriately whilst he was at the table, he was given points on a chart, which went towards earning a treat (see Plate 4 which appears in the unfolioed section between p56 and 57). If Keith became aggressive at the table, he was told to leave at once and received no points. If he refused to leave and continued to be destructive, he was physically removed (see below for discussion on physically moving children). Gradually, the length of time that Keith was able to stay at the table increased.

David (described previously) was disinterested in washing and dressing and could not concentrate on the task. Left to himself, he would avoid washing and throw on any combination of clothes, inside out or back to front. A behaviour programme was established which divided the activity of washing and dressing into small tasks that required a short span of attention. David's key or shadow nurse would help him wash and dress and reward each small task, as it was achieved, by giving praise and awarding him with a token. These tokens were made from discs of coloured card, which David posted into his own token box. Tokens could be exchanged for treats, such as trip to the park or a ride on a train. Gradually, David began to do more of the washing and dressing unaided.

Behaviour can be reinforced by:

✦ *Praise* Simply telling a child that they have done something well, or thanking them for a job well done, can be sufficient reinforcement.

✦ *Incentive charts and rewards* Individual and creative charts can provide a focus for the reinforcement of behaviour (see Chapter 7 – *Points to remember when using incentive charts and rewards*).

✦ *Writing a contract with the child* This can be used to encourage, as well as discourage, behaviour (see Chapter 2 – *Maintaining the child's safety, Writing a contract with the young person*).

Kate, aged 14, would go out with friends straight from school and not return home until late. Apart from failing to do any homework which teachers had set, Kate's parents were naturally concerned for her safety. Figure 3.3 illustrates the contract drawn up between Kate and her parents.

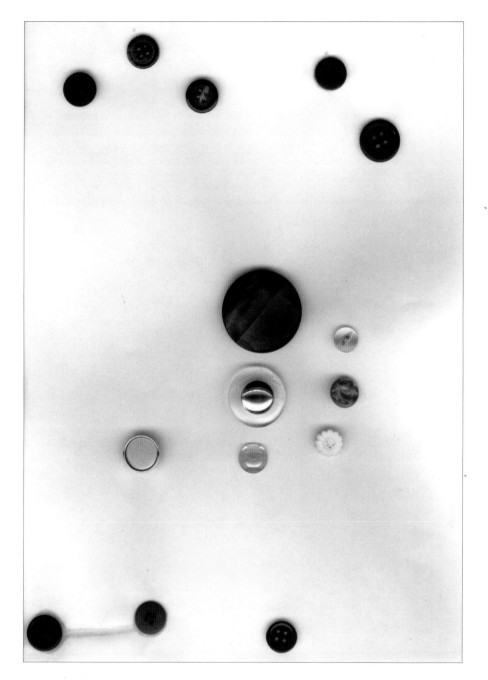

Plate 1 Clarissa, aged 14 years, described herself as someone who had always looked after everyone else, but now felt ill and weak. She chose a button with a 'strong' shiny centre, but 'weak' transparent outer edge, to be herself. Her father was now the main caregiver in the family and so she chose a big, bold, blue button for him (if there had been a suede button, she would have chosen that one, because 'he was cuddly'). Clarissa said that her mother loved pretty things, but was often ill herself. She chose a small pink button for her. Clarissa's younger sister was a 'bright spark', off playing with friends much of the time; Clarissa chose a gold button for her. Small, brightly coloured, buttons represented the family pets, which gave so much pleasure, and 'horrible' brown buttons represented the extended family, who did not believe that Clarissa was ill and offered the family no support.

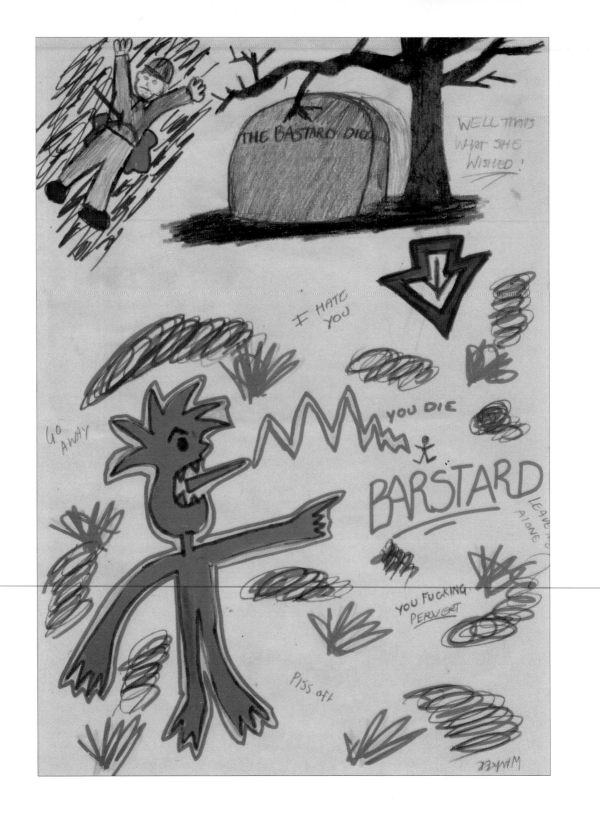

Plate 2 Fiona, aged 14 years, used drawing to express her anger about having been abused. Reproduced with permission from the artist.

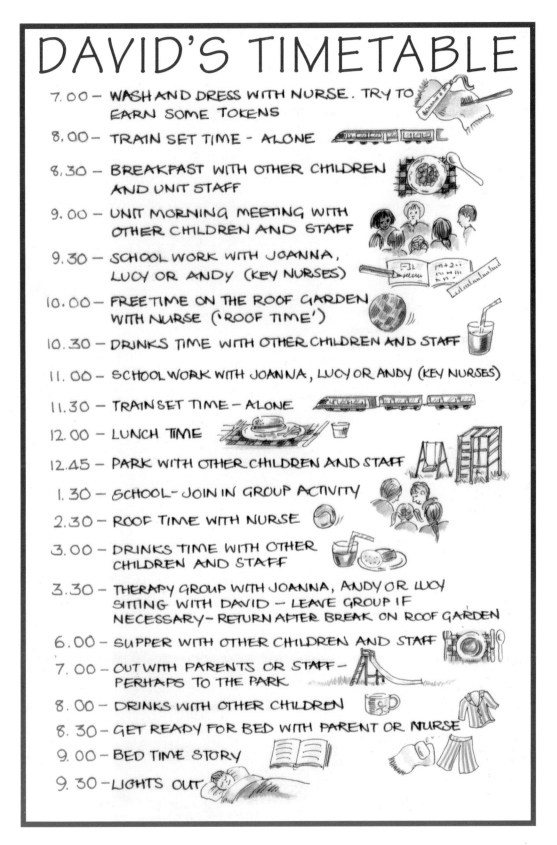

Plate 3 A highly structured daily timetable incorporated into an interesting brightly coloured poster for the child's bedroom.

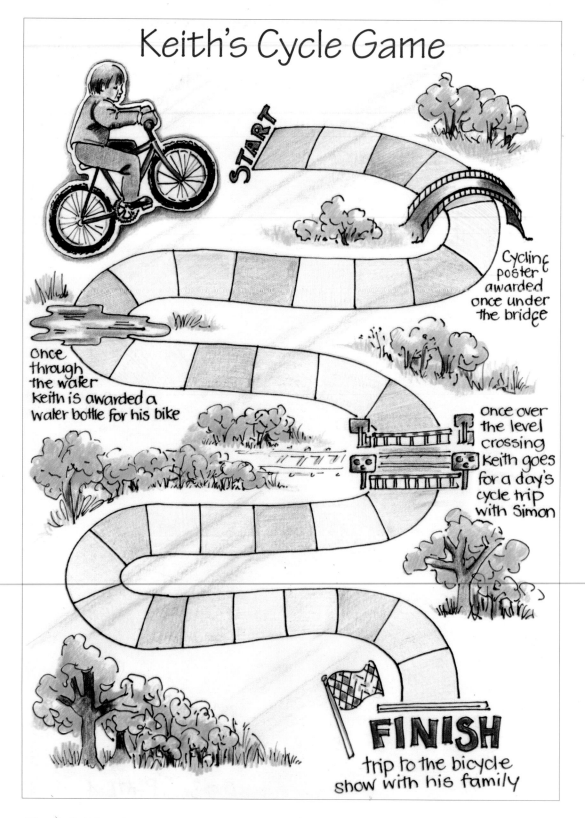

Keith's Cycle Game

START

Cycling poster awarded once under the bridge

Once through the water keith is awarded a water bottle for his bike

Once over the level crossing keith goes for a day's cycle trip with Simon

FINISH
trip to the bicycle show with his family

Plate 4 Keith's cycle course The chart is covered in sticky back plastic and the bicycle made from card, is held in place with blue tac®. As Keith is awarded points he moves the bicycle around the track: two points for remaining at the table throughout the mealtime; one point for removing himself to his bedroom before losing control.

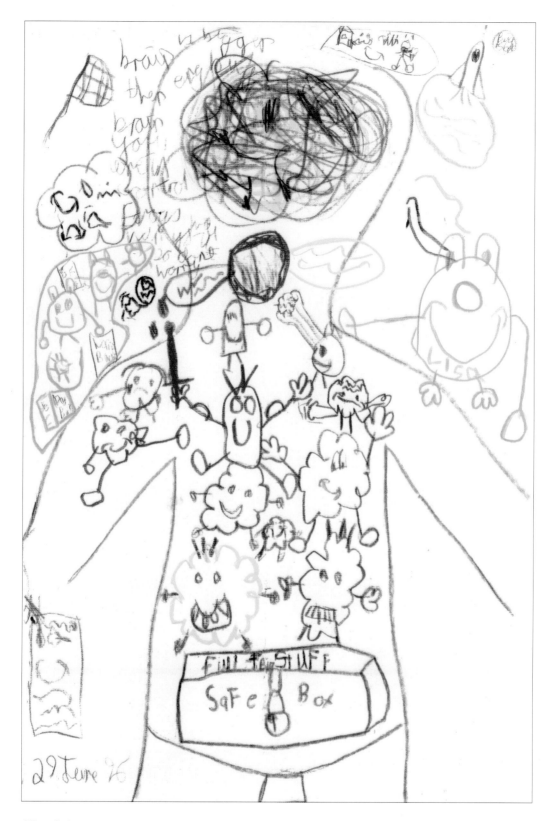

Plate 5 Anna, aged 9, visualised her unpleasent feelings as monsters inside her tummy and those who were helping her to get rid of them as friendly frogs. Reproduced with permission from the artist.

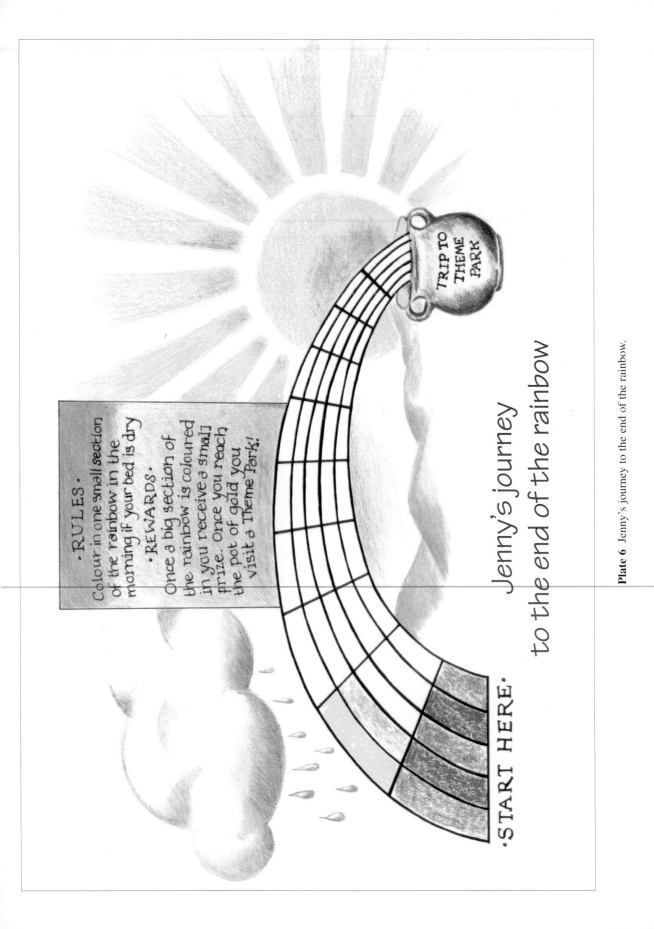

Plate 6 Jenny's journey to the end of the rainbow.

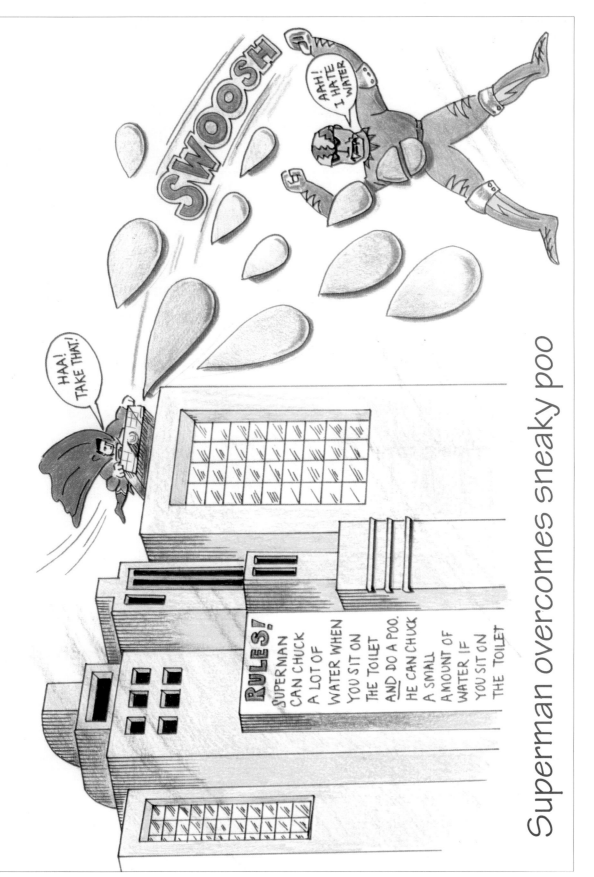

Plate 7 Superman overcomes 'sneaky poo'.

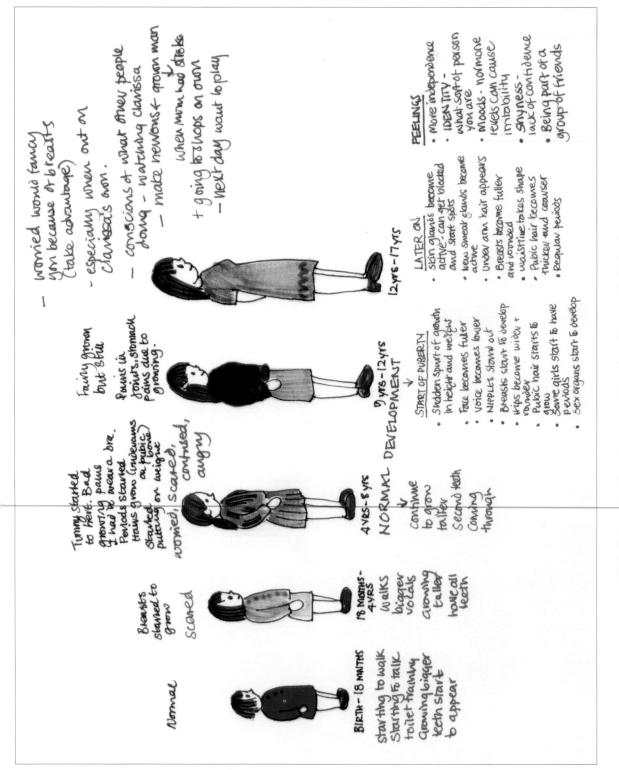

Plate 8 Example of growing up work done by a 12 year old with her key nurse.

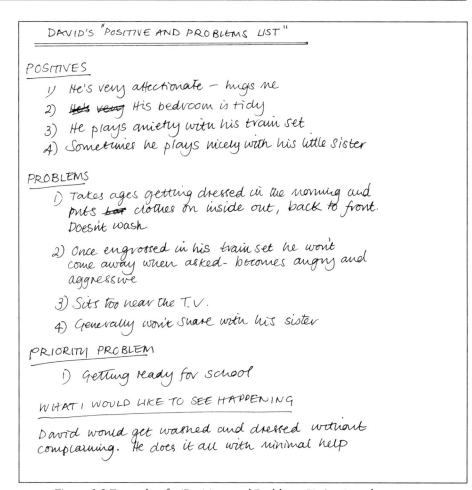

DAVID'S "POSITIVE AND PROBLEMS LIST"

POSITIVES
1) He's very affectionate — hugs me
2) ~~He's very~~ His bedroom is tidy
3) He plays quietly with his train set
4) Sometimes he plays nicely with his little sister

PROBLEMS
1) Takes ages getting dressed in the morning and puts ~~his~~ clothes on inside out, back to front. Doesn't wash
2) Once engrossed in his train set he won't come away when asked- becomes angry and aggressive
3) Sits too near the T.V.
4) Generally won't share with his sister

PRIORITY PROBLEM
1) Getting ready for school

WHAT I WOULD LIKE TO SEE HAPPENING

David would get washed and dressed without complaining. He does it all with minimal help

Figure 3.2 Example of a 'Positives and Problems List' written by a parent.

◆ *Demonstrating the benefits of appropriate behaviour* The child must see that there are inherent rewards for behaving well. For example, it was important for Keith (described above) to see the benefits of staying at the meal table. Nursing staff helped to facilitate a lively discussion; jokes would be told and children were encouraged to talk about themselves.

◆ *Modelling* Children are likely to follow the behaviour of those they like and respect or those who are controlling and dominant. This phenomenon can be used to good effect on an inpatient unit if staff are directive and firm, but, at the same time, kind and able to compromise. Nurses need to demonstrate their respect for children and each other, modelling skills in listening and assertiveness. These are important elements in a therapeutic milieu.

Imitation of peers will occur and, therefore, it is essential to consider the mix of children on an inpatient unit when planning further admissions. Having a number of powerful and aggressive children on one ward is likely to have an escalating effect on negative behaviour. In the author's experience, it is probably most beneficial to have a mix

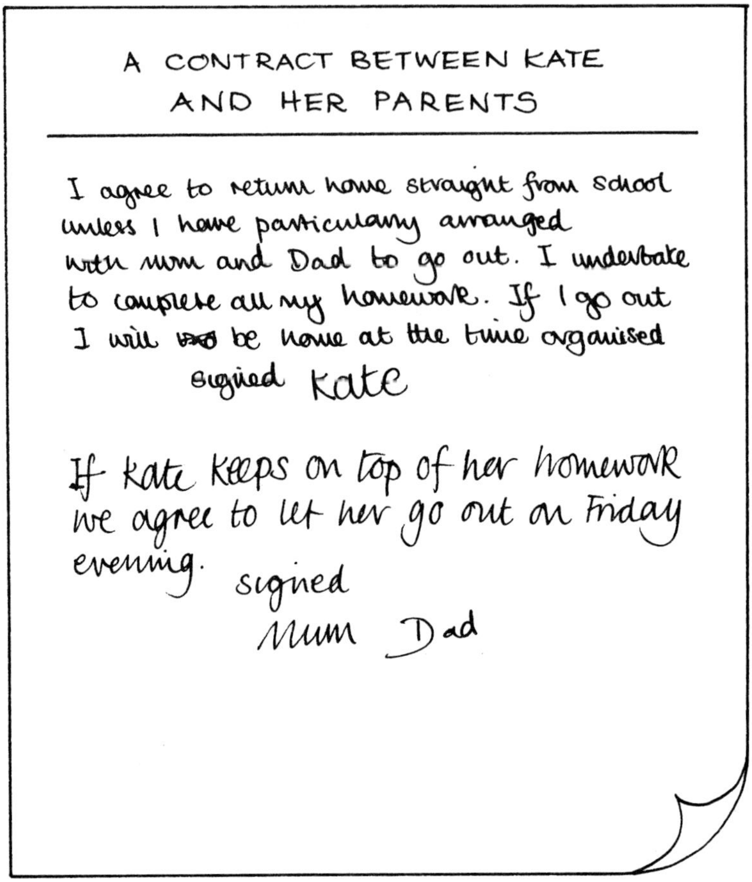

A CONTRACT BETWEEN KATE AND HER PARENTS

I agree to return home straight from school unless I have particularly arranged with mum and Dad to go out. I undertake to complete all my homework. If I go out I will be home at the time organised

signed Kate

If Kate keeps on top of her homework we agree to let her go out on Friday evening.

signed
Mum Dad

Figure 3.3 Example of a contract between a teenager and her parents.

of children with different strengths and weaknesses, and essential to be aware of those who 'lead' the group. If their influence is negative, this must be tackled individually with the particular child and with the group as a whole. Watching violence on television may exaggerate a child's aggressive behaviour, and so careful monitoring and control of the children's viewing is paramount. Education about the reality, or otherwise, of television programmes is also important and can help to immunize against the negative influences of television (Comstock and Strasburger, 1990).

Behaviour can be deterred by:

- *Sanctions* Negative consequences, such as missing an enjoyable activity like swimming or having to stay in after school instead of playing outside with friends, can be useful deterrants to negative behaviour.
- *Withdrawing attention* As giving attention to a child is a key to positive reinforcement, so withdrawing attention is a powerful deterrant. This can be achieved *in situ*, by simply refusing to take notice of the child, having already warned that a continuation of the present behaviour would result in being ignored, or by removing the

child from the situation where they are receiving attention to a place where there is none, such as their bedroom. This is commonly known as 'time out'. Before the Children Act 1989, a practice known as 'seclusion' was used in some psychiatric settings, whereby the child was removed to a bare room which offered no stimulation. This practice sometimes became confused with the practice of 'time out'. The Children Act 1989 has made seclusion unlawful and many institutions have now dropped the term 'time out' to avoid any confusion with the practice of seclusion, and therefore, instead, use terms such as 'sending a child to their room', 'the naughty space', and so on. On a general paediatric ward the principle of 'time out' could be employed, using a spare cubical or a particular bed on which the child must sit. It is obviously important to make sure that the space used for withdrawing attention is safe and that it is possible for staff to observe the child discretely. The length of time that a child is sent away from the attention of others must be long enough to be a deterrant, but not so long that it becomes excessively punitive or the child has time to forget why they are in time out. Time out should occur for 2–5 minutes, after which time the child is told that they can return to the group. When a child is sent to their room, they should be told to go immediately after the undesirable behaviour has occurred. If the child refuses, either the group can move to leave the child alone or nursing staff can physically help the child to move. This may simply require a guiding hand, which could be defined as a form of 'holding' (see above – *Assessing the need for physical restraint or holding*) or may require more force. The latter should be done only after permission has been sought from the child's parents. It is imperative to discuss the use of physical force and restraint with parents before implementation. As the Children Act 1989 states that physical force should only be used if the child is in danger of hurting themself or others, the use of such force for implementing time out is controversial. Parental responsibility is very much a key factor in the principles and practice of childcare laid down by the Children Act 1989. As with the use of restraint, every inpatient psychiatric unit should have a policy regarding the use of time out and a system of audit. If a child is constantly being sent to their room, it is time to look at other more effective ways of changing their behaviour.

Deterrants can have a powerful influence on changing behaviour, but will not be effective in the long term, or their use ethical, without positive reinforcement for appropriate behaviour. Raising the child's self-esteem is a key factor in producing a more permanent change. **Positive reinforcement for positive behaviour should always outweigh negative consequences for negative behaviour.**

When a child has hurt another person or damaged property, it is important that some reparation is made. A positive action, such as a written apology or mending a broken article, will provide a learning opportunity for the perpetrator and help the victim to realise that they were not to blame. If two or more children are involved in a fight, it may be helpful for nursing staff to facilitate a group discussion and apology. Initially, it can be useful for each key nurse to have an individual discussion with their allocated child to prepare them for a group discussion. It is important for each child to realise the part they played in the fight.

INDIVIDUAL WORK

Simply providing the time and place for individual work gives the child a clear message that you are available for them. A child who is restless and has a limited attention span is unlikely to sit down and talk about how they are feeling, but it may be possible to play a game or go for a walk and talk in the process. The areas of individual work that I will focus on in this chapter are cognitive–behavioural work, aimed at helping a child to recognise aggressive feelings and learn to express them in a more acceptable way, and constructive play therapy, to improve attention and provide the child with a sense of achievement. However, individual work with a key nurse is likely to cover a variety of areas, for which the reader will need to consult other chapters, such as 'getting to know' work (see Chapter 2 – *Individual assessment, Getting to know children' and 'beginning a relationship'*).

Cognitive–behavioural work

Kendall et al (1990) demonstrated the effectiveness of cognitive–behavioural treatment for conduct-disordered children. The intervention included training in problem-solving with a system of positive and negative reinforcement. Children were taught a five-step approach to problem-solving: problem definition, problem approach (brainstorming a number of alternative tactics for dealing with the problem), focusing of attention (discriminating between relevant and irrelevant factors), selecting a course of action (deciding which tactic to use) and self-reinforcement for accurate and appropriate performance (giving oneself just praise). During sessions the therapist modelled the process of problem-solving by talking it through (thinking out loud) and the child was asked to do likewise. Over time, the problem-solving process moved from overt talking to covert self-talk. In selecting which tactic to use to overcome a particular problem, the child was encouraged to discuss aloud the emotional and behavioural consequences for each person involved. At the beginning of each session the child was given 20 tokens. Further tokens would be given to the child for appropriate problem-solving in the therapy session and appropriate use of problem-solving outside the session. Tokens would be taken away from the child for inappropriate or ineffective problem-solving in the session, which included missing one of the five steps to problem-solving or rushing the process, and for unacceptable problem-solving outside the session. A bonus token could be awarded by the child him/herself at the end of the session, in agreement with the therapist. At the end of each session the child was required to spend some tokens on a prize. The child picked a reward from a 'prize menu', which had a variety of rewards requiring 3–200 tokens. The child could save tokens by choosing a 'cheap' prize, but had to spend some. The benefit of ensuring that the child always picks one prize is that, even though a child may have lost a lot of tokens during a session, it is concluded with some positive reinforcement. Generally, the author would choose to separate the reward and punishment systems, but the token system instigated by Kendall et al (1990) does ensure that the child is unlikely to loose all their tokens and have no prizes to show for their work. A child who knows that they behave badly may not think they deserve any reward and so the idea of self-appraisal and enforcing prizes is a good one.

An important step in helping a child to problem-solve and gain more self-control is helping them to recognise when they are likely to lose control and become oppositional and perhaps aggressive (in other words, identifying or defining the problem). Keeping a diary or filling in an individualised questionnaire (Figure 3.4) on a daily basis may facilitate the process of gaining insight. Once triggers have been identified, the key nurse can discuss with the child how to avert an aggressive outburst.

Sebastian (aged 15) was admitted to the inpatient psychiatric unit for an assessment. He had been sexually abused by an older boy in his neighbourhood and had since developed behavioural problems. He was overweight, clumsy and found it hard to keep up at school. His self-esteem was at a low ebb. When challenged by adults or peers, he became physically and verbally aggressive, turning over furniture and shouting profanities. For example, on the unit when playing a board game Seb made a simple error, which a peer noticed and commented on. Seb threw the board game on the floor and ran off shouting, 'It's a fucking boring game anyway'. Later in individual work, it became apparent that Seb had felt stupid and assumed that everyone else thought likewise **(the problem)**. Seb wrote in his diary that he felt hot and tense just before an outburst. It was agreed that Seb would run to a nearby park if he felt that he was about to loose control **(selected problem-solving tactic)**. On his way out, he was to let staff know that he was leaving. A nurse would then meet Seb in the park after 10 minutes, to talk about the incident and walk back to the unit with him. Initially being able to 'escape' from a potentially volatile situation was Seb's only way of maintaining self-control. Gradually, he became more able to cope with criticism without having to run off. In individual sessions Seb's key nurse facilitated discussion to develop Seb's insight into the feelings of others and reasons behind their behaviour. She also helped Seb to recognise his own strengths and start to put his 'failures', as he saw them, into perspective.

The way in which a child learns to vent their angry, aggressive feelings in a more acceptable manner must be appropriate for the individual. The nurse can make suggestions but the child may come up with their own idea. **Possible channels for venting angry feelings include:**

✦ Finding space to run around or kick a football

✦ Punching a punch bag, bean bag or pillow

✦ Throwing bottles into a bottle bank

✦ Breaking bubbles in packing plastic

✦ Painting on a large scale, but with clear boundaries (e.g. a designated graffiti board)

✦ Listening to loud music

✦ Jogging

✦ Using puppets to express aggressive feelings with clear boundaries to behaviour

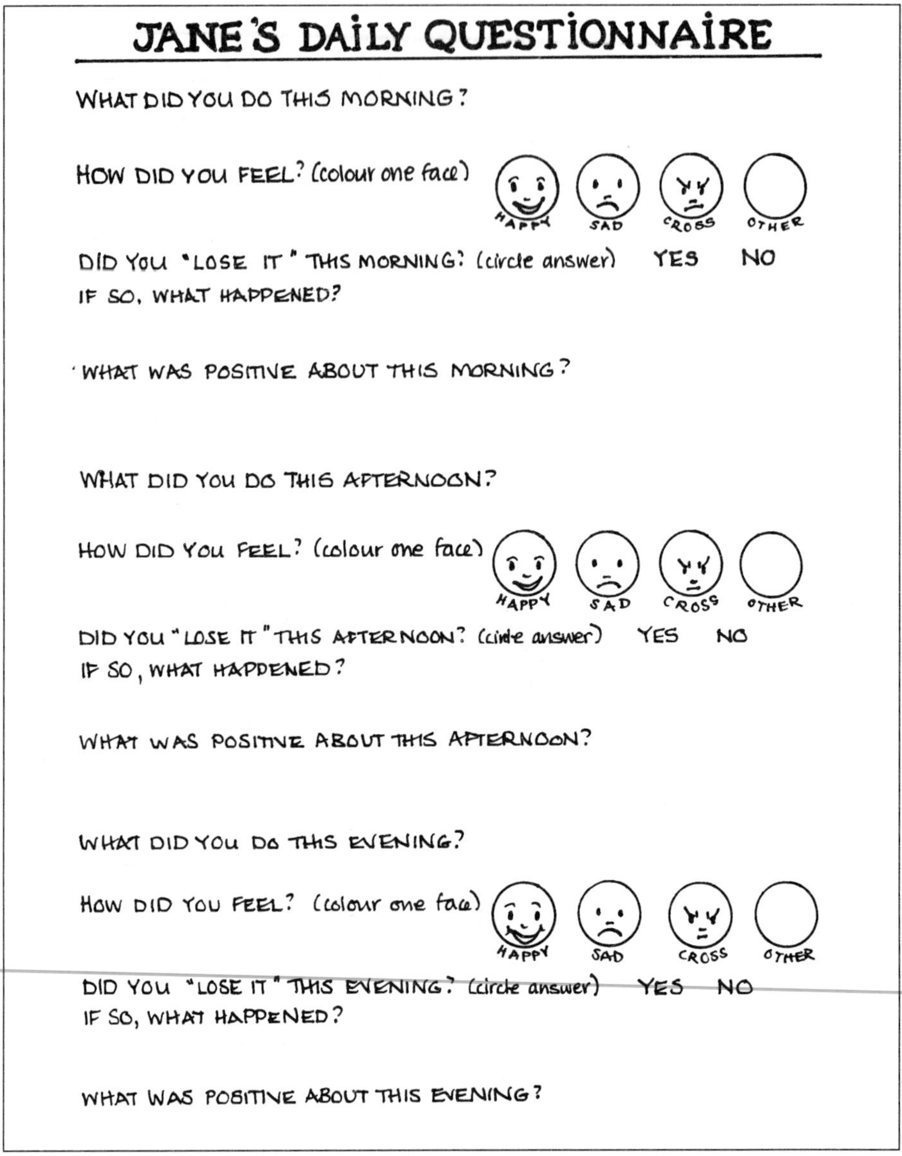

JANE'S DAILY QUESTIONNAIRE

WHAT DID YOU DO THIS MORNING?

HOW DID YOU FEEL? (colour one face)   HAPPY SAD CROSS OTHER

DID YOU "LOSE IT" THIS MORNING? (circle answer)   YES   NO
IF SO, WHAT HAPPENED?

WHAT WAS POSITIVE ABOUT THIS MORNING?

WHAT DID YOU DO THIS AFTERNOON?

HOW DID YOU FEEL? (colour one face)   HAPPY SAD CROSS OTHER

DID YOU "LOSE IT" THIS AFTERNOON? (circle answer)   YES   NO
IF SO, WHAT HAPPENED?

WHAT WAS POSITIVE ABOUT THIS AFTERNOON?

WHAT DID YOU DO THIS EVENING?

HOW DID YOU FEEL? (colour one face)   HAPPY SAD CROSS OTHER

DID YOU "LOSE IT" THIS EVENING? (circle answer)   YES   NO
IF SO, WHAT HAPPENED?

WHAT WAS POSITIVE ABOUT THIS EVENING?

Figure 3.4 Structured questionnaire for a child to record their day.

As mentioned previously, under milieu therapy, some children may benefit from having regular 'angry times', when they are encouraged to vent their feelings. At other times in the day they are taught either to hold on to their angry or aggressive feelings or to ask for an additional 'angry time'. This approach aims to help the child to express their feelings in an appropriate and controlled manner.

Constructive play

Children who are restless, impulsive, inattentive or aggressive are likely to engage in destructive play, such as war games. Children with a short attention span, excess energy, impulsiveness and irritability are likely to find it exceptionally difficult to finish any creative projects and will probably destroy any efforts out of frustration. Individual time with a key nurse can provide a valuable opportunity to help the young person complete a creative project or simply engage in constructive play. Examples of constructive play include:

✦ Jigsaws

✦ Stacking toys

✦ Construction toys, such as Lego and stickle bricks

✦ Model making

It is important to balance time for constructive play with more active pursuits, such as ball games, climbing and swimming, to release and channel energy in a positive way.

SOCIAL SKILLS TRAINING

A social skills training group on an inpatient unit provides a perfect opportunity to help children learn how to express themselves. Using role play and fictitious scenarios, children can practise letting others know how they are feeling and asking for help in a non-threatening and fun atmosphere. Examples of scenarios for children to role play include:

✦ 'Daniel asks Stephen (fictitious names) if he can borrow his bicycle. Stephen had a new bike for his birthday and would prefer not to lend it to anyone at the moment. How will Stephen tell Daniel he cannot borrow it.'

✦ 'Stephen was unable to tell Daniel he could not borrow his bicycle. Daniel has returned with the bike, having had an accident and buckled the wheel. Stephen is angry and upset. Stephen must let Daniel know how he is feeling and ensure that Daniel helps to repair the bike.'

✦ 'Joanna is fed up of being teased by Susan and Jane. She needs help to deal with it. Joanna's class teacher, whom she likes, is in the classroom marking work in break-time. This is a good opportunity to talk with her. How will Joanna go about it?'

✦ 'Joanna's teacher has suggested that one thing that Joanna must do, is talk to Susan and Jane. How will she do this?'

Different groups of children could work on each scenario and show each other the final role plays or have the group facilitator video record them for group discussion.

USING ART, DRAMA, MUSIC AND DANCE

Group work using art, dance, drama and music can provide a safe and non-threatening means of communicating. Creative groups also provide an opportunity for constructive and cathartic exercises, which can take place in a safe and supportive environment (see above – *Individual work, Constructive play*). Creating a short dance or piece of music can give the child a sense of achievement and at the same time provide a means of releasing pent-up feelings.

FAMILY THERAPY AND PARENT TRAINING

Helping parents to develop new skills to manage their child's behaviour may be an important task of family work. The 'parent–child game' is an innovative approach to the teaching of parenting skills (Gent, 1992). Training takes place in a controlled learning environment, using a video suite or one-way mirror and microphone/ear bug link. The parent, and not the child, is able to listen to the therapist speaking from the other room, while engaging in free play with the child. The first phase of treatment is called the 'child game', the emphasis being on the child leading the activity. The parent is taught to be attentive to the child, express warmth and approval when the child's behaviour is acceptable and to ignore inappropriate behaviour. In the second phase, the 'parent game', the parent learns to deliver clear concise commands **(alpha commands)** and use 'time out' for positive reinforcement. **Beta commands** are hesitant, elaborate and vague: 'Your supper is getting cold. I'm really tired and can't be doing with your messing about. You must come and eat, or I'll have to … well, I'll be very cross and I haven't got time for all this; your sister has to be picked up in half an hour and your Dad's not home in time to fetch her, so you'll have to come with me.' Alpha commands address the child by name, use eye contact, are delivered in a firm voice, slightly louder than usual, and are followed immediately by 5 seconds of silence, while the parent waits for the child's response: 'Beth, I want you to sit at the table now'. The therapist uses verbal instruction, prompts, verbal modelling and praise in the training process. A review by Graziano and Diament (1992) suggests that parent behavioural training is a very effective treatment for conduct disorders.

Family therapy can also provide a forum for parent skills training and an opportunity to address family issues that may contribute to the aetiology and/or maintenance of the child's difficult behaviour. Lack of agreement between parents, depression in the mother, minimal involvement of the father (sometimes including alcoholism or a criminal inclination), harsh and inconsistent discipline, little positive involvement with the child and poor supervision of the child's activities are variables that seem important (Lange et al, 1993). Structural family therapy, addressing family boundaries and individual roles, is generally adopted for the treatment of conduct disorders. The need for marital sessions or individual parent counselling may become apparent during the course of treatment. As this work may need to continue long term, such as individual psychotherapy for maternal depression, consideration must be given as to where therapy takes place. If the child is an inpatient some distance from their home, it is probably more appropriate to set up psychotherapy for the mother in the community. However, while the child is an inpatient, keeping all treatment within one team and minimising the number of professionals involved will aid communication. It does seem that, when a number of professionals is involved, the 'whole picture', or system that is creating/aggravating the behaviour problem, may be lost.

GROUP WORK WITH PARENTS

Gill (1989) described a group work approach to helping parents of 2–6 year olds with behavioural problems. Weekly sessions are run by a social worker and health visitor. The group is structured to provide constructive advice but also aims to increase parents' self-confidence. Parents are encouraged to share their feelings of desperation and failure, which are likely to interfere with their successful management of the problem. The group uses peer support and professional opinion to help stop this negative spiral of learned helplessness.

INDIVIDUAL PSYCHOANALYTICAL PSYCHOTHERAPY

Disruptive children, in particular adolescents with conduct disorders, do not generally respond well to psychoanalytical psychotherapy (Target and Fonagy, 1994). Nevertheless, the multi-disciplinary team, including psychotherapist and with the parents, may decide that an individual should be given the opportunity. A receptive child may be able to make the links between their acting-out behaviour and internal conflict.

MEDICATION

Stimulant medication, such as methylphenidate (Ritalin), has been shown to benefit children with ADHD. Some 60–90% of children sustain attention for longer, are less impulsive and display better organisation, are less active, more compliant and less disruptive, and display less covert antisocial behaviour, such as stealing and vandalism. These drugs have a short half-life and so medication is usually prescribed for a morning and noon dose to improve school function. Sustained-release preparations can overcome the need for a noon dose (e.g. Ritalin-SR). Side-effects of stimulant medications include a reduced appetite, disrupted sleep pattern, head and stomache aches. Tics can also be problematic and slight growth decrements may accrue to long-term high dosage. Having breaks in medication should be considered, particularly as the child's behaviour may be less troublesome in different environments. Despite the benefits of medication for the treatment of ADHD, improvements brought about by this means do not generally bring peer relationships and appraisal into the normal range; severe aggression and antisocial behaviour are likely to be rooted in familial and other environmental influences and the long-term course of ADHD does not appear to be altered by medication. Therefore, medication should be used as part of a combined approach to treatment (see review by Hinshaw, 1994).

Children and adolescents with conduct disorders who display aggressive and destructive behaviour can be helped with neuroleptic drugs alongside psychosocial treatments. Lithium chloride, propranolol (beta-blocker) and carbamazepine (anticonvulsant) have also been found to be effective (Campbell et al, 1992).

Finally, it is interesting to note that the use of traditional Chinese medicine has been shown to help in the treatment of hyperkinesia. 'Yizhi' syrup, given to 66 children, produced an effectiveness rate of 84.8%; the children's behaviour and school peformance improved and the appearance of soft neurotic signs decreased (Sun et al, 1994).

FUTURE PLANNING

An essential part of the management of restless, distracted, oppositional and aggressive children will be future planning. Long-term therapeutic placements or changes in schooling may be necessary. Nursing staff can play a vital role in the liaison with community services. A professionals meeting is likely to be set up by the team social worker in which tasks are allocated. After the educational psychologist has helped to find an appropriate school, the child's key nurse can provide teachers with valuable information concerning the most effective approach to facilitate positive behaviour. It may also be useful for the child to visit the school a number of times before starting full time. Having the key nurse available at the school while the child attends one lesson might be considered useful. Odom et al (1994) suggest that school nurses should play a vital role in evaluating the progress of children with ADHD, monitoring the effects and side-effects of medication, providing the child with emotional support, and liaising with other disciplines involved in the child's therapy.

NATIONAL SUPPORT GROUP

The Hyperactive Children's Support Group offers support to parents and children, and advice to professionals.

71 Whyke Lane
Chichester
PO19 2LD
Tel: 01903 725182

CONCLUSION

When children present with 'difficult behaviour', it is important that the problem is defined as accurately as possible. Planning intervention is then made easier and more likely to be successful.

Essentially, the child who is restless, distracted, oppositional and/or aggressive needs structure a high level of individual attention, positive reinforcement, limit-setting, to be taught coping strategies and problem-solving skills, and a great deal of support. However, each child requires an individual programme which targets their specific problem and builds on their particular strengths.

Working with the family and helping parents to develop new skills to manage their child's behaviour must be a key component to treatment. Long-term planning, considering schooling and ongoing support should begin at the outset.

REFERENCES

American Psychiatric Association (1994) *Diagnostic and Statistical Manual of Mental Disorders*, 4th edn (DSM IV). Washington, DC: American Psychiatric Association

Balbernie I (1974) Unintegration, integration and level of ego functioning as the determinants of planned cover therapy, of unit task and of placement. *Journal of the Association of Workers for Maladjusted Children* **2**: 6–46.

Barlow DJ (1989) Therapeutic holding – effective intervention with the aggressive child. *Journal of Psychosocial Nursing* **27(1)**: 10–14.

Biederman J, Faraone SV, Mick E et al (1995) High risk for attention deficit hyperactivity disorder among children of parents with childhood onset of the disorder: a pilot study. *American Journal of Psychiatry* **152(3)**: 431–435.

Bowlby J (1977) The making and breaking of emotional bonds. *British Journal of Psychiatry* **130**: 201–210 and 421–431.

Brown RT, Coles C, Platzman K and Hill L (1993) Parental alcohol exposure and its relationship to externalizing disorders: A longitudinal investigation. In Hinshaw SP (1994) *Attention Deficits and Hyperactivity in Children. Developmental Clinical Psychology and Psychiatry*, Vol. 29, pp. 43–66 London: Sage Publications.

Campbell M, Gonzalez NM and Silva RR (1992) The pharmacologic treatment of conduct disorders and rage outbursts. *Psychiatric Clinics of North America* **15(1)**: 69–85.

Cantwell MD and Baker L (1987) Attention-deficit disorder in children: the role of the nurse practitioner. *Nurse Practitioner* **12(7)**: 38–52.

Cantwell MD and Hanna GL (1989) Attention-deficit hyperactivity disorder. In Hinshaw, SP (1994) *Attention Deficits and Hyperactivity in Children. Developmental Clinical Psychology and Psychiatry*, Vol. 29, p. 62. London: Sage Publications

Comstock G and Strasburger VC (1990) Deceptive appearances: television violence and aggressive behaviour. *Journal of Adolescent Health Care* **11(1)**: 31–44.

Department of Health (1993) *Guidance on Permissible Forms of Control in Children's Residential Care*. London: HMSO.

Gent M (1992) Parenting assessment: the parent/child game. *Nursing Standard* **6(29)**: 31–35.

Gill A (1989) Putting fun back into families. *Social Work Today* **May**: 14–15.

Graziano AM and Diament DM (1992) Parent behavioural training. An examination of the paradigm. *Behaviour Modification* **16**: 3–38.

Hallaway N (1993) From autistic to 'lead toxic. *Canadian Nurse/Infirmière Canadienne* **89(10)**: 53–54.

Hinshaw SP (1994) Attention deficits and hyperactivity in children. In *Intervention Strategies; Pharmacologic Intervention for ADHD*, pp 105–112. London: Sage Publications.

Kendall PC, Reber M, McLeer S, Epps J and Ronan KR (1990) Cognitive–behavioural treatment of conduct-disordered children. *Cognitive Therapy and Research* **14(3)**: 279–297.

LaBarbera JD and Dozier JE (1985) A honeymoon effect in child psychiatric hositalization: a research note. *Journal of Child Psychology and Psychiatry* **26(3)**: 479–483.

Lange A, Schaap C and van Widenfelt B (1993) Family therapy and psychopathology: developments in research and approaches to treatment. *Journal of Family Therapy* **15**: 113–146.

McCormick MC, Gortmaker SL and Sobol AM (1990) Very low birth weight children; behaviour problems and school difficulty in a national sample. *Journal of Pediatrics* **117(5)**: 687–693.

Odom SE, Herrick C, Holman C, Crowe E and Clements C (1994) Case management for children with attention deficit hyperactivity disorder. *Journal of School Nursing* **10(3)**: 17–21.

Pollock I (1991) Do additives make children hyperactive? *Midwife, Health Visitor and Community Nurse* **27(5)**: 132–134.

Rivara JB, Jaffe KM, Polissar NL et al (1994) Family functioning and children's academic performance and behavior problems in the year following traumatic brain injury. *Archives of Physical Medicine and Rehabilitation* **75(4)**: 369–379.

Rowe KS and Rowe KJ (1994) Synthetic food coloring and behavior: a dose response effect in a double-blind, placebo-controlled, repeated measures study. *Journal of Pediatrics* **125**(5 Part 1): 691–698.

Sun Y, Wang Y, Qu X, Wang J, Fang J and Zhang L (1994) Clinical observation and treatment of hyperkinesia in children by traditional Chinese medicine. *Journal of Traditional Chinese Medicine* **14(2)**: 105–109.

Target M and Fonagy P (1994) The efficacy of psychoanalysis for children: prediction of outcome in a developmental context. *Journal of the American Academy of Child and Adolescent Psychiatry* **33(8)**: 1134–1144.

Werbach MR (1992) Nutritional influence on illness. Hyperkinesis: Part 3: Carbohydrates. *International Journal of Alternative and Complementary Medicine* **10(6)**: 17.

Westmacott EVS and Cameron RJ (1981) *Behaviour Can Change*. London: Macmillan Education.

Winnicott DW (1960) *The Maturational Process and the Facilitating Environment*. London: Hogarth.

Wolff S (1985) Non-delinquent disturbances of conduct. In Rutter M and Hersov L (eds) (1985) *Child and Adolescent Psychiatry – Modern Approaches*, 2nd edn, pp 400–413. London: Blackwell Scientific Publications.

Wolkind S and Rutter M (1973) Children who have been 'in-care' – an epidemiological study. *Journal of Child Psychology and Psychiatry* **14**: 97–105.

4   FRIGHTENED AND ANXIOUS

INTRODUCTION

There are many reasons why a child or adolescent might be frightened or anxious and it seems likely that for each individual there will be various contributing factors. Perhaps most obviously, psychological and physical trauma may result in ongoing fear and anxiety, but temperamental and neurological factors in the child and family characteristics are also important.

Children will express their fear in different ways: some may regress to an earlier stage in development and perhaps withdraw totally into their own world, others will experience physical complaints and some may become aggressive, phobic or obsessional. Most children will experience feeling frightened or anxious, but the feelings will be transient and will not interrupt their usual daily activities. However, for others, extreme fear or anxiety may severely disrupt life for the individual and their family. An example is when children experience extreme anxiety on separation from major attachment figures, such as parents. These young people will undoubtedly refuse to go to school and perhaps cannot bear to be left alone even momentarily. The *Diagnostic and Statistical Manual of Mental Disorders* (American Psychiatric Association, 1994) identifies a specific diagnostic category for separation anxiety in children and adolescents. At least three out of the following eight criteria must be met for a duration of at least 4 weeks:

✦ Recurrent excessive distress when separation from home or major attachment figures occurs or is anticipated.

✦ Persistent and excessive worry about losing, or possible harm befalling, major attachment figures.

✦ Persistent and excessive worry that some calamitous event will separate the child from a major attachment figure, such as the child being kidnapped or in an accident.

✦ Persistent reluctance or refusal to go to school, or elsewhere, for fear of separation.

✦ Persistently and excessively fearful or reluctant to be alone, or without major attachment figures at home, or significant adults in other settings.

✦ Persistent reluctance to go to sleep without being near a major attachment figure or to sleep away from home.

✦ Repeated nightmares concerning separation.

✦ Complaints of physical symptoms, such as headaches, stomach aches or nausea.

> Jane, aged 12 years, was so distraught when her mother left her side that she screamed, pleading for her to stay, tried to hit her own head and scratch her face. It became apparent that Jane was convinced her mother would be hurt if she left her alone.

Some children may be severely handicapped by their compulsion to carry out ritualistic behaviour, such as washing, counting and checking. The obsessions of children and adolescents frequently concern contamination or the fear of some traumatic, perhaps fatal, event occurring (Swedo and Rapoport, 1989).

> Mark, aged 14 years, felt that he had to count up to 10 before being able to listen to anything anyone said to him or before answering any question. The problem became progressively worse, so that counting to 10 only once did not alleviate Mark's anxiety and, when limits were set on this behaviour by his parents, he became aggressive. At this point his parents sought professional help. Mark was convinced that some horrific event would occur if he stopped counting.

A phobia, or fear of a specific object or situation, may impinge on many aspects of a child's life. A phobia of hospitals, or perhaps more specifically of needles, may be of serious concern if the child requires ongoing medical treatment, whereas a phobia of toilets is likely to contribute to the social problem of soiling or wetting (see Chapter 7) and a phobia of food may have life-threatening consequences (see Chapter 6).

> Andrew, aged 6 years, required extensive psychological preparation before he could cope with having a tonsillectomy operation. Two previous operations were cancelled because, on one occasion, his mother had been unable to get him into the car to take him to hospital and, on the other, Mark refused to undress or take any preoperative medicine. The nursing team believed that being more forceful with Andrew would have been unethical, causing unnecessary trauma.

Children and adolescents who have experienced severe physical or psychological trauma may experience terrifying nightmares or flashbacks, an indication of post-traumatic stress disorder. Lask et al (1991) described a syndrome of pervasive refusal in children, which often seemed to represent a fearful withdrawal from an abusive situation. The children showed a profound and pervasive refusal to eat, drink, talk or care for themselves.

> Rupinder, aged 12 years, arrived on the psychiatric inpatient unit being carried by her mother. Her limbs were flaccid and she was unable to walk; she was incontinent of urine and faeces, and was not eating or talking. Over a period of weeks, Rupinder had regressed into this totally dependent state. It was more than a year before she was able to start talking about her experiences of sexual abuse and begin to take care of herself again.

Nunn and Thompson (1996) offer another explanation for pervasive refusal syndrome, one of learned helplessness, and report that some children presenting with this syndrome do not appear to have been abused (see Chapter 5 – *Introduction*), and life experiences to date have contributed to a pessimistic outlook and general feeling that nothing they do will make any difference.

ASSESSMENT

The reader will undoubtedly need to consult other chapters to achicvc a holistic assessment, because fear and anxiety are likely to occur concurrently with other problems, such as sadness, physical symptoms, and so on. Certain aspects of the following assessment would also be inappropriate for some children, and so the nurse will need to identify which aspects are relevant for a particular child. For example, it would not make sense to ask parents whether their child experiences flashbacks if they do not believe their child has been traumatised, or to dwell on possible fears if the parents believe the child has a purely physical problem (see Chapter 5 – *Introduction* and *Family assessment* – for some ideas on how to broach emotional issues with parents who see their child's problem as totally physical).

FAMILY ASSESSMENT

The family assessment may involve meeting different combinations of family members, as well as at least one meeting with the whole family. The family therapist may work alongside another member of the multi-disciplinary team, such as the designated key nurse or social worker. One possibility might be for the key nurse to meet the child alone, while the designated family therapist talks with the parents. The two main aims of the family assessment are to discover the areas of concern regarding the child and begin to identify possible family characteristics that contribute to the child's anxiety. Parents may be aware that the child is fearful or they may have brought the child with problems they cannot explain. Equally, professionals may not at first identify fear or anxiety, as this emotion may be masked by other emotions and presenting problems.

Fear and anxiety may present itself in various ways:

◆ *All-pervasive fear* affecting every aspect of the child's life. The young person is likely to have a poor concentration level in school or social activities, as they are constantly watchful in preparation for some disaster or trauma occurring. This vigilance may make the child appear nervous and easily startled by loud noises, their body tensing and shuddering.

◆ *Specific fears* of situations, such as separation or of objects, particular types of people or animals (e.g. medical needles, teenage boys and dogs).

◆ *Sensory triggers that activate fearfulness.* Parents may have noticed that certain sounds, smells, tastes or touches cause the child to panic.

◆ *A general personality change.* Parents may report that the child has become irritable and moody. Siblings may also complain that they can no longer play with their brother or sister. The young person may become aggressive, unable to cope with even minor frustrations, or may be seeking comfort and reassurance constantly.

◆ *Physical symptoms.* It is very common for children and adolescents to develop physical problems as a result of emotional distress, such as headaches, stomach aches and nausea.

◆ *Sleep problems.* The child may not want to sleep alone, might have difficulty getting off to sleep, be woken in the night by nightmares or be sleepwalking. Parents may report blood-curdling screams in the night and find their child wet with sweat and shaking.

◆ *Denial of fear.* Some children may deny feeling frightened of anything, but perhaps become fearful at night or reveal their anxiety in scary drawings or by their fascination with frightening films.

◆ *Developmental regression.* It is not unusual for children and adolescents to regress to an earlier developmental stage when under stress, perhaps having problems with wetting or soiling, or reverting to feeding practices of a much younger child.

◆ *Flashbacks.* The child or adolescent may re-experience trauma, when images and sensations intrude their consciousness. This may occur at random or may be triggered by particular events or sensations.

◆ *Re-telling trauma.* Some children who have been traumatised may constantly want to talk about it, or re-enact their experiences in play or through drawing. Children who have been sexually abused may display sexualised behaviour.

◆ *Obsessional thoughts or compulsive behaviour.* Parents may report that the child has become preoccupied with certain thoughts and developed ritualistic behaviour, perhaps constantly asking the same seemingly meaningless question or touching every door-frame before entering a room.

◆ *Pervasive refusal.* As mentioned previously, some children present with a profound and pervasive refusal, not eating, talking, walking, or moving at all, and perhaps not opening their eyes. This may represent a fearful withdrawal from trauma, although it may be indicative of learned helplessness (see *Introduction* above).

Parents may have ideas as to why their child is fearful and, indeed, there may have been an important traumatic event which they feel is of utmost significance. Examples of possible trauma should be discussed openly with parents, including the possibility that someone has hurt their child and other less obvious forms of traumatisation, such as the young person's access to horror films. Simons and Silveira (1994) described the cases of two 10-year-old boys who developed post-traumatic stress syndrome after watching a ghost film on Halloween night. The boys experienced sleep problems, including nightmares and a fear of sleeping alone, persistent intrusive thoughts and images of the traumatic event, poor concentration, depressed mood, panic attacks, and raised levels of anxiety and irritability.

Parents may be less aware of how they contribute to, or alleviate, their child's anxiety or, where there has been trauma, how they influence their child's coping style. During the course of assessment and treatment, the multi-disciplinary team will need to look at factors within the family that reinforce the child's fear and anxiety.

Family characteristics and dynamics that may influence the child's fearfulness are:

◆ *Learnt fears.* Some phobias have a traumatic origin and are learnt through conditioning, whereas others may be learnt through the acquisition of information or modelling. The traumatic event may be related directly to the subsequent fear, such as a child being afraid of dogs who has been bitten by one, or may be related indirectly, where a traumatic experience occurred in the presence of the subsequent object of fear, such as the family dog barking whenever the child was hit by a parent. Having been repeatedly exposed to the fearful or phobic reaction of parents, siblings or peers in response to a particular stimulus (an object or situation), a child may imitate this behaviour when confronted with a similar stimulus. Alternatively or additionally, a child may be given repeated information concerning another's fear, such as horrific stories of visiting the dentist (King et al, 1988).

◆ *Learnt coping strategies.* Children will look to parents to learn how to cope with trauma. Parents may talk openly about their concerns and worries, or may deny any difficulties, but reveal their distress through altered behaviour or the development of physical symptoms. Children learn whether it is acceptable to talk about worries and seek support, or the reverse.

◆ *Family turmoil.* If there are family problems, such as marital difficulties, the child may believe that they should cope with their own worries alone, added to which a family experiencing problems may be less likely to pick up on an individual child's worries. Alternatively, or additionally, the child's fears may be directly linked with the family problems.

◆ *Anxiety disorders in other relatives.* Anxiety disorders tend to run in families (Klein and Last, 1989b). It seems that certain individuals are more vulnerable genetically to develop an anxiety disorder, although environmental factors also play an important part. A mother who is over-protective and has separation anxiety issues of her own may reinforce the dependency and lack of autonomy in her children.

◆ *Post-traumatic stress reactions in parents.* Parents of children who have been involved in a major trauma or disaster may show signs of post-traumatic stress disorder, even though they were not directly affected themselves (Parker et al, 1995). It is therefore important to screen these parents for stress reactions in order to provide treatment and the support that they will need to help their own child.

INDIVIDUAL ASSESSMENT

A member of the multi-disciplinary team who is likely to continue working with the child, such as a designated key nurse, should begin to form a therapeutic relationship with the child whilst assessing the young person's fears (see Chapter 2 – *Individual assessment, 'Getting to know children' and 'beginning a relationship'*). Specific questions covering areas highlighted in the *Family assessment* (above) may be asked directly or fun questionnaires can be created (Figure 4.1). Observation of a child's play or drawing may give valuable insight into the child's fears or the trauma they have experienced, which perhaps cannot yet be spoken about.

Characteristics of the play of a traumatised child include:

◆ A part, or the entirety, of a traumatic scene may be re-created.

◆ The play is likely to be repetitive.

◆ There will be a lack of pleasure for the child.

◆ The child may try to gain a sense of mastery over the trauma by acting as the aggressor rather than the victim, or introducing a hero to rescue the victim.

(see Chapter 10 – *Individual assessment, Facilitating disclosure of abuse* for the characteristics of drawings by children who have been sexually abused).

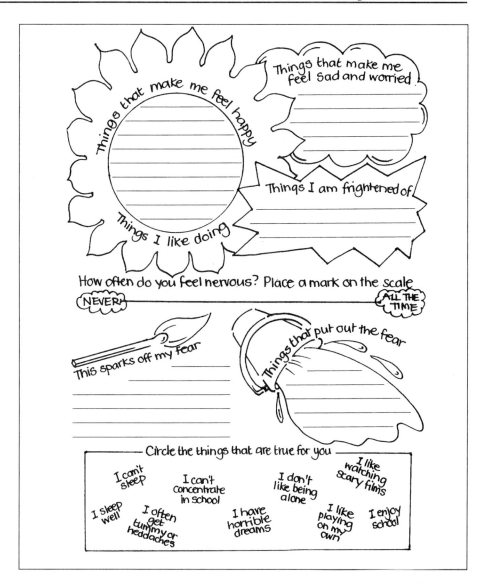

Figure 4.1 Fun questionnaire to help a child start to describe his or her fears.

BASELINE RECORDING

It may be useful systematically to record episodes of fearfulness. This task could be performed by parents, nursing staff on an inpatient unit or the young person. An 'ABC' chart, which establishes **antecedents** to the child's fearfulness, changes in the child's **behaviour** as a result of fear and the **consequences** of this change in behaviour, may help to identify factors that reinforce the fear (Figure 4.2). King et al (1988) described the benefits of children self-monitoring, many children showing an improvement in their own anxiety management before treatment has begun. From an assessment point of view, self-monitoring with supervision enables the nurse to gain some insight into the child's thoughts surrounding their fear (Figure 4.3).

DATE & TIME	PLACE	PERSONS PRESENT	ANTECEDENT	BEHAVIOUR	CONSEQUENCES
May 6th 6.00pm	Outside super-market	Myself and Jenny	Dog jumped out of the back of a car as owner put shopping in hatch back and bounded onto pavement where we were collecting a trolley	Jenny screamed and froze, said she felt sick.	I shouted at the owner to collect her dog and said that the dog could have bitten us — it looked angry. The woman called her dog back into the car and we continued with shopping once Jenny felt able.

Figure 4.2 ABC chart completed by a parent.

Where a child is showing compulsive behaviour it will be important to establish a baseline recording of just how often this is occurring and whether there are any significant factors associated with it (Figure 4.4). Sometimes it may become apparent that a child displays a certain type of behaviour in a particular situation, which may or may not be indicative of fear, such as soiling. In these situations it is often helpful to pursue this hunch by recording whenever the change in behaviour occurs and the circumstances surrounding it.

INDIVIDUAL ASSESSMENT BY A PSYCHOANALYTICAL PSYCHOTHERAPIST

An assessment by a child psychotherapist may help to shed more light on the underlying cause(s) of the young person's fear. If the child experiences separation anxiety, it may be helpful for the child to be accompanied into the session(s). This can sometimes prove to be a useful start to therapeutic work, particularly if much of the child's anxiety is connected to worries regarding the significant attachment figure.

MEDICAL ASSESSMENT

A psychiatrist should make a medical assessment and, if necessary, call upon paediatric colleagues for consultation.

DATE AND TIME	PLACE	WHO WAS PRESENT	WHAT HAPPENED		BEHAVIOUR	WHAT HAPPENED AFTERWARDS	
			THE EVENT	MY THOUGHTS		MY THOUGHTS	ACTIONS AND EVENTS
April 4th 4.30pm	Walking home from school	Helen and Jane (school friends)	dog came running towards us. Owner of dog walking quite a way behind dog walking.	the dog is going to attack me, dogs don't like me.	I froze, shaking and gave out a short scream — more of a gasp. I started breathing fast.	I felt embarrassed in front of Helen and Jane. I felt angry with the dog owner and thought he should have called his dog back or better still, not let it off the lead	Helen and Jane patted the dog and said it wouldn't hurt me. They waited for me to move after the dog had gone. They looked shocked by my reaction to the dog.

Figure 4.3 Self-monitoring by a child who is afraid of dogs.

◆ If the child or adolescent is experiencing physical symptoms, obviously these must be investigated thoroughly to exclude an organic cause (see Chapter 5).

◆ A neurological examination may reveal signs of brain damage. Shaffer et al (1985) identified a strong relationship between anxiety disorders in late adolescence and neurological 'soft signs', such as difficulty in performing rapid alternating movements (dysdiadochokinesis) and finger–nose and thumb–finger apposition. Discovery of any neurological abnormality may require further investigation to exclude the need for medical treatment. It may not be possible to treat a brain dysfunction that is detected, but being aware of its presence may help parents to come to terms with their child's problem and start to look at other contributing factors, such as psychological trauma.

◆ Certain drugs may induce anxiety and so any medication the child is currently taking should be looked at. Pimozide, a neuroleptic used in the treatment of Gilles de la Tourette syndrome, has been linked with the development of school phobia (Linet, 1985).

HOME AND SCHOOL VISIT

A home and school visit by the nurse may provide further useful information regarding the child's fear and factors that contribute to it. Forming a link with the child's school will be essential if school phobia or separation anxiety is the presenting problem; if the young person is to be

DATE AND TIME	ANTECEDENTS	BEHAVIOUR	CONSEQUENCES
May 7th 3.30pm	We were all sitting around the table having tea - staff and children. We were talking about family holidays. Some of the older children were saying they liked taking friends on holiday and meeting other young people. Others were saying they liked to stay with their family	Susan reached into her pocket for her hand cream and started vigorously rubbing cream into her hands. She seemed in a world of her own and didn't seem to hear/or ignored a question asked of her about holidays	She stopped after about 1 minute. I (S/N Brown) asked Susan to come and talk with me in the playroom. I suggested that she had found the conversation at tea difficult. Susan did not answer but looked anxious and sad.

Figure 4.4 ABC chart completed by nursing staff, aimed at establishing a base line of compulsive behaviour and identifying any significant factors associated with it.

admitted to hospital for treatment, a home visit will be invaluable for preparation.

Examples of particular things to look out for include:

✦ Does the fear seem to be located solely in the child or is another member of the family particularly anxious?

✦ Does the child sleep in their own room or have sleeping arrangements been changed to accommodate the child's anxiety and, if so, does this change appear also to alleviate parent's anxiety?

✦ At school, does the child appear more or less relaxed than at home?

✦ If there is school phobia or separation anxiety when a parent leaves the child at school, how does this present itself and does any particular approach appear to help?

(See Appendices A and B for general checklists for *Home visits* and *School visits*).

NURSING/MULTI-DISCIPLINARY INTERVENTION

Following the assessment a decision will be made regarding appropriate treatment. This may take place on an outpatient or inpatient setting, depending on the severity of the young person's problem and the family's ability to care for the child. If there are concerns regarding possible abuse within the family, an inpatient admission will enable further clarification of the child's needs as well as affording their safety.

INDIVIDUAL WORK

Individual work by nursing staff will vary considerably depending on the severity of the child's fear and anxiety. A child showing signs of pervasive refusal will need a very different approach to the young person who is able to talk openly about their particular fear. It is probably helpful to point out at this stage that, in the author's experience, children with pervasive refusal take a long time, sometimes as long as a year in treatment before they are able to function normally, let alone begin to talk about things that worry them. It can be very disheartening for the nurse if goals are set unrealistically high. The following ideas for individual work encompass a range of approaches, which may or may not be suitable at different stages of treatment.

Addressing sensory delays

Following severe trauma, it is not unusual to experience a feeling of numbness, temporarily not seeing, smelling, tasting, hearing or touching with the same degree of awareness as before. The speed at which the senses return to their full function will depend on the severity of the trauma, the help that is provided in addresssing the sensory delay and the assurance to the child that the trauma will not recur. Nurses can use sensory play with children who are totally 'shut down' as well as those who are nearer to recovery. The following are some examples of sensory games:

◆ Record different sound tracks on to a cassette tape, such as the noise at a public swimming pool, in a station, in a park, and so on. Make a game and ask the child to guess what each track is and to identify three individual sounds in each track. This game can be played with a child who is mute, but the nurse should comment on what she/he hears rather than put pressure on the child to talk.

◆ Ask the child to close their eyes and listen to all the sounds around them. Slowly focus the child's attention on to the sound that is the furthest away, such as birds singing, to that which is nearest, such as the child's own breathing.

◆ Place objects of different textures in a bag or pillow case, such as a furry pencil-case, a smooth-surfaced ball, some scrunched sweet paper, and so on. The child places their hand in the bag and guesses what each object is, describing its shape and texture, before removing it. The nurse can play the game with a child who is mute or unable to use their hands, by holding the child's hand and describing what is felt. Some toy and educational manufacturers produce sensory games, such as 'feely boxes' from Nes Arnold.

◆ Make up or purchase smelling pots and play a similar guessing game to those described above. The small pots must either be unrecognisable by sight or the child should be blind-folded or close their eyes (some children may find being blind-folded too frightening). Pots could contain Marmite, cotton wool soaked in perfume, tobacco, and so on. Nes Arnold produce a smelling game called 'Perfumemaster'.

◆ If the child is eating, a fun game could be guessing ice-cream flavours or different drinks.

Sensory games can trigger off flashbacks if a particular smell, sight, feel or sound has been associated with a traumatic event, for example the sound of a public swimming pool if this is where the child was sexually abused. The distress caused to the child may provide useful insight but, once discovered, the particular trigger should be avoided so as not to re-traumatise the child. Further into treatment it may be possible to desensitise the young person to the trigger, for example by taking the child to a public swimming pool and ensuring that they both feel and are safe.

Play therapy

Through play, children can express feelings that may be too frightening to talk about. Following trauma, play therapy can enable the child to gain a sense of mastery, correct any misconceptions regarding the trauma, increase their self-esteem and allow the safe expression of feelings, such as anger. Some adolescents may find the idea of play too 'childish', but for some it can be a relief to be given permission to express themselves in this way. The nurse must assess whether play is a useful channel of communication for each individual. The ways in which play can be used are inexhaustable, but here are a few examples:

◆ Allow the child to play freely with all manner of toys, such as a dolls' house, soft toys, puppets, toy telephones, and so on. Ideally, it is helpful to have a playroom where all these things are readily at hand, but the nurse must ensure that there are no interruptions from other children wanting to come and join in. Some children will readily act out their memory of trauma, whereas others may reveal the thoughts and feelings about their experience in a less direct way. Allowing free play can provide the child with space to gain a sense of mastery over their experience of trauma. At other times it will be important for the nurse to join in playing in order to facilitate the safe expression of strong feelings, perhaps by introducing a character (in the form of a doll or puppet, for example) who gets very angry and shouts on behalf of the victim; to correct misconceptions, such as trauma being the fault of the victim, by introducing a character who disagrees with the child's character who is apportioning blame and raising the child's self-esteem, by recognising her/his strengths and acknowledging these, again through a fictional character.

◆ A child who feels frightened may be given strength by an imaginary superhero, such as 'batman', who fights against their fear. In individual sessions the nurse can help to build up this character, by asking the child to paint a picture of their superhero, make a list of the hero's positive attributes and perhaps tell stories of how this character has helped other children. Together, the nurse and child decide how this superhero can be summoned to rescue the child when she/he feels frightened, and this scenario can then be rehearsed through play. It may be helpful for the child to have a visual representation of their fear, such as a monster, and to draw their idea of how the hero overcomes the 'fear'. Outwith individual sessions, whenever nursing staff observe that the child is frightened, perhaps on seeing a dog or experiencing a flashback of a traumatic event, they can remind the child to call on the superhero and offer their assistance. If treatment is occurring on an outpatient basis, the nurse may ask the child who could help them at home and then bring that person, perhaps one parent, in on the plan.

Anna, aged 9 years, was admitted to the psychiatric unit with pervasive refusal syndrome. Several months after admission, she began to draw pictures of the 'monsters' inside her tummy, which stopped her from doing things. Anna saw her key nurse and other staff members as 'helpful frogs', who could help her to get rid of the monsters (see Plate 5 which appears in the unfolioed section between p56 and 57). At the time of Anna's discharge, her drawings revealed no monsters left in her tummy. Her key nurse wrote a short story about the monsters and the frogs, which was read at Anna's leaving tea and given to her to take home. In the ensuing weeks, Anna could read the story if she felt that the monsters were threatening to come back.

✦ One way of coping with frightening flashbacks is to take control of them rather than the other way around. A child's mind may be intruded upon by the sight or voice of a scary figure when they least expect it, perhaps whilst working in school. Together, the nurse and child can decide what the child should do when the flashback occurs. The child could have an imaginary or real box to put the 'figure' in, which is then locked in a room that the child feels is a secure place. A drawing of the figure could facilitate this process and give the child something tangible to place in the box. Obviously the child must realise that it may escape, but she/he can always put it back where it belongs (draw another picture and place it in the box). Individual sessions can be used to discuss strategies and practise this scenario. The nurse or a parent can help the child to put the plan into action when they recognise that a flashback is occurring. Children experiencing flashbacks will often freeze, staring into space. If the child is an inpatient, other staff, such as the teacher, can call upon the key nurse when help is needed. The child will need to come out of the classroom to act out the ritual.

Cognitive therapies

Self-monitoring of fears by older children and adolescents can provide the nurse with a useful tool for cognitive therapy (see *Assessment* above and Figure 4.3). Through discussion of frightening situations, including the thoughts, feelings and behaviour surrounding them, the nurse can help the young person to re-evaluate and adjust their reactions. Using the example depicted in Figure 4.3, the nurse might ask the child to think of all the other reasons why the dog ran towards her, apart from the intention of attack, such as it wanted to be patted or to play. The nurse could then go on to discuss the reaction of the child's friends and what could have been said to relieve her embarrassment, such as, 'I'm terrified of dogs because I was badly bitten once, but I am trying to overcome my fear. Thank you for staying with me'. The child also recorded feeling angry with the dog's owner, but did not appear to do anything with these feelings. The nurse could ask the child whether she feels that her anger was justified and, if so, what she could have said to the dog's owner. It might be useful to re-run the whole situation in role play, the nurse acting all other parts, to help the child gain a sense of mastery and to practise for similar situations that may occur.

Obsessions and rituals can also be challenged using a cognitive approach. As well as questioning the reality of obsessions and the necessity of compulsions, a technique known as thought-stopping can be effective. Thought-stopping is designed to interrupt obsessions. The young person uses their own special word or phrase to interject and halt the obsessive thought.

Relaxation

Relaxation techniques can be taught effectively to children and can be beneficial in reducing stress and anxiety (Lamontagne et al, 1985). Initially the nurse will need to facilitate relaxation, but the ultimate aim is to teach the child how to use relaxation techniques on their own.

A common way to achieve a state of relaxation is for the subject systematically to tense and relax the major muscle groups of the body. This encourages a sense of body awareness and therefore allows areas of tension to be identified. Relaxation should take place in a room that is dimly lit, at a pleasant temperature and free from any distraction. The child should be wearing loose clothes, no shoes and either sitting or lying comfortably, with a light blanket over them if they wish. The nurse talks the child through the relaxation process in a calm and soothing voice. Guided imagery can be used to make these exercises more fun and easier for the child to remember for themselves (Figure 4.5).

Figure 4.5. Example of a relaxation script for children using guided imagery alongside muscle tension–relaxation exercises.

'Push your feet down so that you are pointing your toes like a ballerina. Push as hard as you can, using your whole legs to help you. Imagine your dance teacher is telling you to point more and more. Feel the muscles in the front of your legs working. Now hold it there' (*for a count of 5*) … 'and now relax, letting your legs and feet go floppy. Now pull your feet up towards you and splay your toes out as widely as you can. Pretend you are pushing against a wall using all the strength in your legs. Feel the muscles in the back of your legs working. Hold … and now let it go. Your legs are feeling warm and tingly … and relaxed.

Now tighten your bottom as hard as you can, so that it raises slightly off the chair. Hold … and now let it go, so that your bottom spreads out like jelly over the chair. Tighten your tummy, pulling it in as far as you can … hold it there … imagine a glass of water is being balanced on your tummy … if you let those muscles go, the water will spill. The glass has been taken away, you can relax and let your tummy go. Feel how soft your tummy and bottom feel.

Tighten your fists as if you are squeezing a soft ball … squeeze as hard as you can … hold it … now let the ball go and feel your fingers relax into a natural position … your hand will probably fall half open, fingers curled over slightly. Imagine you are a sleepy cat, just waking to stretch. Stretch out your arms in front of you. Raise them above your head … reach up … stretch out your claws, which are your fingers … now let your arms drop

continued

Figure 4.5 continued

quickly on to the cushions beside you and relax your hands. Your arms feel heavy and relaxed. Now stretch your arms out again and have a big yawn … now let your arms flop down again.

Pull your shoulders up and try to touch your ears with your shoulders. Feel the tension in your neck and shoulders. Hold them there … and now let them drop. Do it again … pull your shoulders up … hold … and let them go. Feel how relaxed and heavy your shoulders feel and how your neck feels as if it is sinking into your body.

Now imagine you have a sweet in your mouth which has a hard shell and lovely soft centre. Bite into it to get to the centre … you'll have to bite hard. Feel the tension in your jaw. Now relax and let your jaw drop and your tongue drop to the floor of your mouth. It's time to try to get into that sweet again. Bite down hard … You've got through! Let the sweet dissolve in your mouth. It tastes good. Your mouth feels soft and relaxed. Your teeth are slightly separated and your tongue is resting on the bottom of your mouth. A dandelion seed has floated on to your nose. Scrunch up your nose and wriggle it around to move the seed off. Now relax your nose and breathe out of your nose. Your nose feels relaxed … but the seed tickles again … it's still there. Scrunch up your nose again … now let it go. The seed has blown away. The sun has become very bright … close your eyes. That's not enough … the sunlight is painful … scrunch up your eyes as tightly as you can. A cloud has passed over the sun … you can open your eyes and relax the muscles around them. The sun has moved into the open again … scrunch up your eyes and keep them tightly closed. A larger cloud has appeared and covered the sun … you can relax and open your eyes. Open your eyes as widely as you can and make wrinkles in your forehead. Feel the tension in your forehead and over the top of your head … hold. Now imagine a friend is brushing your hair … making smooth strokes over your head, from your forehead to the back of your neck. Feel the tension being taken away with the brush. The wrinkles in your forehead have gone.'

Following the tension–relaxation exercises, guided imagery can be used to enhance the state of relaxation. The child is asked to close their eyes gently and the nurse talks them through a short story (Figure 4.6). The scene conjured up should be personally significant for the individual child. The nurse should discuss with the child the sort of story they would like; an older child may write their own with some help. If the story is recorded on to a cassette tape, the child can use it on their own at other times.

After a number of relaxation sessions with the nurse facilitating, the child should be encouraged to practise alone.

Desensitisation

Desensitisation is frequently used to tackle children's phobias. A clinical psychologist is usually involved in implementing this form of treatment, but it may be part of the key nurse's role, so long as they are trained in the procedure or working under supervision. Systematic desensitisa-

---

Figure 4.6. Example of guided imagery to enhance relaxation.

'I want you to close your eyes and imagine you are going on a trip to the beach. Imagine the chair that you are sitting on is turning into a magic carpet. It feels very special and your body is sinking into its thick, soft pile. Slowly and gently the carpet is rising into the air. You feel perfectly safe, comfortable and relaxed. The carpet drifts out of a wide open window into the warm air outside. The sky is blue and the sun is warming your face. The carpet floats gracefully through the sky. Every now and then you open your eyes to see the birds fly past and reach out to touch a soft cloud. After a while, the carpet starts to descend, floating slowly downwards. You can hear seagulls and smell the salt in the air. The carpet lands gently on a beautiful beach. The sea is blue and the waves are breaking gently on to the shore. You reach out to feel the warm sand. It is dry and fine and slips through your fingers. You feel perfectly relaxed and happy. Listen to the cry of the seagulls and the rhythm of the waves crashing on to the beach. In the distance you can hear children play-ing and laughing. Just lie there for a while … '(*a tape of seaside sound effects could be introduced at this point, slowly bringing up the volume to a pleasant, soft level. Pause for a few minutes, no longer talking.*) 'Now you feel ready to return to the hospital. All you have to do is tap the carpet and it starts to rise. Gently it drifts up into the warm sky and floats away towards the hospital. (*If a tape of sound effects has been used, this can slowly be faded out.*) Soon you are floating through the wide open window and the carpet lands on the chair you left a while ago. Magically, the carpet disappears, leaving you sitting on the chair, feeling calm and at peace.'

---

tion involves the establishment of an anxiety hierarchy, consisting of 15 to 25 anxiety-provoking situations (Figure 4.7), followed by the systematic exposure of child to these situations with the aid of a coping strategy involving relaxation.

To help the young person produce their own hierarchy, it can be helpful to ask them to write down different anxiety-provoking situations on separate index cards and to rate each one on a scale of 1–100, where 1 represents very little anxiety and 100 extreme anxiety. For a younger child, a visual scale could be used, where a mark is placed on a line. The index cards can then be put into sequence and the hierarchy constructed. The child is taught relaxation techniques (see above) and in the first desensitisation session, once in a state of relaxation, is either exposed to situation number 1 on their anxiety hierarchy or asked to imagine it. Pictures or objects can be used to help stimulate the child's imagination. The young person is then helped to maintain their relaxed state whilst being exposed to the anxiety-provoking stimulus for 10–15 seconds. If extreme anxiety is felt during this time, the child can indicate this, perhaps by raising one finger. At the next desensitisation session, a less anxiety-provoking situation should be tried. The speed at which progress is made through the hierarchy will depend on the child's response to treat-ment. If imagery has be used rather than live situations, the process must be tested out in reality at some stage.

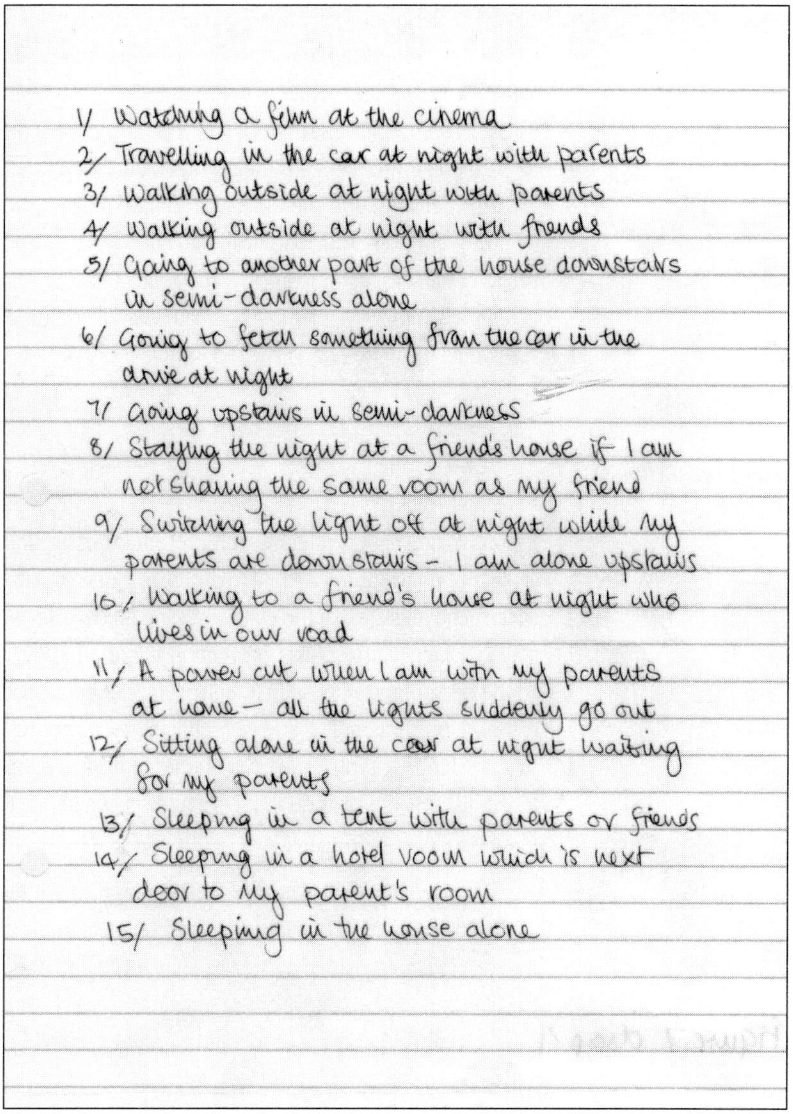

1/ Watching a film at the cinema
2/ Travelling in the car at night with parents
3/ Walking outside at night with parents
4/ Walking outside at night with friends
5/ Going to another part of the house downstairs in semi-darkness alone
6/ Going to fetch something from the car in the drive at night
7/ Going upstairs in semi-darkness
8/ Staying the night at a friend's house if I am not sharing the same room as my friend
9/ Switching the light off at night while my parents are downstairs - I am alone upstairs
10/ Walking to a friend's house at night who lives in our road
11/ A power cut when I am with my parents at home - all the lights suddenly go out
12/ Sitting alone in the car at night waiting for my parents
13/ Sleeping in a tent with parents or friends
14/ Sleeping in a hotel room which is next door to my parent's room
15/ Sleeping in the house alone

Figure 4.7 Hierarchy of anxiety-provoking situations written by a teenager.

'Worry times' and paradoxical approaches to compulsive behaviour

Children and adolescents who are constantly in a state of worrying, and perhaps feel the need to talk about their concerns to everyone at every possible moment, may benefit from prescribed 'worry times'. Set times in the day are allocated for the child to talk about worries with a key nurse. The number and length of these times should depend on the individual's capacity to hold on to worries between 'worry times'. Every 'worry time' must be used to the full, even if the child considers it is not necessary and, equally, discussion of worries is not allowed between 'worry times'. If holding on to worries is too difficult, the number of 'worry times' should be increased, or the young person encouraged to write down their worries, which can then be discussed at the next 'worry time'. Some children may like to write their worries on slips of paper which are then posted into a 'worry box', whereas others may prefer to use a diary. If the child still attempts to talk to staff between 'worry times', it must be explained that worries cannot be listened to now, but must be kept for the next 'worry time' with their key nurse. This approach helps the child to 'contain' their worries and therefore feel more in control. Insisting that the 'worry time' is used to the full may also have a paradoxical effect. In a similar way, children who behave compulsively or habitually in other ways can be encouraged actively to perform their rituals or habits at certain times. A child with a habitual facial tic may be encouraged to sit in front of a mirror and exaggerate their particular facial contortion at set times in the day; at other times tics would be ignored. The child should be involved in the decision to use this particular approach.

Response prevention

Response prevention refers to the prevention of an unhealthy response, that is compulsive or avoidant behaviour, to an underlying fear. Nursing staff must be prepared for the backlash of anxiety and anger when the child's 'coping mechanism' is taken away and indeed, in many cases, may consider that response prevention is not ethically acceptable. The level of distress for the young person and oppositional behaviour can be reduced if they have entered voluntarily into response prevention. It is also very difficult to enforce response prevention, for example compulsive washing, without supervising the individual constantly (see review by March, 1995). Individual sessions provide the space to discuss and practise response prevention.

> Sally, aged 13 years, who had a compulsion to ask the same question repeatedly, despite having received an answer, was given only one reply and when she repeated the question, was reminded that an answer had already been given and that she was now asking a ritual question. Sally was given a small treat every time she succeeded in stopping her compulsive questioning without becoming oppositional or aggressive.

Fighting nightmares

See Chapter 8.

Preparation for medical procedures

An important role of the paediatric nurse is to prepare children psychologically for medical procedures. Even if a child does not have a specific fear, such as needle phobia, they will quite possibly have misconceptions regarding their treatment. Providing information and correcting misconceptions is essential for the mental well-being of the child. There is a wealth of literature concerning the psychological preparation of children for medical procedures (e.g. Sharman, 1985) and most paediatric nurses are expert in this area of mental health.

MILIEU AND GROUP WORK

The main aim for nursing staff who are caring for children who are frightened or anxious is to ensure that they feel safe; only then can they be encouraged to express their worries more openly. Here are some examples of how to help a child feel safe and encourage healthy coping behaviours.

The environment must be made as safe as posssible

If there has been abuse by a known perpetrator, this person should not have access to the child. If there are suspicions of abuse involving a person who is close to the child, a decision may be made to supervise access. Telephone calls and letter reading may need to be supervised if there are concerns that the perpetrator will attempt to intimidate the child from a distance. These decisions must be made in the context of the multi-disciplinary team and involve the family. Legal action may be required to secure the child's safety. It is important for the nurse to explain to the child why certain measures are being taken, i.e. to ensure that the child is safe. Hopefully the parents will be in agreement and should convey this to the child themselves with the support of staff. The child will need a great deal of reassurance that they are not causing difficulties.

If a child has a specific fear of an object or situation, it is obviously essential to protect them from exposure, unless part of a controlled behaviour programme. A child who is frightened of dogs should not be left alone in a place where dogs are likely to be, such as a park. A child who is afraid of sleeping alone in the dark could perhaps share a room with another child or have a night light in the room.

Anna, aged 9, who was diagnosed with pervasive refusal syndrome, became extremely distressed when nursing staff attempted to clean her teeth. She would scream, close her mouth tightly and tears would roll down her cheeks. The dentist reported that Anna was in danger of developing dental caries if her teeth were not cleaned at least once in 48 hours. Therefore, a care plan was drawn up which limited the frequency of teeth cleaning and restricted the number of nurses involved. This approach aimed to give Anna the message that staff cared enough about her to look after her teeth, but also wanted to cause her as little distress as possible.

The child must be helped to develop healthy coping strategies and give up disabling behaviours

Much of the work that is started in individual sessions can be consolidated in the wider therapeutic environment. 'Homework' from cognitive therapy sessions might be put into action using the ideas of other children and staff. The child who is being teased at school could gather ideas from others as to how to deal with it, or could practise friendship skills, such as initiating games. Desensitisation work will at some point need to continue outside individual sessions, and response prevention, or a decision to ignore compulsive behaviour, will need the support of the whole nursing team.

Nursing staff should be alert for cues that indicate how the child is feeling

Nursing staff can attempt to guess how the child is feeling by observing his/her behaviour. Sometimes it can be helpful to comment on what is observed to the child. In this way the child learns that you are interested and that it is appropriate and safe to express feelings openly.

Using peer interaction

Children who find a particular situation frightening may be convinced more easily by other children that it is actually harmless, than by adults. It may be possible to set up situations where modelling by peers can occur. A child who is frightened of going swimming may be helped by observing others enjoying themselves in the water, and may be enticed more easily into the pool by peers, than by adults.

Children who find it relatively easy to express their feelings openly can act as important role models for those who find it more difficult. Group therapy sessions can provide a useful opportunity to facilitate this learning process and enable young people to share old and learn new coping strategies to deal with anxiety.

LIAISON WITH SCHOOLS

Where children have a phobia of school or separation anxiety from parents, health professionals need to work closely with the school to achieve the young person's re-integration. Nursing staff are often the most appropriate team members to fulfill this task, as they are likely to have been involved in teaching the child coping strategies and will have a good idea of the child's strengths and weaknesses.

From the author's experience, a gradual re-introduction into school seems to work better than a rapid forced re-entry, although the latter may be more effective where the problem is less severe. Research has highlighted the benefits of both (see review by Klein and Last, 1989a). A gradual re-introduction into school might start off with a visit to the school with a key nurse and an informal meeting with the class teacher. Together, the nurse, child and teacher plan further visits, gradually incorporating some lessons. It may be helpful for the nurse to be present in these initial lessons or at least to remain in the school building. Management of difficulties must be planned for, in conjunction with the teacher. Perhaps the child develops physical symptoms, such as stomach aches, when anxiety reaches a certain pitch. The planned intervention might intially include diverting the child into an activity that she/he finds non-threatening, such as drawing, and if this fails a specified time lying down in the 'sick room'. The aim is to keep the child in school, rather than be sent home or back to the inpatient unit.

INDIVIDUAL PSYCHOANALYTICAL PSYCHOTHERAPY

Individual psychotherapy may be helpful in identifying the underlying origins of the child's fear and the internal psychic mechanisms that re-activate anxiety. Children who experience separation anxiety may need to be accompanied to sessions with a parent or key nurse. Therapeutically, it may be very useful to include the parent for whom separation is most difficult. The therapist is likely to talk about how children with these difficulties have often been traumatised in some way, threatened with separation or been separated, perhaps because of parental ill-health, or harbour a great deal of resentment towards parents internally and, as a defence against these frightening feelings, develop feelings of dependency and become reliant on the parent's presence.

FAMILY THERAPY

Working with the family is an essential part of treating the anxious or frightened child. Frey and Oppenheimer (1990) identified enmeshment or disengagement in family boundaries and an inability to cope with change, in families where a child had been diagnosed as having an anxiety disorder. These family characteristics may be part of the cause or the effect of the child's anxiety but, whatever the reason for these family dynamics, effective treatment of the child will depend on the parents' current ability to manage their child's emotional upset.

White (1989) describes how childhood fears can be inadvertently maintained by the family. Parents may assume greater responsibility for protecting the child and, in so doing, reinforce the fear and reduce their child's confidence in tackling the problem alone. White describes an intervention using imagery, similar to that described above in individual work, which disrupts this negative process (see Chapter 8 – *Family therapy*).

Where a child has been traumatised, the whole family will be affected. Parents and siblings will often experience many of the same reactions as the child who was directly affected. They, too, may have difficulty sleeping, feel depressed and be intruded by their own images of the trauma. Family members will find their own ways of coping: some become over-protective of the affected child and outwardly emotional, whereas others may find activities to divert their attention and avoid talking about their feelings. Siblings are likely to feel a mixture of emotions: fear and distress, but also jealousy of the child who is getting so much attention, and subsequent shame. Parents will undoubtedly feel guilty for not preventing the catastrophe even when it was totally out of their control. Family reactions need to be addressed in family therapy, in order to help parents care for their traumatised child and the siblings. Sometimes different coping styles can cause family rifts and leave individuals feeling isolated and unsupported. It may be important to consider individual therapy for a particular family member who needs additional support – marital therapy, where marital conflict has been aggravated by the family's current situation, or work with siblings, to address the impact on brothers and sisters. Individual therapy should be provided by a separate therapist. On an inpatient unit, it may be helpful for the key nurse to take group sessions with siblings. When a number of therapeutic approaches are being used, it is essential that team communication is effective. From the author's experience, it can be detrimental to have too many different professionals working with one family.

Dadds et al (1992) demonstrated an improvement in childhood anxiety disorders after a 12-week programme of family therapy. Treatment focused on how the parents interacted with their child during displays of anxiety, their management of emotional upsets, family communication and problem-solving skills. Burgess and Hinkle (1993) illustrated the effective use of strategic family therapy for a school-avoidant adolescent. Strategic family therapists work on the premise that dysfunctional family dynamics, rather than individual psychopathology, result in problem behaviours. In the case example described, it became apparent during treatment that the mother checked on her daughter each morning, and began crying if her daughter expressed any degree of anxiety or somatic complaint. Her father waited outside school anticipating that she would become ill and need to be taken home. The family therapist hypothesised that the parents' extreme level of attentiveness reinforced their daughter's anxiety and served to keep the family together. Paradoxical interventions included symptom prescription (instructing the teenager to be as anxious as possible at school, 'in order to gain greater understanding of her problem', regardless of her parents' emotional reaction), reframing (suggesting that the parents' unwillingness to demand that their daughter attend school was an indication that they wished her to be placed elsewhere; the juvenile court had raised this possibility) and predicting a relapse after some improvement in school attendance. These strategies gave the teenager permission to be worried and relieved her of the burden of worrying for her parents' sake (she had stated that she could not go to school if her mother was upset) and encouraged parental control to be re-established. The natural hierarchy between parental and child subsystems was restored, which allowed the teenager to discontinue her phobic avoidance of school.

March and colleagues (1994) suggested that working with families where a child has an obsessive–compulsive disorder provides a helpful adjunct to individual work. Typical concerns in the family are: the involvement of parents and siblings in rituals, parental difficulties in dealing with aggressive or sexual obsessions, and differences in opinion between parents concerning how they should deal with the obsessive–compulsive behaviour.

MEDICATION

Some children may benefit from medication. Treatment may influence recovery directly and/or may enable the child to benefit more fully from other therapies. However, there is limited evidence to support the efficacy of drug treatment in children with anxiety disorders.

Research has looked at the effects of benzodiazepines, such as alprazolam, but findings are not promising (e.g. Simeon et al, 1992). However, fluoxetine appears to have beneficial effects in treating a variety of anxiety disorders in children with no significant adverse side-effects (Birmaher et al, 1994). Obsessive–compulsive disorder appears to respond well to the tricyclic antidepressant clomipramine (Flament et al, 1985).

LONG-TERM THERAPY

Children demonstrating more severe signs of fear and anxiety, such as those with pervasive refusal or obsessive–compulsive disorder, will undoubtedly require long-term therapy. During an inpatient admission to a child psychiatric unit, the multi-disciplinary team must plan for long-term treatment. Some young people may benefit from a long-term placement in a psychiatric unit or therapeutic community.

CONCLUSION

A child's fear or anxiety may present itself in many different ways. Social withdrawal, somatisation, obsessional thoughts and compulsive behaviour, phobias, irritability, flashbacks, developmental regression and sleeping difficulties are possible indicators. Subsequently, intervention will take many forms.

Addressing sensory delay, using play to facilitate the expression of feelings and enable children to gain a sense of control, teaching healthy coping strategies and using desensitisation are possible nursing interventions.

Inadvertently, fears may be maintained by the family. Parents may be over-protective or deny any problems and avoid talking about feelings. Family therapy will need to address such family dynamics and facilitate change.

REFERENCES

American Psychiatric Association (1994) *Diagnostic and Statistical Manual of Mental Disorders*, 4th edn (DSM IV). Washington, DC: American Psychiatric Association.

Birmaher B, Scott Waterman G, Ryan N et al (1994) Fluoxetine for childhood anxiety disorders. *Journal of the American Academy of Child and Adolescent Psychiatry* **33(7)**: 993–999.

Burgess TA and Hinkle JS (1993) Strategic family therapy of avoidant behavior. *Journal of Mental Health Counseling* **15(2)**: 132–140.

Dadds MR, Heard PM and Rapee RM (1992) The role of family intervention in the treatment of anxiety disorders: some preliminary findings. *Behaviour-Change* **9(3)**: 171–177.

Flament M, Rapoport JL, Murphy D et al (1985) Clomipramine treatment of children with obsessive–compulsive disorder: a double-blind controlled trial. *Archives of General Psychiatry* **42**: 977–986.

Frey J and Oppenheimer K (1990) Family dynamics and anxiety disorders: a clinical investigation. *Family Systems Medicine* **8(1)**: 28–37.

King NJ, Hamilton DI and Ollendick TH (1988) Aetiology of children's phobias. In *Children's Phobias: A Behavioural Perspective*, pp 30–49. Chichester, UK: John Wiley.

Klein RG and Last CG (1989a) Behavioural treatments.

Separation anxiety disorder and school phobia. In *Anxiety Disorders in Children*, pp 67–71. London: Sage Publications.

Klein RG and Last CG (1989b) Risk factors. In *Anxiety Disorders in Children*, pp 84–98. London: Sage Publications.

Lamontagne LL, Mason KR and Hepworth JT (1985) Effects of relaxation on anxiety in children: implications for coping with stress. *Nursing Research* **34(5)**: 289–292.

Lask B, Britten C, Kroll L, Magagna J and Tranter M. (1991) Children with pervasive refusal. *Archives of Disease of Childhood* **64**: 346–351.

Linet LS (1985) Tourette syndrome, pimozide and school phobia: the neuroleptic separation anxiety syndrome. *American Journal of Psychiatry* **142**: 613–615.

March JS (1995) Cognitive–behavioral psychotherapy for children and adolescents with OCD: a review and recommendations for treatment *Journal of the American Academy of Child and Adolescent Psychiatry* **34(1)**: 7–18.

March JS, Mulle K and Herbel B (1994) Behavioral psychotherapy for children and adolescents with obsessive–compulsive disorder: an open trial of a new protocol-driven treatment package. *Journal of the American Academy of Child and Adolescent Psychiatry* **33**: 333–341.

Nunn P and Thompson SL (1996) The pervasive refusal syndrome: learned helplessness and hopelessness. *Clinical Child*

Psychology and Psychiatry **1(1)**: 121–132.

Parker J, Watts H and Allsopp MR (1995) Post-traumatic stress symptoms in children and parents following a school-based fatality. *Child: Care, Health and Development* **21(3)**: 183–189.

Shaffer D, Schonfeld I, O'Connor PA et al (1985) Neurological soft signs: their relationship to psychiatric disorder and intelligence in childhood and adolescence. *Archives of General Psychiatry* **42**: 342–351.

Sharman WJ (1985) Tonsillectomy through a child's eyes. *Nursing Times* **81(8)**: 48–52.

Simeon GJ, Ferguson BH, Knott V and Roberts N (1992) Clinical, cognitive and neurophysiological effects of alprazolum in children and adolescents with overanxious and avoidant disorders. *Journal of the American Academy of Child and Adolescent Psychiatry*. Special section: New developments in psychopharmacology **31(1)**: 29–33.

Simons D and Silveira WR (1994) Post-traumatic stress disorder in children after television programmes. *British Medical Journal* **308**: 389–390.

Swedo SE and Rapoport JL (1989) Phenomenology and differential diagnosis of obsessive–compulsive disorder in children and adolescents. In *Obsessive–Compulsive Disorder in Children and Adolescents*, pp 13–32. Washington, DC: American Psychiatric Press.

White M (1989) Fear busting and monster taming – an approach to the fears of young children. Selected papers. *Dulwich Centre Review* 107– 113.

5 PHYSICAL SYMPTOMS THAT CANNOT BE DIAGNOSED MEDICALLY

INTRODUCTION

Children commonly develop physical symptoms that cannot be given a medical diagnosis. However, if a holistic approach to diagnosis is taken, the range of possibilities to explain such phenomena broaden considerably. Because our mind and body are linked inextricably, it is perhaps not surprising that mental distress can result in physical symptoms (see Chapter 1). The term 'psychosomatic' was first used to describe disorders in which a psychological component was thought to be important, such as asthma and diabetes. Now it is frequently used to describe disorders for which no physical cause can be found, such as unexplained recurrent abdominal pain. Implicit in both these definitions is the idea that there are some disorders for which psychological factors are unimportant. A holistic approach to medicine requires us to consider the relationship between physical and psychological factors in all disorders. Unfortunately, because historically we have adopted a reductionist approach to medicine in the Western world, there is a still a tendency to describe disorders as wholly physical or psychological. Lask and Fosson (1989) suggest that it is more logical and sensible to think in terms of a continuum of illness causation, with predominantly physical at one end and predominantly psychological at the other (Figure 5.1).

Debating whether a disorder has a physical or psychological cause is not only futile, but also unlikely to help the child's recovery. The notion that mental distress may contribute to a child's illness is often difficult for parents to contemplate. They may believe that this would apportion blame to them, and the feelings of guilt and shame would be unbearable. Similarly, the stigma of mental illness, which is multi-cultural, would encourage many families to look for a physical cause to their child's illness. If professionals adopt a holistic approach from the start, giving equal consideration to physical and psychological factors, parents may find it easier to accept important mental health care for their child (see *Assessment* below).

Research has required an artificial line to be drawn between disorders that are predominantly psychological and those that are essentially physical in origin. Terms such as psychogenic (having a psychological origin) and organic (having a biological basis) are used to separate disorders of the mind and body. In reality, all disorders are likely to have a multi-factorial aetiology, involving some physical and some psychological factors (see Chapter 1 on Myalgic encephalitis).

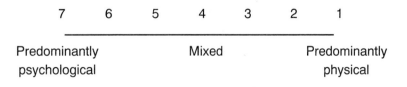

Figure 5.1 Spectrum of aetiology. Reproduced with permission from Lask and Fosson (1989).

Therefore, it is important that the reader holds on to a holistic view, because crude dividing lines and terminology are unavoidable in reviewing the literature.

Children are perhaps more prone to present with physical, rather than psychological, symptoms because of their limited verbal skills and immature localisation of pain. A review by Ryan-Wenger (1994) suggests that 10–15% of all children experience psychogenic headache, abdominal, chest or limb pain. Abdominal and limb pains occur more often in girls than boys and primarily during the school-age period. Headaches and chest pains are more often reported in adolescents, headaches more commonly in girls and chest pain in boys. The sensation of pain can be explained by the response of the autonomic nervous system to emotional arousal.

The psychiatric diagnosis of a 'dissociative' or 'conversion' disorder refers to the presentation of symptoms for which no organic cause has been found and where there is evidence of psychological causation (ICD-10; World Health Organisation, 1992). Conversion disorders may include sensations, such as pain, mediated by the autonomic nervous system, but also involve another set of symptoms, not referrable to the autonomic nervous system. These include paralysis, incoordination, blindness, deafness, seizures, anaesthesia, fugue states and amnesia. Conversion disorders are more common in adolescents than pre-adolescents and are rare in children under 9 years of age. Most studies report a prevalence of between 0.5% and 10% (Lehmkuhl et al, 1989). Seizures and gait problems are the most frequent problems, whereas hearing and visual disturbances are rare.

Other examples where physical symptoms may baffle the paediatrician include: the exacerbation of an existing chronic illness, such as asthma, and its resistance to stabilise with drugs; the fabrication of symptoms and/or precipitation of symptoms by a parent, usually the mother (Munchausen by proxy); the prolongation and deterioration of a disorder usually receptive to treatment (e.g. reflex sympathetic dystrophy); the loss of several activities of living (e.g. walking, eating, seeing, talking) in a previously healthy child (pervasive refusal syndrome); and chronic loss of energy and physical strength without an understandable biological basis (myalgic encephalitis or chronic fatigue syndrome).

This chapter is essentially concerned with the process of 'somatisation'; that is, the expression of psychological distress through bodily symptoms. All the disorders mentioned so far can be seen as forms of somatisation, perhaps with the exception of Munchausen by proxy, although somatisation may become a part of this disorder.

It is important to understand the factors that increase the likelihood of a child somatising, in order to ensure a comprehensive assessment and to plan effective therapeutic intervention. Lask and Fosson (1989) talk about predisposing, precipitating, perpetuating and protective factors, and the author has used this framework to describe the aetiology of somatisation.

Factors that predispose a child to somatise their distress, and which determine the form that somatisation will take, include:

◆ *A biological vulnerability* Most people have organs or body systems that are physiologically vulnerable and therefore likely to be targeted by distress. For example, children with asthma have bronchial hypersensitivity and, under stressful conditions, such children are likely to have an asthmatic attack.

◆ *Physiological response to stress* Stress produces a number of autonomic responses, including breathlessness, sweating and increased heart rate. Children tend to focus on these normal bodily responses rather than report the underlying distress. For example, muscle tension may be perceived and reported as pain.

◆ *Family characteristics* Enmeshment, over-protectiveness, rigidity, lack of conflict resolution and involvement of the sick child in parental conflict have been identified in families of children with psychosomatic disorders (Sargent, 1983). (See *Family therapy* below, where this will be explained further.)

◆ *Early life experiences of illness* Children may identify with a sick parent and model their illness behaviour, or develop symptoms that previously had led to parental concern (Lask and Fosson, 1989). Several studies have found that a family history of chronic pain or other symptoms is more typical of children with psychogenic pain than asymptomatic children (see review by Ryan-Wenger, 1994).

◆ *Personality characteristics* Although there is no clear agreement on personality traits predisposing to somatisation, it seems likely that those who find it difficult to express their feelings are more likely to demonstrate physical symptoms. Such children will probably come from families where expression of emotion is inhibited (Lask and Fosson, 1989).

◆ *Cultural factors* Some societies discourage the expression of feelings and are therefore perhaps more prone to develop somatic symptoms. The Chinese culture, for example, values self-control and considers the expression of strong emotional feelings as rude and disgraceful (Kuo and Hopkins Kavanagh, 1994).

Factors precipitating somatisation are those that cause stress for the individual. Depending on their biological and psychological dispositions and their previous life experiences, different individuals will experience varying levels of stress in response to similar circumstances (Lask and Fosson, 1989). Some children will see a stressful life event as a challenge, whereas others will view it as a threat. Stressors might include:

◆ Death of grandparents or other loved ones
◆ Abuse
◆ Disturbed family relationships such as marital discord
◆ Birth of a sibling
◆ Migration of the family
◆ Illness or accidents involving the child or a parent
◆ Parental unemployment
◆ Change of school, in particular entry into secondary school

Nunn and Thompson (1996) suggest that pervasive refusal syndrome is the result of the child's perception that they have no control over their future and/or the future of their family. A sense of helplessness or hopelessness moves between the child and parents, as each watch the other struggling with uncontrollable life events. The child is therefore learning directly and indirectly, through watching his or her parents, that nothing can be done to change the situation.

Factors that precipitate somatisation may also help to maintain it. However, additional factors may also come into play which help to perpetuate the symptoms. These include:

◆ *Primary and secondary gain* Somatisation produces a primary gain, which is the release of unpleasant emotions, and a secondary gain through the consequences that follow illness, such as missing school, additional parental attention, and so on. The primary and secondary gains then serve to reinforce somatisation.

◆ *Family functioning* The somatic symptoms of one family member can deflect attention from other family problems, such as marital discord, financial difficulties or substance abuse, which would ordinarily result in conflict. The maintenance of somatisation in one individual may therefore help to maintain family equilibrium (Ryan-Wenger, 1994)

◆ *Stigmatisation of mental health problems* In most cultures mental illness carries with it stigmatisation. This discourages families from exploring the possibility that mental distress may be contributing to physical symptoms and, indeed, encourages the family's search for a physical cause. This denial of emotional distress can only help to perpetuate the problem.

◆ *Over-investigation* Excessive medical investigation can be the cause of iatrogenic illness, by reinforcing somatisation and/or causing physical harm.

Factors that help to buffer the effects of stressful events and therefore protect against somatisation include (Aro et al 1989; Lask and Fosson, 1989):

◆ Having a parent as a confident

◆ Peer support

◆ Temperamental attributes, such as adaptability

A common mistake amongst professionals is to assume that, if no organic cause can be found for physical symptoms, they must be psychogenic and, therefore, somehow 'put on'. 'Malingering', which refers to the feigning of illness, is in fact exceptionally rare in children. Nevertheless, an obvious degree of conscious control, such as a child with a limp seen walking more easily out of the sight of nursing staff, can lead to misunderstanding these children. The whole story, however, is likely to be more complicated and involve conscious and unconscious processes. For example, the parents may deny painful feelings, such as anxiety, anger and fear, which the child has picked up on and internalised as 'rules' for acceptable behaviour. Initially they will have consciously suppressed their feelings, but, in time, this pattern of behaviour will have become so habitual that feelings are repressed automatically and unconsciously. Therefore, when under stress, the child will somatise distress; the symptoms being beyond conscious control. The primary and secondary gains of illness may then reinforce the limp at a conscious and unconscious level. Perhaps during therapy, this child has become more aware of a tendency to somatise and/or symptoms have abated as underlying conflicts are expressed. However, the child still experiences some symptoms and has other worries that he or she is still unable to talk about and therefore is concerned that, if nursing staff see an improvement in walking, discharge will be imminent.

In summary, somatisation is an unconscious process, although some additional illness behaviour may occur at a conscious level. However, it is important to remember that, whatever control the child has over symptoms, there will be important psychological reasons for the maintenance of symptoms and therefore the child requires help.

ASSESSMENT

The importance of a holistic approach to assessment and treatment is made all the clearer when physical symptoms start to elude medical diagnosis. Offering a psychiatric assessment after medical assessment has failed to find a cause is likely to cause an obstacle to successful treatment. It reinforces the notion that disorders are either physical or psychological, rather than a mixture of the two, and it perpetuates the stigma of mental illness, leaving this possibility as a last resort. Assessment must therefore have a multi-disciplinary approach and include paediatric and child psychiatric involvement from the start.

MEDICAL ASSESSMENT

Medical and psychiatric staff must work together to determine the extent of physical investigations. Over-zealous medical examination can lead to iatrogenic illness but, equally, inadequate investigation can mean organic pathology is missed. Abdominal ultrasonographic examinations of children with recurrent abdominal pain have shown that, in 80–90%, results are within normal limits (Shanon et al 1990; van der Meer et al, 1990). However, Goodyer (1981) found that 27% of children and adolescents initially diagnosed with a conversion disorder were later found to have an organic illness. Nevertheless, it is important to remember that physical and psychological factors interact together to produce the final picture and that there is no reason why an essentially psychogenic disorder cannot occur simultaneously with a predominantly organic disease. Although the frequency in children is unknown, Lazare (1981) reported that organic illness accompanies conversion disorders in 63.5% of adults.

Clarissa, aged 14, had a 9-month history of abdominal pain, which had deteriorated to such an extent that she was unable to walk and required a wheelchair. The pain was spasmodic and, when Clarissa experienced an 'attack', she felt shooting pains down her arms and legs and developed a splitting headache. She had become so handicapped by the pain that her parents had moved her bedroom downstairs and Clarissa required help to wash, dress and go to the toilet. Initial medical investigation found no organic cause for Clarissa's symptoms and, indeed, there were many factors that pointed to a conversion disorder. Clarissa had experienced precocious puberty at the age of 6 and suffered considerable teasing at school. Her mother had a history of undiagnosed illness, in particular back pain, and as a result Clarissa had become a significant carer for her younger sister, looking after her while her father was at work and her mother in bed. Recently, her father had been made redundant and was suffering from depression. Clarissa was now caring for her father as well, providing emotional support and a listening ear. Clarissa was admitted to the inpatient psychiatric unit and made striking progress. During the admission, an ultrasonographic scan of her abdomen revealed a massive ovarian cyst which required surgery.

This case vignette highlights how inadequate investigation earlier in Clarissa's admission allowed organic pathology to be missed. However, Clarissa's history and the nature of her symptoms suggested that a conversion disorder was probably occurring simultaneously with organic pathology. One could postulate that stress played a significant part in the development of the ovarian cyst. Research has shown that an exaggerated and prolonged somatic response to stress may result in structural changes and tissue damage (Ryan-Wenger, 1994).

William, aged 12, suffered recurrent vomiting from the second day of life. At the age of 2 years he swallowed a coin. After this had been removed from his oesophagus, William developed choking fits, which persisted for 4 years. At the age of 6, reflux oesophagitis and an oesophageal stricture were identified and surgical dilatation was performed. Over the following years, numerous gastrointestinal operations were carried out, including further surgery for oesophageal stricture and partial resection of William's stomach. The vomiting persisted and developed a cyclical pattern. For about 4–5 days every 2–3 weeks, William would experience abdominal pains, vomiting and generally feel weak and unwell. Despite important psychological factors, which could have been contributing to William's illness (William and his parents having been understandably sensitised to gastric symptoms in William, concerned for his long-term health, the parent's tendency to reinforce William's position in the sick role and general tension at home), the medical profession continued to operate on William. Eventually a psychiatric referral was made, which the parents accepted reluctantly. Unfortunately, although considerable improvement was achieved on the psychiatric unit, the parents discharged William and resumed a purely medical approach. Perhaps if a joint assessment, including paediatric and psychiatric expertise, had been instigated from the start, a more favourable outcome would have been possible.

It is possible that the continued surgery described in this case exacerbated the very problems that it set out to cure. Detrimental psychological, and perhaps physical, consequences seem inevitable.

Unexplained physical symptoms may be the result of Munchausen by proxy. Other signs that might indicate this syndrome include: signs and symptoms incongruous with the child's history or apparent only when the mother is present; treatment is proving ineffective or poorly tolerated; the child is alleged to be allergic to a great variety of foods and drugs; the mother seems unconcerned with her child's illness; and the family reports an unusually high incidence of serious illness. Meadow (1985) suggests important areas for investigation when Munchausen by proxy is suspected:

◆ A careful study of the child's history to identify events likely to have been fabricated or inflicted, an association between illness and the presence of the mother, and incongruous or fantastic details in the personal, social and family history, which are likely to have been fabricated.

◆ Contacting other family members, which may reveal discrepancies in the information about the child's illness or the family.

◆ Contacting the family doctor to discuss episodes of illness within the family. In about 20% of cases, the mother has a history of Munchausen syndrome.

◆ Trying to identify a motive for the mother's actions. There is generally some gain for the mother, such as emotional support from their child being in hospital.

◆ If the child is hospitalised, it is important to ensure that the mother does not alter charts or records.

◆ Careful surveillance of the mother will be required by nursing staff, in order to identify any link between her presence and the appearance of symptoms in the child.

◆ Any samples that are collected should be tested to ensure they are what they appear to be. For example, if there is haematuria, is the blood of human origin or has it been extracted from meat.

◆ Samples resulting from unexplained bouts of illness, such as serious gastrointestinal upsets, should be tested for poisons.

◆ Examination of any substances that the child is being administered.

INDIVIDUAL ASSESSMENT BY A PSYCHOANALYTICAL PSYCHOTHERAPIST

Psychoanalytical theories suggest that unconscious conflicts may be converted into physical symptoms, resulting in a conversion disorder, and that these symptoms serve a function in communicating feelings that the individual is unable to express verbally (Sullivan and Buchanan, 1989). The conversion symptom is said to symbolise the underlying conflict. This last idea is somewhat incongruous with the notion of biological vulnerability, which suggests that most people have organs or body systems that are more sensitive to stress than others. Whether or not the symptoms have a symbolic function, an assessment by a psychoanalytical psychotherapist is valuable to start trying to understand the child's present psyche.

INDIVIDUAL ASSESSMENT

It is paramount that the nurse accepts the child's description of their physical symptoms and their individual method of coping. Unfortunately, many professionals are under the false impression that symptoms that are somatised are somehow not real and therefore not felt. Most people will have felt 'butterflies' before an examination or whilst sitting in the dentist's waiting room, or experienced a throbbing headache when tense. Those same people would undoubtedly reject any suggestion that they were imagining their symptoms.

The nurse should try to ascertain when the symptoms are less pronounced and/or whether the child has found a means of reducing their severity. This is an important starting point for treatment, as it helps to build a trusting relationship with the child, who may have previously felt that their symptoms were not believed. It also establishes a method of giving some immediate relief. It may be useful, particularly if the child is adamant that nothing helps, to ask them to keep a diary of events (Figure 5.2).

Discussion of the child's physical symptoms will need to form the basis of the nurse's assessment, as this will undoubtedly be the main concern of the young person. However, some

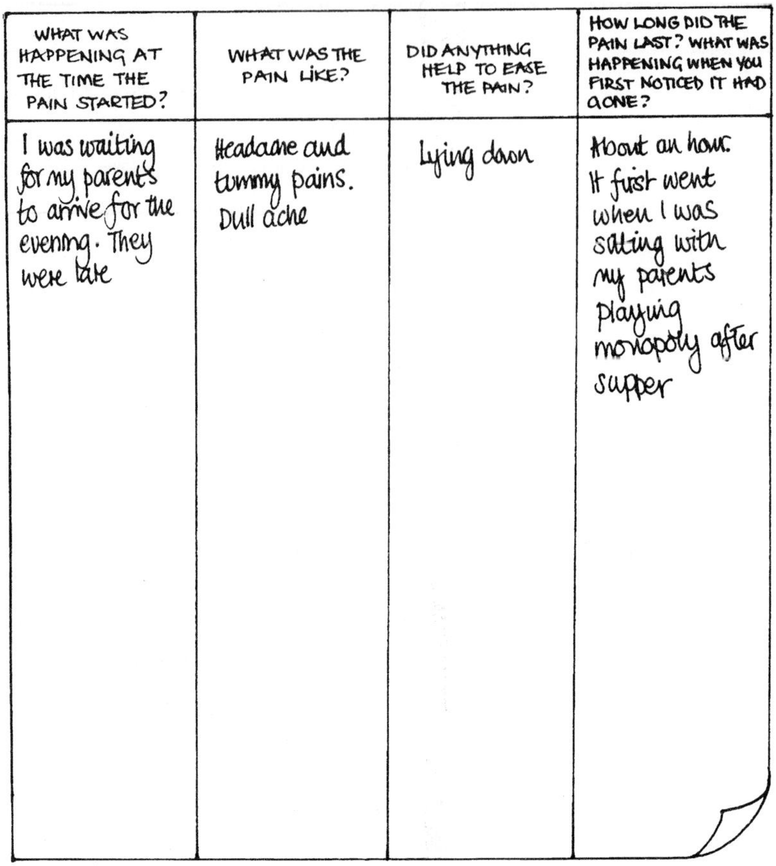

WHAT WAS HAPPENING AT THE TIME THE PAIN STARTED?	WHAT WAS THE PAIN LIKE?	DID ANYTHING HELP TO EASE THE PAIN?	HOW LONG DID THE PAIN LAST? WHAT WAS HAPPENING WHEN YOU FIRST NOTICED IT HAD GONE?
I was waiting for my parents to arrive for the evening. They were late	Headache and tummy pains. Dull ache	Lying down	About an hour. It first went when I was sitting with my parents playing monopoly after supper

Figure 5.2 Diary, completed by Clarissa, aged 14, aimed at identifying factors which may contribute to or ease her pain.

more general 'getting to know work' (see Chapter 2 – *Individual assessment*) should also start in the assessment phase and, indeed, will provide a more holistic picture of the child.

Clarissa (mentioned above) found that resting in a darkened room helped her when she experienced a pain 'attack'. She also explained that, if the person handling her wheelchair was rough and bumped into things, this 'hurt a lot'. Her key worker explained that she would take great care when pushing Clarissa in her chair and would relay this important message to other staff. Arrangements were also made for Clarissa to rest when necessary.

FAMILY ASSESSMENT

Joining with the family, rather than entering into a debate on whether the problem has a physical or psychological origin, is essential if any progress in treatment is to be made. Assessment is therefore about listening to the family's account of the current situation. The idea that 'worrying' or 'sadness' can sometimes contribute to physical symptoms can be introduced into the discussion. Giving common examples, such as 'butterflies' before an exam, can help to normalise this phenomenon. It is also important to acknowledge that any severe physical illness, or one requiring hospitalisation, will have emotional sequelae. Pain, unpleasant treatment, missing home and school will all take their toll. At the same time, the family therapist will need to reassure the family that all contributing factors must be looked at, which will include a thorough medical examination of the problem. It can be helpful to include the paediatrician in this initial meeting, so that the family can see paediatric and mental health professionals working together.

Identifying characteristics of family functioning that typically contribute to somatisation will obviously be the other part of a family assessment (see *Introduction* above and *Family therapy* below).

HOME AND SCHOOL VISIT

A home and school visit will give the nurse a more vivid picture of how the child functions at home and in school (see Appendices A and B). The school nurse may be able to provide valuable information concerning the frequency and severity of symptoms occurring at school, and the timing of visits to the 'sick room' may shed some light on precipitating factors.

Clarissa (mentioned previously) had slept downstairs since she had been unwell. Her bedroom had the feel of a 'sick' room, with dim lighting (the curtains drawn), a commode by the bed, and wash bowl and toiletries nearby. Clarissa's father had managed to acquire the commode through social services and was currently fighting a battle to have Clarissa recognised as disabled, so that hand rails and a ramp could be installed in the house.

Clarissa's schoolteacher reported that Clarissa was a bit of a loner. She seemed old for her age and uninterested in teenage things. The teacher thought that Clarissa had very few friends; other teenagers seemed to avoid her. She tended to be with her younger sister at break times. Clarissa was absent from school a great deal and often appeared distracted from her work when in class. The teacher was aware that Clarissa's mother was often unwell and thought that Clarissa worried about her. Consequently, her school work was poor. The teacher was aware that Clarissa had been badly teased in primary school because of her precocious puberty, but felt sure that she was not currently being bullied.

PSYCHIATRIC ASSESSMENT

Assessment by a child psychiatrist will be important to establish the young person's mental state. While research is divided concerning the relationship between depression and psychogenic pain, there is considerable evidence linking anxiety with somatic symptoms (Ryan-Wenger, 1994).

MULTI-DISCIPLINARY INTERVENTION

Children who present with severe and/or chronic physical symptoms are likely to be admitted to a paediatric ward for assessment. Early collaboration with psychiatric colleagues will help to introduce families to the idea that psychological factors may be important and facilitate a transition to mental health care if appropriate. For some children, admission to a psychiatric unit may be appropriate.

INDIVIDUAL WORK

Supportive and insight-oriented work

◆ *Non-threatening games and conversation* If asked directly, the child is likely to deny having any concerns or worries, either because they are not consciously aware of them or because the feelings are too painful to mention. The nurse will need to establish a relationship in which the young person feels safe. Starting with games, activities and general non-threatening conversation may be necessary.

◆ *Using stories* Reading stories with the young person may help to facilitate discussion about feelings, or simply arouse the child's thoughts and emotions, and give the child hope. *The Secret Garden* by F. Hodgson Burnett may be particularly pertinent.

◆ *Using non-verbal forms of communication* Because somatisation can be viewed as a form of non-verbal communication, the nurse must be prepared to utilise non-verbal communication skills in her or his individual work. What children do not say may be more significant than what they do say. Tone of voice, moments of hesitation or an averted gaze may be important indicators of painful feelings being withheld. The nurse may need sensitively to hypothesise what the child is feeling, acknowledging that he/she may be wrong and asking the child to indicate verbally or non-verbally whether the hypothesis is correct. A wide variety of non-verbal means of communication can be explored and utilised whilst building a relationship with the child, getting to know more about them and facilitating the child's awareness of their feelings and possible connection with symptoms. The possible channels of communication are endless: drawing, puppets, a dolls' house, sand tray and so on (see Chapter 2 – *Individual assessment, 'Getting to know children'* and *Individual work, Helping the child to recognise and express their own thoughts and feelings*).

William (mentioned previously), aged 12, had a long history of abdominal pain and vomiting. Before referral to the psychiatric unit he had numerous intrusive medical investigations and extensive treatment, including surgery, all of which failed to improve his condition. William drew a picture depicting how he felt (Figure 5.3). The impressive cruise liner and its wreck poignantly represent how awful he felt when ill, but also suggested a glimmer of hope of how he could be, if well.

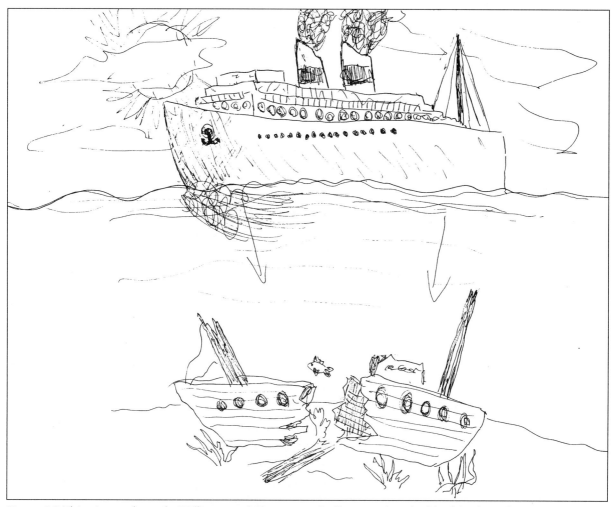

Figure 5.3 This picture drawn by William, aged 12, poignantly illustrates how bad he felt when ill. Reproduced with permission from the artist.

Children who have been physically or sexually abused often develop somatic symptoms. Alper et al (1993) found a high correlation between non-epileptic seizures and childhood sexual and physical abuse, and Lask and colleagues (1991) suggested that sexual abuse is frequently indicated amongst children with pervasive refusal syndrome. The nurse will need to be sensitive to any signs of possible abuse communicated by the child and discuss these in multi-disciplinary team meetings. Both the nurse who lacks expertise in exploring such issues and the experienced nurse will require supervision to facilitate such delicate individual work. In the author's experience, exploration of abuse is best continued with the person to whom the child first discloses, rather than introducing a 'stranger' to the child. Sometimes this may, of course, be unavoidable; for example, if the nurse in question, or multi-disciplinary team, believes that a more experienced colleague is needed.

◆ *Using diaries* It may be helpful for the young person to keep a diary of their symptoms and the context in which they occur, similar to the assessment diary (see Figure 5.2). This can provide useful material for discussion in individual sessions, including problem-solving work.

Problem-solving work

Using self-monitoring (as mentioned above), the nurse can help the child to identify events that appear to precipitate symptoms and formulate strategies to tackle them. Such strategies might include:

◆ Finding a significant adult, perhaps a key nurse or parent, to talk to about possible worries. Aro and co-workers (1989) found that adolescents who had a parent as a confidante were less likely to develop somatic symptoms when under stress than those who lacked parental support.

◆ The use of relaxation techniques (see Chapter 4 – *Individual work, Relaxation*). Based on the assumption that psychological distress causes muscle tension, several researchers have looked at the effect of relaxation on psychogenic pain and it would appear to have a positive effect (Ryan-Wenger, 1994). Using biofeedback that involves a changing computer image can make relaxation training more fun and a greater challenge for the young person. It can also provide a face-saver for the child who is reluctant to comply with treatment, because they are adamant that nothing will help their pain. If the nurse explains the physiological theory on which it is based and is optimistic about its success, relaxation can indeed be effective through the release of muscle tension, as a placebo or as a face-saver for the child to get well (see below).

◆ Using visual imagery to fight against the symptom; putting 'a face' to the symptom and creating 'a hero' to fight it.

> William (mentioned above) visualised his symptoms as a dragon with vicious claws (Figure 5.4) and created a warrior, Arnold, to fight against it whenever it appeared. In individual work, he drew these figures fighting (Figure 5.5) and talked about each of their characteristics. Time was spent discussing how William would call on his hero and what help he would need. He decided that he would ask his key nurse to assist him in summoning Arnold, as the pain would make it difficult for him alone. William drew a comic strip to consolidate his plan (Figure 5.6).

Improving self-esteem

Research suggests that children who suffer frequent headaches or recurrent abdominal, limb or chest pain have lower self-esteem than asymptomatic or chronically ill children (Ryan-Wenger, 1994). An important part of the nurse's individual work should therefore aim to improve the child's self-image (see Chapter 2 – *Individual work, Improving self-esteem*).

Massage and exercise

If physiotherapy is prescribed (see *Physiotherapy* below), the key nurse can provide continuity of treatment. These sessions can also provide an opportunity for talking.

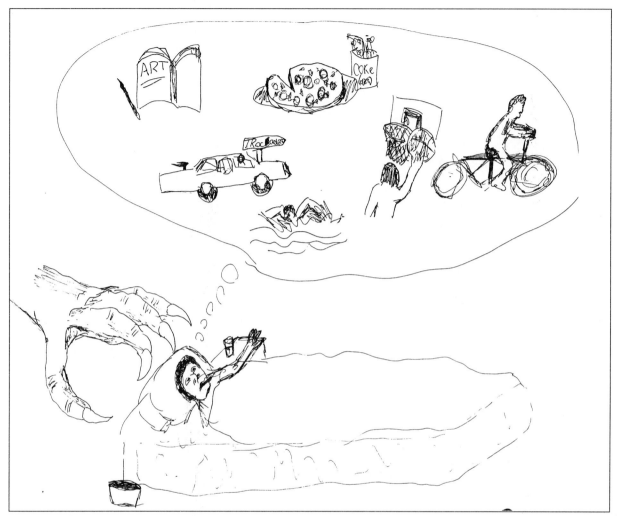

Figure 5.4 William visualised his illness as a dragon with vicious claws which dragged him down preventing him from doing all the things he enjoyed. Reproduced with permission from the artist.

MILIEU AND GROUP THERAPY

Children and adolescents with more complex and challenging physical problems may require admission to a psychiatric unit. This will allow a more thorough assessment and provide valuable milieu therapy. If there are concerns about abuse, admission may be essential to protect the child and to confirm suspicions. For example, the mother of a child with Munchausen by proxy can be closely observed and the young person with pervasive refusal syndrome may start to communicate more openly about possible abuse, once in a safe environment, separated from her or his family.

In the author's experience, the therapeutic milieu plays a very important part in the rehabilitation of children with conversion disorders and those with pervasive refusal. Several potentially significant elements of the therapeutic environment can be identified:

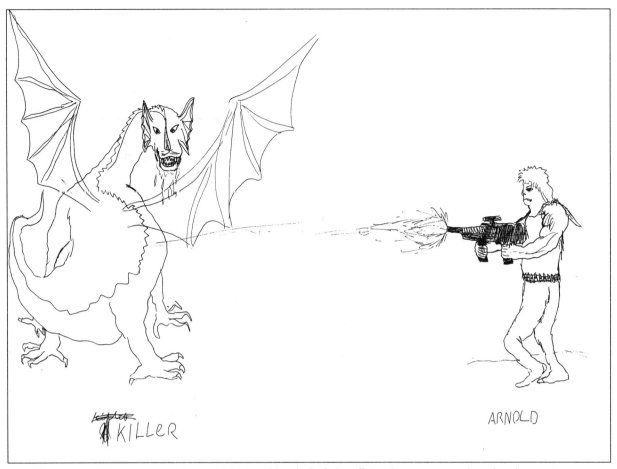

Figure 5.5 William created a hero called Arnold to help fight off the dragon. Reproduced with permission from the artist.

◆ *Peer support* The importance of empathy and support from others who have had similar experiences and are of a similar age should not be underestimated. Aro et al (1989) highlighted the significance of peer support in mediating the impact of adverse life events on psychosomatic symptoms. Adolescents who had experienced adverse life events and lacked the support of friends were more likely to develop somatic symptoms.

◆ *A structured daily timetable* The structure of the day, including periods of activity and rest, individual time with staff and time spent in group activities, will be important for the rehabilitation of these children. Young people with myalgic encephalitis (ME) or chronic fatigue syndrome, for example, seem to benefit from a gradual, prescribed, increase in activity, and those with pervasive refusal appear to derive great strength from group activities and contact with peers.

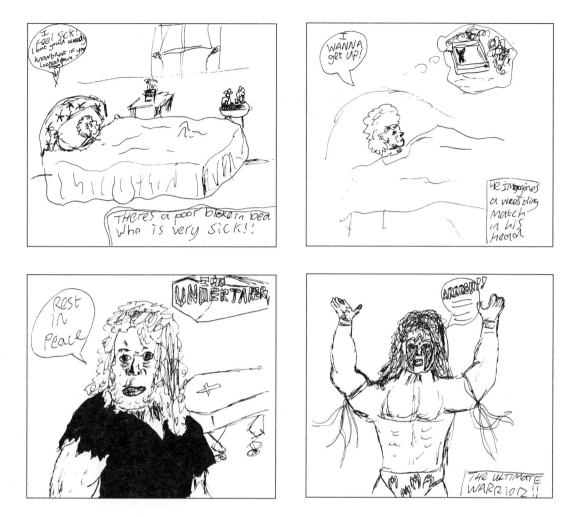

Figure 5.6 William drew a comic strip to tell the story of his fight against illness. Reproduced with permission from the artist.

Fiona (aged 13) was admitted to the psychiatric unit with a diagnosis of ME. She was in a wheelchair and needed to rest on her bed for long periods during the day. Once on the unit, a programme was set up to increase gradually the time she spent joining in group activities and to reduce resting time. Fiona was given three stretchy red hair bands each morning, which she wore on her wrist; these could be handed to staff, each in exchange for half an hour's bed rest. This allowed Fiona to maintain some control in her rehabilitation, as she decided when to take her rests, but at the same time ensured some activity. After a while, the number of bands issued reduced to two, and then one.

◆ *An environment in which there is a sensitivity to non-verbal communication* An important role of the nursing staff is to observe the children's behaviour and pick up and respond to non-verbal cues. Demonstrating a willingness to try to understand is a fundamental component of a therapeutic environment.

◆ *An environment in which it feels safe to disclose strong and painful feelings* Children may go through a phase of acting out strong and negative feelings, which may be too painful for the family to cope with alone, at home.

◆ *Acknowledgement of physical symptoms and the provision of face-savers* Admission to hospital, including a thorough medical assessment, can help to give the child the important reassurance that they need. As there may be a conscious element to the illness behaviour (see *Introduction* above) and due to the stigmatisation attached to mental illness, it is also helpful to take the approach that some physical treatments will be necessary to get the child better, such as physiotherapy and rest. It should be explained to the child that you would expect their symptoms to improve slowly with the various treatments being utilised. Encouraging the child to 'take it easy' and not expect too rapid an improvement may be reassuring. It is also generally helpful to explain that, even when the symptoms have disappeared, the child may need to remain in hospital, because staff are aware that they have other concerns needing attention. In the author's experience, many children seem fearful that their 'worries' will be forgotten once they are symptom-free.

PHYSIOTHERAPY

Physiotherapy, including hydrotherapy, can play an important physical and psychological role in treatment of movement disorders. It can be a valuable face-saver for the child, but will also be essential to prevent the development of contractures, which are inevitable if the young person is immobile for a long time. Reflex sympathetic dystrophy (RSD) is a syndrome characterised by severe regional pain with swelling, dysaesthesia to light touch and vasomotor instability. It is thought to result from the abnormal firing of peripheral nerves, due to their increased sensitivity, and research suggests that psychological stress may be an important underlying factor in its development (Sherry and Weisman, 1988). Mobilisation and massage are essential for successful treatment. Immobilisation can result in chronic trophic changes in soft tissues, contractures and osteoporosis. Sometimes the routine treatment of mobilisation and massage in a paediatric setting proves to be inadequate and a psychiatric referral will be necessary to look more closely at the underlying psychological factors, which are perhaps maintaining the disorder.

FAMILY THERAPY

A research study by Salvador Minuchin and colleagues identified five prevalent characteristics of families of children with somatic disorders (Sargent, 1983):

◆ *Enmeshment* A high level of involvement and responsiveness between family members, to the extent that there is poor differentiation between the perception of self and other family members.

✦   *Over-protectiveness* An excessive degree of concern for other family members, so that individual competence and autonomy is inhibited.

✦   *Rigidity* The family clings to its usual way of functioning, even when ineffective, especially when change threatens the status quo, such as a child entering adolescence.

✦   *Lack of conflict resolution* When relationships are enmeshed and there is a high level of over-protectiveness, the usual conflicts of family life tend to threaten family stability and are therefore avoided.

✦   *Involvement of the symptomatic child in parental conflict* There is a tendency for parents to put the child in the position of siding with one or other of them; for there to be a strong coalition between the child and one particular parent; and for both parents to focus on the child in order to cease their own conflict, either by protecting or attacking the child.

The family is likely to present itself as a 'normal', if not an extremely close and loving, family and to deny any need for change. The initial stages of therapy will therefore need to establish a climate of trust and collaboration, in which the family members feel able to open up and express themselves. Positive aspects of family functioning will need to be utilised in order to avoid the family coming into conflict with the therapist, which will help only to strengthen their enmeshment. An important function of family therapy must be to strengthen family boundaries and allow each family member develop a sense of self. Resolution of conflicts requires each family member to have a degree of autonomy and be respected as an individual. Ensuring that parents work together in helping the child to get better, and, in particular, encouraging involvement of the parent who has been more peripheral, will help to undermine the role of the child's symptoms.

Clarissa had become a parental figure for her younger sister, cared for her mother when she was sick and her father was out at work, and now that he was unemployed, provided him with emotional support. Since Clarissa had become ill, her father had taken on the role of helping her to wash, dress and sit on the commode. During family therapy, Clarrisa's mother was encouraged to become more involved in the care of her sick daughter and Clarissa's father, who had complained that he could not look for work because his family needed him at home, was encouraged to do so. The months that he had spent caring for his daughter were acknowledged and his decision to seek professional help commended. Clarissa was unhappy about being left alone in the house and would not allow anyone else to look after her, apart from her parents. Gradually, through discussion in family meetings, the family was able to identify someone in whom they would have confidence in as a 'babysitter'. The parents were encouraged to make plans to go out together as a couple, something they complained could no longer happen. Clarissa's younger sister, who now stayed at home to keep her sick sister company, was encouraged to resume contact with her own friends.

Onnis et al (1994) described the value of 'sculpting' as a family therapy technique for use with psychosomatic families. Similar to somatisation, sculpting is a non-verbal form of communication. Each family member is asked to arrange the rest of the family into a live sculpture, which represents how he or she perceives family relationships (Burnham, 1986). The position of their bodies in space, in terms of closeness or distance, their posture and facial expression all contribute to the spatial metaphor. Onnis and colleagues (1994) suggested that a sculpture of the present and future allows exploration of the family's evolutionary capacity with the objective of 'stimulating therapeutic evolution'. Some families may see no change in their sculpt over time, demonstrating little capacity to evolve; others may see a different sculpt in the future, but be unsure of how they will reach it.

Sculpts seem to work at a number of levels (Onnis et al, 1994):

◆ Sculpting, which involves the metaphorical utilisation of the body, introduces the idea that the symptom can have a metaphorical significance.

◆ As individual family members represent their own perception of the family, sculpting encourages individual identity.

◆ The sculpture of the future is likely to reveal singularly different views amongst family members, which will dispel the family myth of togetherness.

◆ At a basic therapeutic level, the therapist acts like a mirror, receiving and transmitting information about the family, so that the family can see itself not only through the image it projects, but also in its image as reflected by the therapist.

Meeting with parents alone or as a couple, and meeting siblings together without parents, may form a part of working with the family. For example, the mother of a child with Munchausen by proxy may respond more positively to help if initially confronted with her actions away from the rest of the family. If the subject is first broached with the father present, he is more than likely to become exceedingly angry and deny any such accusations, as he is probably unaware of the mother's deception. Taking the approach that the nurse knows what the mother is doing, understands it, and wishes to help her and the child will probably be most productive (Meadow, 1985). Siblings of a child with a chronic conversion disorder or pervasive refusal syndrome are likely to be worried about their sick brother or sister, jealous of the attention they are attracting, and guilty of the negative thoughts they are holding. A sibling meeting, perhaps with the key nurse, either including or excluding the sick child, can bring some relief. In the author's experience, parents are usually relieved that someone is giving their other children some 'special' time, which they are currently unable, or at least struggling, to do.

INDIVIDUAL PSYCHOANALYTICAL PSYCHOTHERAPY

Individual psychotherapy may help the child to gain some understanding of, and deal with, internal conflicts. Lehmkuhl et al (1989), in their study of children and adolescents with conversion disorders, found that treatment outcome was improved considerably where the young person agreed to individual psychotherapy. Just as the nurse will need to use non-verbal means of communication, so the psychotherapist will need to explore different avenues. It may be helpful to include the mother in therapy sessions. This can help to build on the mother–child relationship, which in turn may help to protect the child from somatising their distress. As previously mentioned, having a parent as a confidante can reduce the impact of stressful life events and protect against the development of psychosomatic symptoms (Aro et al 1989).

MEDICATION

The psychiatrist may prescribe medication if, for example, the child is considered to be clinically depressed or handicapped by feelings of anxiety (see Chapters 2 and 4 – *Medication*). Drug therapy will not be the solution, but may enable other therapies to be utilised by the child and family.

Children who have a chronic illness, such as diabetes, which is failing to respond to treatment, will require admission to stabilise their condition. In addition to the unsettling effects of stress on their physical state, it may become apparent that the child is not complying with treat-

Carol, aged 14 years, was admitted to the psychiatric unit with unstable diabetes mellitus and chronic non-compliance with treatment. She had developed diabetes 2 years after her mother's death. Carol had had a turbulent relationship with her mother, who had a drinking problem and died very suddenly from liver failure. During the admission, it became apparent that Carol's father was unaware that Carol or her siblings knew of his wife's drinking problem. Carol later disclosed that an older cousin had abused her sexually. She had told her mother, who had played down the incident and suggested that Carol must have encouraged him. Since her mother's death, a negative relationship had developed between Carol and her siblings, and between her and her father. It seemed as though the family had been unable to grieve for the wife and mother, and that Carol, who wanted to talk about her, had become a scapegoat in the family. The family was unable to talk about the mother's drinking, although Carol's siblings suggested that Carol was partly to blame, because she was always arguing with their mother. It soon became clear that Carol had many good reasons for refusing to monitor her blood sugar level, administer her insulin or eat a sensible diet. She had developed a chronic and potentially handicapping disorder just as she was entering adolescence, with all the developmental hurdles that this entails; at this difficult time, when she needed support, her mother was no longer around and her father was busy, working and looking after three other children (one only 5 years old); she felt disgusted with herself, that she had allowed or perhaps, as she now thought, encouraged her cousin to abuse her; and she felt guilty and to blame for arguing with her mother and now considered her mother's death to be her own responsibility. Nursing staff on the psychiatric unit had to restrain Carol in order to monitor her blood sugar level and administer insulin. In close collaboration with the paediatricians, Carol's diabetes management was stabilised. However, this was a long and arduous task, and required nursing staff to be consistently firm, but caring.

ment. It will be essential that the nurse closely supervises the child's self-care and, if necessary, takes over this role until the young person is ready to resume the responsibility. This will not be easy if the child is set on harming themselves. However, it is paramount that staff maintain a firm, but kind, approach, explaining that they do appreciate the child has valid reasons for non-compliance and demonstrating a willingness to understand.

TREATMENT OUTCOME AND FUTURE PLANNING

Collaboration between psychiatry and paediatrics is probably significant in promoting the family's compliance with treatment. Lehmkuhl et al (1989), who reported a 22% drop-out rate in their study of children with conversion disorders, suggest making a therapeutic contract with the child or adolescent and their family. Setting specific goals for treatment will give the child and family something concrete to work on, similar to a physical diagnosis.

Turgay (1990) found that a positive outcome to the treatment of conversion disorders seemed to depend on the following:

◆ *Age* The younger the child, the better the response to treatment. Another characteristic of younger children is the tendency for symptoms to change more frequently (it is not uncommon in conversion disorders for a different symptom to appear as another is 'successfully' treated).

◆ *Child's strengths* A child's ego strength seems to be correlated with a positive treatment outcome.

◆ *Insight* The child or adolescent's capacity to gain insight into the development and meaning of their symptoms appears to be related to an early response to treatment.

◆ *Cooperation* Cooperation of the child and their family correlates with a positive and early response to treatment.

◆ *Family functioning* The presence of serious family dysfunction has a negative effect on treatment success and lengthens the time needed for recovery.

◆ *Denial by the family* The child's denial and non-compliance with treatment strongly correlates with the family's denial of the psychological component to their child's symptoms.

◆ *Internal and environmental conflict* Internal and environmental conflict is thought to play a part in causing and maintaining conversion symptoms, and children who seem to have more severe internal conflict appear to be more resistant to treatment.

◆ *Chronicity* The longer an individual has a conversion symptom, the longer it takes to recover.

In Turgay's (1990) study, all 89 children who were followed recovered and only three required more than 4 weeks' treatment. Lehmkuhl et al (1989) reported a very different picture, with 48% showing significant improvement, 30% showing a slight improvement and 22% having no change or a change for the worse. Perhaps it is not surprising, with the multitude of factors contributing to somatisation and the various factors influencing successful treatment outcome, that the success rate and length of treatment required for recovery actually vary considerably.

Depending on circumstances, some children may require long-term treatment away from their home environment. In the author's experience, children with pervasive refusal syndrome need months of therapy on an inpatient unit and possibly long-term care in a therapeutic community. For others, ongoing therapy and support in the community will be important. The child's return to school will require careful planning. Nursing staff and parents should liaise with the class teacher to ensure a continuity of approach to symptoms. For example, a plan may be set up whereby the teacher initially offers relief from academic work, perhaps drawing a picture, when the child first complains of symptoms. If this fails to bring the child relief, the child could be taken to the school 'sick room' for a rest. The aim would be to avoid sending the child home, which might reinforce symptoms. It seems to be helpful if there is a designated person in school, to whom the child can talk about any worries or concerns they are experiencing.

Some children will benefit from ongoing psychotherapy and family therapy, and some will require continuing physiotherapy. The future planning should be made by the multi-disciplinary team and parents, in collaboration with local services.

CONCLUSION

Both physical and psychological factors are significant in the aetiology of most, if not all, illnesses. It is too simplistic to see illness as being purely physical or purely psychological in origin, and perhaps more helpful to think in terms of a continuum, with predominantly physical at one end and predominantly psychological at the other.

Somatisation is the unconscious expression of emotional distress through bodily symptoms. A common error that many nurses make is to assume that physical symptoms with a psychological component are somehow 'put on' and not experienced as if they had an identified physical cause. The reality is that the child is experiencing the symptoms as they are reported. As a child begins to recover, they may partly feign delay of this recovery for fear that treatment will be terminated before they feel sufficiently well and/or because underlying emotional issues, which have been brought to the fore, have not been resolved.

Assessment and intervention are all about 'finding the right balance'. Inadequate investigation into possible organic pathology may result in the child being deprived of appropriate and potentially effective physical treatment, and over-zealous investigation may reinforce somatisation as well as having serious ethical implications. Intervention must strike a balance between physical treatments, such as physiotherapy and rest, and psychological treatments, such as teaching coping strategies and encouraging a healthy expression of feelings. It is also important to be led by the child and family in terms of listening to their needs as they see them, while pushing them to achieve goals towards recovery.

REFERENCES

Alper K, Devinsky O, Perrine K, Vazquez B and Luciano D (1993) Nonepileptic seizures and childhood sexual and physical abuse. *Neurology* **43**: 1950–1953.

Aro H, Hanninen V and Paronen O (1989) Social support, life events and psychosomatic symptoms among 14–16 year-old adolescents. *Social Science and Medicine* **29(9)**: 1051–1056.

Burnham JB (1986) Sculpting. In *Family Therapy,* pp 135–141. London: Tavistock.

Goodyer J (1981) Hysterical conversion reactions in childhood. *Journal of Child Psychology and Psychiatry* **22**: 179–188.

Kuo C-L and Hopkins Kavanagh K (1994) Chinese perspectives on culture and mental health. *Issues in Mental Health Nursing* **15**: 551–567.

Lask B and Fosson A (1989) A search for meaning. In *Childhood Illness: The Psychosomatic Approach – Children Talking with their Bodies*, pp 1–12. Chichester, UK: John Wiley.

Lask B. Britten C, Knoll L, Magagna J and Tranter M (1991) Children with pervasive refusal. *Archives of Disease in Childhood* **64**: 346–869.

Lazare A (1981) Conversion symptoms. *New England Journal of Medicine* **13**: 745–748.

Lehmkuhl G, Blanz B, Lehmkuhl U and Braun-Scharm (1989) Conversion disorder (DSM-III 300.11): symptomatology and course in childhood and adolescence. *European Archives of Psychiatry and Neurological Sciences* **238**: 155–160.

Meadow R (1985) Management of Munchausen syndrome by proxy. *Archives of Disease in Childhood* **60**: 385–393.

Nunn P and Thompson SL (1996) The pervasive refusal syndrome: learned helplessness and hopelessness. *Clinical Child Psychology and Psychiatry* **1(1)**: 121–132.

Onnis L, Di Gennaro A, Cespa G et al (1994) Sculpting present and future: a systematic intervention model applied to psychosomatic families. *Family Process* **33**: 341–355.

Ryan-Wenger NM (1994) Psychogenic pain in children. *Annual Review of Nursing Research* **12**: 3–31.

Sargent J (1983) The family and childhood psychosomatic disorders. *General Hospital Psychiatry* **5**: 41–48.

Shanon A, Martin DJ and Feldman W (1990) Ultrasonographic studies in the management of recurrent abdominal pain. *Pediatrics* **86**: 35–38.

Sherry DD and Weisman R (1988) Psychologic aspects of childhood reflex neurovascular dystrophy. *Pediatrics* **81**: 572.

Sullivan MJL and Buchanan DC (1989) The treatment of conversion disorder in a rehabilitation setting. *Canadian Journal of Rehabilitation* **2(3)**: 175–180.

Turgay A (1990) Treatment outcome for children and adolescents with conversion disorder. *Canadian Journal of Psychiatry* **35**: 585–584.

van der Meer SB, Forget PP, Arends JW, Kuijten RH and van Engelshoven JMA (1990) Diagnostic value of ultrasound in children with recurrent abdominal pain. *Pediatric Radiology* **20**: 501–503.

World Health Organisation (1992) *The ICD-10 Classification of Mental and Behavioural Disorders – Clinical Descriptions and Diagnostic Guidelines.* Geneva: WHO

6 PROBLEMS WITH EATING

INTRODUCTION

The act of eating goes far beyond the provision of energy and nutrients. It provides an important channel of communication. It facilitates the bonding process between parent and child, and harnesses relationships later in life; it communicates our religious beliefs and cultural identity to others. The young infant derives nourishment and comfort while being fed and learns to rely on the parent to be satisfied. The attachment process begins. As we grow up, we learn that sharing food plays an important part in fostering relationships. It seems that in all cultures eating with others, rather than eating alone, is highly significant. Offering food to others is often a sign of friendship or respect and in some cultures, such as the Cewa African tribe, the ritual of eating together is an explicit sign of attachment.

The type of food we eat, the way in which it is prepared and the style in which we eat it reflect our culture and possibly our religious beliefs. Certain foods have acquired a national identity, such as Italian pasta or Japanese suchi. Religious laws may forbid the consumption of particular foods, such as pork and shellfish in Judaism. Special feasts may mark events of cultural or religious significance, such as the wedding breakfast or Christmas lunch, and in certain religions, as in the Muslim faith, fasting is important. In India the caste system determines the type of food to be eaten, who should prepare it and with whom it can be eaten.

Body shape also reflects the culture in which we live. In developing countries, where food may be sparse, a rounded figure signifies health and prosperity. Among certain African tribes, fatness is a sign of beauty. This was also the case in the Western world until the turn of the twentieth century, when thinness became associated with beauty. Our body shape portrays a certain image of the type of person that we are, albeit incorrect. In the Western world many assumptions are made about the person who is obese; laziness is one attribute commonly given (Gilbert, 1986).

To help children and their families where there are problems with eating, it is essential that we understand the significance of food and eating for those individuals. Eating problems may take many different forms but, in order to plan treatment, can be divided into two basic categories: **refusing to eat** or **eating excessively**. However, it must be remembered that this is a somewhat artificial division, as some people will suffer from both, either at different times or concurrently.

CHILDREN AND ADOLESCENTS REFUSING TO EAT

The experiences of young people refusing to eat will obviously vary between individuals, but there do appear to be quite distinct differences between age groups. A young child's motivation not to eat is likely to differ from that of a teenager. Anorexia nervosa and related eating disorders do not appear to occur in very young children, although they have been seen in those as young as 8 years (Fosson et al, 1987). However, there are some similarities throughout childhood, such as refusing food as a protest. Nevertheless, to plan nursing care it is important to consider developmental differences, and so the problem of young people refusing to eat will be divided into two sections: **early childhood** and **middle childhood to teens**. There is no clear dividing line between these age groups and some of the problems presented, for example food phobias, may occur at any age.

EARLY CHILDHOOD

Feeding difficulties in the first few months of life are very common and usually transient. Advice and support from the midwife or health visitor will be invaluable in helping parents overcome these problems. However, feeding difficulties are sometimes more persistent and require multi-disciplinary assessment and management.

Failure to thrive occurs in 1–5% of children aged under 5 years (Berwick et al, 1982) and where there is no medical cause, such as malabsorption, feeding problems are likely to be associated (Woolston, 1983). Failure to thrive is said to occur when there is a **'failure to grow or gain weight either from birth or after a period of normal physical development'** when children **'are consistently below the third centile in weight'** on standardised growth charts, **'who have documented weight loss over time, or who have a reduction in growth velocity'** (Graham, 1991). A delay in growth can occur throughout childhood into adolescence, but will generally start and be picked up in early years. If there is no medical cause, the failure to thrive is said to be non-organic. In these cases the child is generally consuming inadequate calories, although there is some suggestion that emotional deprivation may stunt growth in children who are eating adequately. This phenomenon is sometimes referred to as psychosocial dwarfism (Green et al, 1984). It is probably too simplistic to attempt to separate organic and non-organic failure to thrive, or to distinguish between nutritional and emotional deprivation in non-organic failure to thrive. Failure to grow is probably always directly related to a dysfunctional secretion of growth hormone, although the cause for this may be emotional; where emotional abuse is linked with failure to thrive, there are often feeding difficulties. Therefore, a combination of factors is likely to cause a failure in growth (Homer and Ludwig, 1981; Skuse, 1985, 1989).

It is essential that nurses recognise children who are failing to thrive because there may be long-term detrimental effects, including impaired intellectual functioning, emotional problems and behavioural difficulties (Oates et al, 1985), as well as continued growth retardation. Furthermore, children who have been, or are continuing to be, abused may have delayed growth, and failure to thrive may be the first sign to arouse suspicion (Skuse, 1989). A Children's Society project revealed that health visitors were failing to recognise children with poor weight gain in one in three cases (Hampton, 1993). This research also discovered that parents of professional status were less likely to have their child diagnosed as failing to thrive. Because nutritional and emotional deprivation are associated with non-organic failure to thrive, perhaps some professionals make inappropriate assumptions related to social class. Failure to thrive is found in children of all social classes.

Feeding difficulties may be the result of a number of factors including:

◆ Physical problems or ill-health in the child (e.g. cleft palate, ear infection)

◆ Emotional problems

◆ Temperamental characteristics of the child

◆ Parental ignorance regarding the calorific requirements of their child or appropriate feeding techniques

◆ Disorganisation surrounding mealtimes, so that the parent is unaware of how much the child has consumed

♦ Depression, anxiety or anger in the parent feeding the child

♦ Family stress (e.g. marital conflict, unemployment)

ASSESSMENT –
EARLY
CHILDHOOD

A multi-disciplinary assessment of feeding difficulties will need to identify risk factors, including characteristics in the child, the parent(s) feeding the child, the parent–child interaction, family and social factors. Different parts of the assessment may be allocated to different members of the multi-disciplinary team, depending on individual professional skills.

PHYSICAL AND DEVELOPMENTAL ASSESSMENT OF THE CHILD

Physical examination must include accurate measurement of the child's height or supine length, if under 2 years of age, head circumference and weight in underwear or naked, if a baby. The diagnosis of failure to thrive is made on evidence of low or decreasing growth velocity (Figure 6.1). Further medical investigations should be undertaken if medical staff are concerned that there may be an organic cause for the growth retardation.

Some children have physical or developmental problems that affect feeding. Neuromotor dysfunction may result in poor coordination or hypotonia of facial and oral muscles, and so affect the act of sucking, chewing and swallowing, whereas tactile hypersensitivity in the mouth area may provoke strong negative reactions to feeding (Wolke and Skuse, 1992).

Developmental delay is often associated with failure to thrive and therefore an assessment

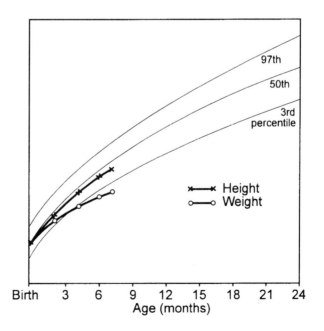

Figure 6.1 Growth curve in children with failure to thrive.

of developmental skills, using a standardised tool, such as the Denver scale, is essential (Skuse, 1985). If a child is not growing well and has a delay in skills that depend on environmental stimulation, for example language, it is likely that the failure to thrive is resulting from a combination of emotional and nutritional deprivation.

FAMILY ASSESSMENT

Meeting the whole family will provide a picture of how the family functions, what the nature of parent–child interaction is, how siblings interact with the identified child, what stressors the family is experiencing, such as marital tensions or unemployment, and how the family is affected by having a child with eating problems. Fosson and Wilson (1987) believe that a focal family assessment identifying factors that may have produced or exacerbated the feeding problem can enable successful brief family therapy interventions.

Some useful questions to ask parents are:

◆ How long have the parents seen eating/feeding as a problem?

◆ What do they see as the problem?

◆ Do they have any thoughts on why the problem has arisen?

◆ What are the parents' expectations of the child?

    Texture of food they expect their child to eat

    Varieties of food

    How much?

    Whether the child should be feeding her/himself

    What level of skill the child should have

    How long a meal should take

◆ What is the family's style of eating?

    Number of meals eaten each day

    Time of eating

    Who eats together

    Where do they eat ?

    What do the family eat?

◆ What methods have the parents tried to overcome the problem?

    What has been helpful?

◆ Who is most concerned about the child's eating?

Similar questions can be asked in relation to the child who has not yet been weaned, in order to build a picture of the family's attitude to breast or bottle feeding, their perception of the problem and what has been helpful, albeit small, in tackling the difficulties.

INFORMATION TO ESTABLISH FROM MEAL OBSERVATION

As well as talking with parents, it is extremely useful to observe the parent–child interaction during a meal.

Questions to ask yourself:

◆ How does the parent organise the mealtime?

◆ What food is being offered to the child?

> Quantity
>
> Content
>
> Texture

◆ What fluid is being offered?

> Type
>
> Quantity
>
> Temperature

◆ What is the child's first reaction to food?

◆ What is the child's behaviour during the course of the meal?

◆ What is the child's mood like?

◆ How does the parent react to the child?

◆ What is the parent's mood?

◆ How much eye contact is there between parent and child?

◆ Is there much verbalisation between parent and child?

◆ How much food has been eaten by the end of the meal?

◆ How long was spent over the meal?

After observation, it is important to explore with the parents what you have noticed. In one case described by Fosson and Wilson (1987) where the child had a facial cleft, it was observed that the mother held the baby loosely during feeding and gave little eye contact. On exploration, it became apparent that she lacked confidence in her feeding skills, her abilities were undermined by the father and maternal grandmother, and her anger with them was being displaced on to the child.

FOOD DIARY

It is often helpful to ask the parents to keep a diary of everything the child eats over the course of a week. This not only provides useful information but can sometimes reduce parents' anxiety if it becomes apparent that the child is eating more than they had realised.

NURSING/MULTI-DISCIPLINARY INTERVENTION – EARLY CHILDHOOD

A thorough assessment will enable a comprehensive management plan to be established.

FAMILY THERAPY

In meetings with a family therapist the parents may be helped to identify family processes that have contributed to, or maintain, the feeding problem. Rivalry between siblings may result in disruption of feeding or, in a chaotic family, individual children's needs or cues for attention may be ignored. In these situations it may be helpful to identify specific times when the parents can give each child attention and plan for the siblings to be otherwise occupied while the identified child is being fed.

When there is anger or a lack of feeling towards the child with feeding problems, the parent is unlikely to respond to cues for attention or food. A parent who was placed in a parental role as a child may feel resentful of their own child, and a mother who is suffering postnatal depression may feel very little towards her child (Fosson and Wilson, 1987). Family therapy may enable change, perhaps through mobilising the support of a spouse. Alternatively, negative feelings towards another member of the family may be displaced on to the child and family therapy may enable these feelings to be redirected and resolved.

Mothers who have suffered from eating disorders themselves may be so concerned that their own child does not develop a problem that one is created by an over-intrusive and critical approach to feeding (Stein et al, 1994). Family therapy addressing parent–child interaction, together with advice concerning mealtime management, may help the mother to put her own worries to one side whilst feeding.

EDUCATION

Education regarding diet and feeding techniques may be an important part of the nurse's and/or dietician's intervention. A number of feeding practices will help to maintain feeding problems, such as allowing the child unlimited access to food. Parents who are desperate to get their child to eat may leave biscuits or crisps in easy reach. The child may 'graze' constantly but have an inadequate diet for growth and health.

> Martin, aged 2, refused to eat at mealtimes, clamping his mouth tightly closed and becoming restless and irritable. His mother was exasperated and concerned that her child would starve. She decided to leave open packets of biscuits in low-level cupboards, so that he could help himself when he felt hungry. Martin soon found the sweet biscuits and picked at them throughout the day. He was not hungry at mealtimes and resented having to sit at the table.

A parent who is over-concerned about mess and insists on feeding the child her/himself, instead of allowing self-feeding, may set up a conflict so that child then refuses to eat at all (Stein et al, 1994).

MEALTIME BEHAVIOUR PROGRAMME

Some children will refuse to eat, struggling to create autonomy from the parent (Chatoor and Egan, 1983; Woolston, 1983). The relationship between parent and child is usually angry and negative. A behaviour programme at mealtimes can help to diffuse anger and be effective in correcting behavioural problems.

Points to consider when devising a behaviour programme:

◆ It is important to decide with the parents who should feed the child. If a parent is particularly anxious about the child's eating, it may be helpful for the other parent or another adult to be more involved for a period of time. This will give the anxious parent a break and reduce the level of tension surrounding mealtimes, which may in itself help the feeding process.

◆ Encourage the parents to establish a routine for mealtimes within the context of their own culture. It is helpful if children are seated comfortably and there are minimal distractions at mealtimes. The parents may wish to feed the child separately or eat together as a family; either way, a matter-of-fact attitude to mealtimes should be fostered.

◆ A time limit for mealtimes is generally helpful: 20 minutes per course should be adequate. After the time limit, any remaining food should be taken away. Feelings of hunger later on should encourage the child to eat more quickly at the next meal.

◆ The food presented to the child must be age-appropriate, in quantity and texture. If the child has become a faddy eater, it may be necessary to start with foods that the child likes and slowly introduce new foods. It is important to strike a balance between allowing the child some choice but also ensuring a balanced diet, avoiding complicated food preparation for the family and the expense of wasting uneaten food. It can be effective for parents not to replace food that the child has left with an alternative and to persist in offering the particular food at further mealtimes. Eventually hunger should overcome the fad (Douglas, 1989).

◆ Many children enjoy having their own cutlery and crockery, and it may help them to gain more confidence in feeding themselves. Children should be allowed and encouraged to feed themselves, but, if they are being fed, small amounts of food should be offered on a spoon with adequate time allowed for swallowing.

◆ The child must be allowed to play with food. Through this experience, the child learns about the texture of food and eating becomes fun. Parents may need practical advice on how to cope and manage with mess, such as placing some protective covering on the floor and avoiding the constant wiping of the child's face during a meal.

◆ Parents should talk to the child during the meal and include topics other than food.

Encouraging the child to eat may be helpful, but only if in a relaxed manner. Coercive feeding techniques, including force-feeding, are not helpful and are likely to be counter-productive (Sanders et al, 1993).

◆   Encourage parents to give the child a lot of praise when a mouthful of food is taken. A child with more extreme difficulties will need encouragement to take smaller steps, such as sitting in a high-chair without fighting. Some older children may respond well to star charts, for example, one star on their chart for each course eaten. Alternatively, parents could create a colouring chart, where one part is filled in for each course (Figure 6.2). It is essential that the child is involved in sticking on stars or colouring in. Some children may not want attention drawn to their eating and in these situations it is obviously better to play down their success.

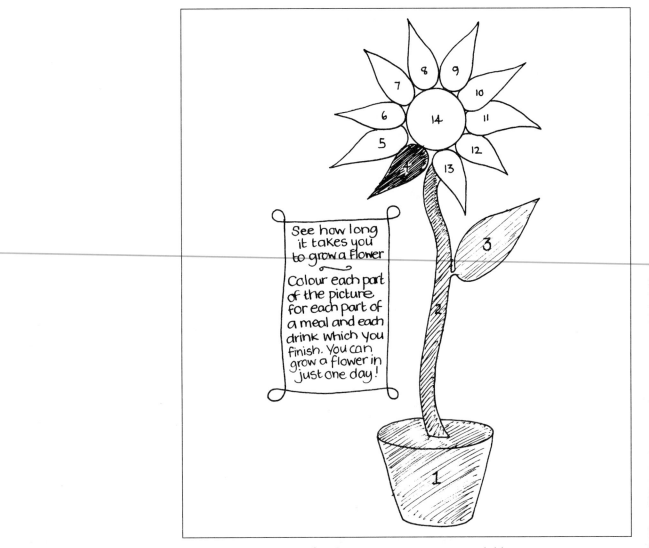

Figure 6.2 Chart to encourage a young child to eat.

◆   If the child is crying or spitting out food, parents should stop their interaction with the child until she/he is calm. Parents must avoid displays of anger, and should look away from the child. The parent can resume interaction as soon as the child is calm.

DESENSITISATION PROGRAMME

During assessment it may have become apparent that the child is afraid of swallowing, having previously experienced choking. A desensitisation programme, coupled with relaxation techniques, has been shown to be helpful (Chatoor et al, 1988). A hierarchy of food types should be drawn up with the child and parents, starting with the most easily swallowed food to the most difficult imagined. The child is taught simple relaxation techniques which can be used before meals. During relaxation, the child is asked to imagine eating a particular food which is difficult to swallow and then taken through the steps of relaxation again, while still thinking about eating the food. This food is then incorporated into the meal that follows (see Chapter 4 – *Individual work, Relaxation* and *Desensitisation*). Gradually new foods are introduced in an ascending order of difficulty. Initially the texture of food eaten is likely to be puréed, slowly progressing through lumpy foods, eventually reaching hard or crispy food. It may even be necessary to introduce new flavours in a puréed form, before building up the texture of the food. An older child may find it helpful to keep a diary of their progress, which includes reflection on how it felt eating the new food (Figure 6.3). Some children may appreciate time to let off steam after the meal, perhaps punching a pillow or kicking a football around (see Chapter 3 – *Individual work* on possible channels for venting angry feelings). It is important to be led by the child: find out what they find helpful and adapt your programme accordingly.

WHAT I ATE	WHAT NUMBER ATTEMPT WAS IT	COMMENTS: HOW DID I FEEL ABOUT IT? WOULD IT BE BETTER TO TRY IT IN A DIFFERENT FORM, AT A DIFFERENT TIME ETC.? CAN I SUCCESSFULLY ADD IT TO MY DIET?
Fruit yogurt	First attempt	I liked the taste but didn't like the bits of fruit in it. Next time I'll try a smooth variety. Later I could try this variety again but on my own – not with people watching

Figure 6.3 Teenage diary to reflect on desensitisation.

ENCOURAGING HEALTHY PARENT–CHILD INTERACTION

The depressed or distant parent is unlikely to respond to cues for attention from the child. Helping parents to enjoy being with their child may be the first step to improving the relationship between them. Encouraging parents to talk about moments when they have felt close to their child or memories of closeness to their own parents can help to arouse feelings in the present. Modelling physical signs of closeness, such as holding, cuddling and stroking, positively reinforcing attempts by parents and pointing out the child's positive responses to attention, such as smiling, can facilitate a healthy relationship between the parent and child (Klein, 1990).

Encouraging play between the parent and child is an essential part of enriching their relationship. A mother who was deprived herself as a child will need to be taught how to play. Joining the mother and child in play provides an opportunity for modelling.

In some families where there are eating problems, there may be separation difficulties between a parent and child, rather than a lack of closeness. The child who has had a frightening experience, such as choking, may regress to a more clingy, dependent age and need help to regain self-confidence, while the parent may have become over-protective and need help to give the child more independence. Reduced anxiety in the parent–child relationship, together with the child's enhanced confidence, should enable eating difficulties to be overcome.

Refusing food is one way in which a child may attempt to assert their autonomy (Chatoor et al, 1988). The child may feel unable to depend on his or her parents and so aims to become self-sufficient. When parents are inconsistent in responding to cues from the child, sometimes being neglectful and at other times particularly controlling, the child is likely to be confused and frustrated. Using play, parents may be taught how to identify their child's cues and respond in a non-controlling manner.

PLAY TECHNIQUES TO ENCOURAGE EATING

Parents and/or nurses can use specific play to help eating become more enjoyable and meaningful. Some examples include:

✦ Help the child to grow their own plant. Buy the seeds together, prepare the pot in which to sow them and teach the child how to look after the plant, watering and feeding it, to enable growth.

✦ Messy play may help the child who becomes distressed with mess at mealtimes. Finger painting, using clay, pots of play slime, are possibilities.

✦ Role play with pretend food, perhaps shopping or a scene in a café.

✦ Playing with feeding utensils in the bath, where they may be perceived as less threatening.

> Anna, aged 7, was failing to thrive. Both her parents had learning difficulties and were deprived themselves as children. The parents looked to Anna for support. Anna, who was bright, had an ambivalent relationship with her parents, sometimes 'looking after them' and at other times being angry with them. She was admitted to the psychiatric unit. Anna's key nurse helped her to grow her own plant. Anna nurtured her plant and became excited when it showed signs of growth. The plant became a useful analogy to talk about the need to eat in order to grow.

INDIVIDUAL THERAPY FOR A PARENT

Sometimes individual therapy should be recommended for parents. A mother suffering from post-natal depression needs individual therapy and possibly medical treatment. However, many more parents will need individual support or counselling, simply to help boost their self-esteem, which is likely to be low if they feel to blame for their child's eating problems.

MEDICAL TREATMENT AND PHYSICAL REVIEW

Physical investigation may have identified medical problems receptive to treatment. Disorders of gut motility are sometimes associated with feeding problems and can be helped with cisapride, a drug that increases gut motility.

Multi-vitamin supplements with zinc and iron should be prescribed to children who are failing to thrive. Iron deficiency is common in these children and can be associated with irritability and short attention span; it could therefore hinder behavioural feeding approaches (Wolke and Skuse, 1992). Addressing the underlying causes of failure to thrive will be a lengthy process and so growth hormone may also be prescribed to help the child catch up more quickly.

Where children are frightened of eating for fear of choking, medication may be prescribed to lessen anxiety, such as the benzodiazepine alprazolam. However, this should be considered only in conjunction with behavioural and psychodynamic therapy.

During the course of treatment, children should be weighed and measured weekly and a weight chart used to record progress. The daily calorific requirements for a child who is failing to thrive are approximately 1.5–2.0 times the expected intake for their age, to ensure optimal catch-up growth (Wolke and Skuse, 1992). It is generally helpful to set a daily calorific target even if the child is not failing to thrive, and to record intake. This will enable concrete evaluation of the multi-disciplinary intervention.

CHANGE OF ENVIRONMENT

It has often been observed that children affected by psychosocial dwarfism show a dramatic increase in linear growth once they have been removed from home (Skuse, 1989). Therefore, an important part of the multi-disciplinary intervention will be to establish where the child can best thrive. Obviously it is preferable to keep the family together, but in some instances this will not be in the child's best interests. Case conferences, including psychiatric and paediatric specialists, and the parents, will be held and legal proceedings may be required.

MIDDLE CHILDHOOD TO TEENS

A number of studies have shown that anorexia nervosa can occur in prepubertal children as young as 8 years (e.g. Fosson et al, 1987; Higgs et al, 1989). The disorder is characterised by a determined food avoidance, weight loss or a failure to gain the weight during the adolescent growth spurt, and two or more of the following: preoccupation with body-weight, preoccupation with calorie intake, distorted body image, fear of fatness, self-induced vomiting, excessive exercising and laxative abuse (Lask and Bryant-Waugh, 1993). Some children may avoid food and have associated symptoms of emotional disturbance, but not be concerned with body shape or use energy-purging activities. Higgs and co-workers (1989) described these children as having food avoidance emotional disorder (FAED), which should be recognised as overlapping with early childhood problems. Selective eating or extreme food faddiness is another problem that can present at any age. Bulimia nervosa has not been reported in children aged less than 13 years. This disorder is characterised by regular episodes of binge eating, which is considered by the young person to be out of their control, followed by self-induced vomiting, laxative abuse, vigorous exercise or fasting (Lask and Bryant-Waugh, 1993). Multi-impulsive bulimia nervosa is characterised by other compulsions as well as bingeing, such as cutting, stealing or drug abuse. Sometimes, refusal to eat can accompany other mental health problems, such as depression, or be part of a much wider problem, as in pervasive refusal syndrome where there is also a refusal to talk, walk or engage in self-care (Lask et al, 1991; Nunn and Thompson, 1996).

The incidence of anorexia and bulimia nervosa is largely unknown, but appears to be relatively rare in children compared with adults. However, if the problem is identified early, prognosis will be improved and it is important to remember that a proportion of children will die from eating disorders. Unlike the adult population, where only 5–10% of patients will be males, amongst children as many as 30% are likely to be boys (Higgs et al, 1989). Anorexia nervosa and related eating disorders may occur in all social classes, although possibly there is a bias towards 'middle' and 'upper' class (Lask and Bryant-Waugh, 1993), and in different ethnic backgrounds. Although it was commonly thought that anorexia and bulimia occurred only in people of white ethnic origin, more recent studies have identified the problem amongst those of Asian and African racial background (Holden and Robinson, 1988; Bhadrinath, 1990; Timimi and Adams, 1996).

ASSESSMENT – MIDDLE CHILDHOOD TO TEENS

Parents may not recognise that their child has a problem and so it may be a school or paediatric nurse that initiates referral for assessment and treatment.

PHYSICAL ASSESSMENT

The child should be weighed in underwear, after being asked to pass urine. Some children attempt to feign weight by hiding heavy objects under clothes or by drinking excessive quantities of water. The child must be measured so that their percentage weight for height can be calculated, that is the percentage of the 'ideal' weight for their age, where 100% represents the 'ideal' or average. This calculation can be performed on Cole's growth assessment slide-rule, which is based on Tanner–Whitehouse norms (Lask and Bryant-Waugh, 1993).

Due to low weight and poor peripheral circulation, some children develop skin ulceration. It is important to examine the child's skin closely, particularly the pressure points, such as along the vertebrae. Lanugo hair is commonly seen. The teeth of a bulimic child may have been eroded by gastric acid because of repeated vomiting; if this seems likely, an appointment with a dentist should be arranged (Robb et al, 1995).

To establish whether growth has been retarded, radiography of the hand may be arranged to measure bone age. Examination of bone density may detect the signs of osteoporosis, a long-term effect of anorexia nervosa. Anorexia nervosa can delay sexual maturation in females, and ultrasonography of the pelvis will reveal the degree of ovarian maturity. The ultrasonographic picture will be much clearer if the bladder is full and so the child must drink 1.5–2 litres of fluid beforehand. Computed tomography (CT) has revealed cerebral atrophy in patients with anorexia nervosa and so cranial CT may be organised. Early reports of simple photo emission computerized tomography (SPECT) scanning suggest that blood perfusion in the brain may be affected by anorexia nervosa (reported at 'Eating Disorders '95', a major conference on eating disorders held in London), and hepatic steatosis has been identified by means of ultrasonography of the liver. The importance of some of these investigations for treatment purposes is not yet known; research is at an early stage. Blood samples will definitely be taken, as there are many biochemical changes that are likely to occur, some of which must be treated immediately, such as dehydration or hypokalaemia. Bulimic patients are particularly prone to low potassium levels because of excessive vomiting.

INDIVIDUAL ASSESSMENT

If possible, the team member who will continue to do some form of individual work, such as the key nurse, should carry out the individual assessment. Tranter (1993) identifies important areas to explore with the child:

◆ *Perception of illness* Children with eating disorders often do not recognise that they have a problem, although will sometimes acknowledge feeling sad or depressed.

◆ *Body image* It is important to establish how the child feels about their size and shape. The drawing in Figure 6.4 was drawn by a very thin boy. A silhouette chart could be used to establish how the child sees her/himself now and how she/he would like to look (Figure 6.5) and/or the child could be asked to draw a picture of themselves.

◆ *Perception of self in relation to family* Who does the child feel closest to, who is most worried about them, what effect has the illness had on the family and what views does the

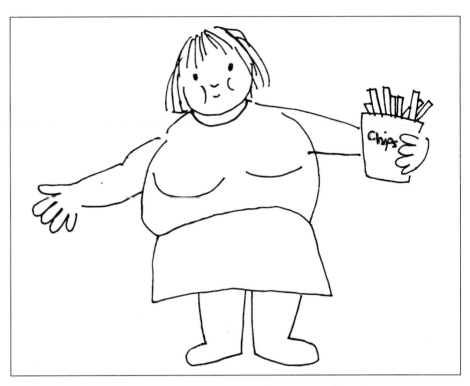

Figure 6.4 Self portrait by girl with an eating disorder

young person hold regarding her/his family? Previously unspoken worries may be disclosed.

◆   *School* Are there any concerns, such as bullying or not coping with work?

◆   *Interests and activities* Has the child become socially isolated or preoccupied with certain activities, such as school work or exercise, like ballet or gymnastics?

◆   *Anxieties* Is there anything in particular on the child's mind related to home, friends, school?

◆   *Attitude towards growing-up* What feelings does the child have regarding the physical and emotional changes in adolescence and the social expectations placed on them?

◆   *Exploring adverse sexual experiences* A number of adult women with eating disorders have reported sexual abuse in their childhood (Hall et al, 1989) and so it is important to bear this in mind during assessment. The child can be gently asked about sexual experience during the discussion on growing up.

It may be a long time before the child with pervasive refusal is able to talk about these issues and the nurse must stretch her/his communication skills to the full (see Chapter 2 – *Individual assessment, 'Getting to know children' and 'beginning a relationship'*).

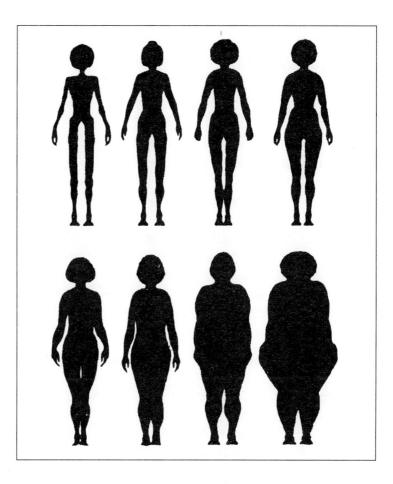

Figure 6.5 Silhouette chart. Reproduced from Bell et al. (1986) Body image of anorexia, obese and normal females. Journal of Clinical Psychology 42, 431–439, with permission from John Wiley and Sons, Inc.

FAMILY ASSESSMENT

As well as establishing the history of the disorder and its impact on family members, meeting the family may help to identify family dynamics that are helping to maintain the illness. The relationship between family members can be observed, together with family boundaries. Often, there is an over-involved or spouse-like relationship between the child with anorexia and one parent. The ease with which family members can express feelings openly can be noted. Minuchin et al (1978) described the anorectic family as being one in which there is a difficulty in resolving conflicts so that unexpressed feelings are channelled through one particular child and somatised. However, in some more chaotic families, conflict may be expressed overtly in the form of frequent arguments, which the child may find unbearable to cope with and becomes ill.

As well as meeting the family in a clinic setting, a home visit can be particularly enlightening and provides a forum for hospital preparation, if the child is to be admitted (see Appendix A).

SCHOOL ASSESSMENT

It is extremely useful to visit the child's school, (see Appendix B) to establish how the child is coping academically and the nature of peer relationships, and to gain an understanding of the school's philosophy. During treatment a change in school may be recommended. Additional information may be obtained by asking teachers to complete a standardised questionnaire (Rutter, 1967).

OBSERVATION OF MEALTIME BEHAVIOUR

Although family meals can be contrived in an outpatient setting or on a home visit, observation of mealtime behaviour is best achieved when the child is an inpatient and less aware that their actions are being noted. What and how much the child eats should be recorded, together with related behaviour, such as hiding food, eating particularly slowly, becoming withdrawn or talking excessively during the meal. On an inpatient setting, behaviour away from the table can also be observed, such as vomiting, laxative abuse and excessive exercising. However, it must be noted that these children are very discrete and so assumptions should not be made on the absence of evidence.

NURSING/MULTI-DISCIPLINARY INTERVENTION – MIDDLE CHILDHOOD TO TEENS

WEIGHT RESTORATION

Malnutrition is thought to have both physical and psychological sequelae (American Psychiatric Association, 1992). Physical symptoms, such as dehydration and electrolyte imbalance, obviously require immediate treatment to preserve life, and attention to nutritional status is important to allow healthy development. Weight restoration may also improve psychological symptoms such as depression. The process of helping the child to gain weight may in itself contribute to psychological treatment. Many children seem to experience some relief when parents and professionals take away some of their 'addictive' control over eating. Some children with eating disorders can be treated successfully as outpatients, whereas others require hospitalisation if their weight is dangerously low or a more comprehensive assessment of the problem is required.

Target weight

It is preferable to establish a realistic target weight range rather than a specific weight. The child's notion of a healthy weight is likely to be very different from that of parents or professionals, and a weight range will allow the child to feel they have some control. It also demonstrates a more healthy and less obsessional attitude to weight. A weight chart should be drawn up, clearly demonstrating the target weight range of 95–100% (Figure 6.6). Menstruation is unlikely to occur below 95%, but those with anorexia nervosa will be determined to be below average weight. Occasionally girls menstruate below 90% or need to be above 100% to achieve sexual maturity. It is important at the outset to explain that the target weight range will increase with age and it may be helpful to set weekly targets for weight gain of between 750 g and 1 kg.

Individual diet sheet

Divide the daily intake into small meals and snacks (Figure 6.7). The calorie content should be discussed with the dietician, but is likely to be at around 1500 kcal, slowly building up to 2000–3000 kcal. Refeeding a starving individual too rapidly may lead to gastric dilation or even perforation (Browning, 1977). Some choice in food types should be allowed, so that the child has some control over what is eaten. It is probably better not to discuss calories, but to talk in terms of a healthy diet. A diet sheet can be given to the young person which indicates portion size rather than energy values. The 'faddy' child may require a diet that accommodates a desensitisation programme (see *Early childhood* above).

Restricted or supervised access to food

Children with bulimia nervosa will need help to control binge eating. Restricting access to the kitchen, hospital cafeteria, local sweet shop and so on will be important in the early stages of treatment (Cahill, 1994). Those with anorexia nervosa must have limits set around food preparation, or at least close supervision. Time and energy may be used to feed others, rather than feed themselves, and vital ingredients such as fat and sugar may be rationed in the preparation of their own food.

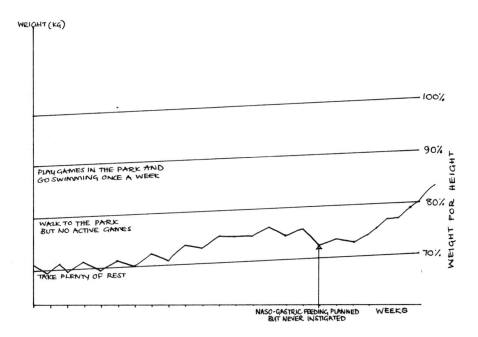

Figure 6.6 Example of a young girl's weight chart.

Figure 6.7 Example of a diet sheet to produce weight gain.

On waking
A glass of 'build-up' (a fortified milk drink)

Breakfast
2 Weetabix with milk (full fat)
A glass of fresh orange juice

Mid-morning
A glass of cordial made with Caloreen (a calorie additive)
A digestive biscuit

Lunch
A portion of meat or vegetarian alternative
A portion of potato, rice or pasta (4 tablespoons)
A portion of vegetable (3 tablespoons)
A dessert (if fruit is chosen, it must be supplemented with a biscuit)
A glass of water

Mid-afternoon
A glass of cordial made with Caloreen
A digestive biscuit

Supper
A sandwich (1 round)
A yogurt
A piece of fruit
A glass of water

Bedtime
A glass of 'build-up'

Portion size

There is some evidence that patients with anorexia nervosa may perceive food items as being larger than they actually are (Yellowlees et al, 1988) and that gastric emptying is impaired, resulting in an early sensation of satiety (Ravelli et al, 1993). It may therefore be helpful to start by giving small portions more frequently.

Psychodynamic approach to mealtimes

Anorexia and bulimia can be thought of as taking over part of the individual, so that part of the child wants to stay strictly in control of their eating and remain thin, while another part, albeit small, wants to eat healthily and return to a more normal home and school life. At mealtimes you can use this idea to encourage the child to fight against the anorectic side and give strength to their healthy side.

Using analogies

Helping to mobilise a young person's imagination can give them strength to fight against the 'voice in their head' telling them not to eat. Children with anorexia, bulimia and pervasive refusal sometimes describe such a voice. Imagining that this comes from a silly little monster which can be shut in a box during mealtime might be one helpful analogy to use. In another way, analogies can be used to encourage the child to keep struggling through the meal, for example imagining that each mouthful represents a step along the road back to school.

Recognising counter-transference

Commenting on how you are feeling while sitting with the child eating, and wondering out loud whether that is how they are feeling, can help the child to feel understood. For example, 'I'm sitting here feeling stuck and helpless. I wonder if that is how you are feeling'. Do not expect the child to answer.

Limit-setting

At mealtimes the child is likely to become upset and angry, possibly running away from the table. It is important to be firm but kind, and either insist that they return to the table or make a compromise, allowing the child to eat elsewhere but with an adult present. This firm approach demonstrates that you care about the child, which includes ensuring that they eat adequately. For many sufferers of anorexia nervosa, food intake may be the only area in their life that they feel in control of and therefore it will be very frightening to give this up. However, as their diet control is not compatible with health, it is essential that adults predominantly take charge. The child who has been abused may not feel worthy of being fed and so, again, adults must take over to prove otherwise. At all times there needs to be structure coupled with flexibility and compromise. In this way the child hopefully feels looked after but also maintains some independence. Compromise can also provide a valuable face-saver for the young person.

Goals for mealtimes are negotiated with the child, and may be anything from touching their lips with food, to eating three-quarters of the meal. Limit-setting must also include observing the child closely during the meal and immediately afterwards, in case food is hidden and then disposed of after the meal. Children may hide food in their clothes, stick food under the table or simply spread it over the plate.

> Mark, aged 14, was admitted to the child and adolescent psychiatric unit with anorexia nervosa. He was so malnourished that he had developed sores on his ankles and the beginnings of gangrene. As Mark started to put on weight and to recover emotionally, he talked about his initial experiences of being ill. In one family therapy meeting, he shouted at his parents: 'Why didn't you notice when I stopped eating and do something about it!' Mark's parents had, of course, noticed, but had decided that the best approach was not to draw attention to the problem or pressurise Mark to eat in any way.

Professionals and parents working together

Any disagreement between parents, or between parents and professionals, regarding food intake or mealtime approach should not be dealt with in front of the child. Children with eating disorders frequently split adults caring for them and this needs to be acknowledged.

Incentives

A lenient behavioural approach to weight restoration seems to be most effective (American Psychiatric Association, 1992). As children gain weight, they may be allowed to participate in more activities, such as swimming or dancing. However, a child who is in the 'wasting' weight range (below 80%), will require their activity to be restricted considerably. Activity goals can be clearly marked on the child's weight chart (Figure 6.6).

Control of vomiting, laxative abuse and excessive exercise

Vomiting repeatedly will result in electrolyte disturbance, in particular hypokalaemia, ulceration of the oesophagus and dental decay, as well as undernutrition. Children with anorexia or bulimia nervosa will need to be escorted to the toilet and required to stay with an adult for at least 2 hours after a meal. Helping to distract the child after a meal may allay their anxiety about not being allowed to vomit.

Laxative abuse will also lead to an electrolyte imbalance and, in the longer term, a dependence on medication to prevent constipation. Due to poor diet and possibly depression, children with eating disorders are likely to suffer from constipation. There must be an attempt to treat this with diet alone, but laxatives may need to be prescribed after abdominal examination or radiography. If the child is an outpatient, parents must be responsible for looking after and giving the medication. Parents and nursing staff should not allow children to go shopping alone and may need to check through their belongings to remove any laxatives after unsupervised periods. Gaining weight is so frightening for these children that they will go to great lengths to prevent it. Talking openly about the problem, without reprimanding, is important.

In the anorexic patient, excessive exercise will exacerbate the state of undernutrition, through expending energy and reducing appetite. Undernutrition may increase hyperactivity and so a dangerous vicious circle ensues which can lead to serious physical complications, such as cardiovascular problems (Beumont et al, 1994). It is therefore important to restrict excessive exercise, but as the child gains weight a moderate amount of 'healthy' activity should be encouraged. Total restriction is not likely to be successful and is not health inducing, unless the child is seriously malnourished. Part of the child's treatment should include education regarding diet, exercise and the dangers of laxative abuse and vomiting.

Nasogastric feeding

Sometimes it will be necessary to feed children artificially if they are dangerously malnourished or dehydrated. At other times it may be helpful to use nasogastric feeding if treatment has become 'stuck' – if the child's weight persists at a level below the target range. Given that weight increase in undernourished patients can improve psychological symptoms, such as obsessionality and mood, helping the child to move above a static weight may also move them into a state that is more receptive to psychiatric treatment. These particular children may respond well to bolus feeding after each meal, where the calorie content of the feed 'tops up' the energy value of food eaten. Bolus feeding has the advantage of mimicking a normal pattern of eating, so that appetite patterns are hopefully retained. Children who are dangerously malnourished may require a period of continuous feeding. When children refuse to be fed, careful consideration must be given to the ethical and legal problems presented. It is important to establish whether the child has the mental competence to make a decision to refuse treatment (see Chapter 1 – *Ethical issues*). If there is any uncertainty regarding the ethical or legal situation, such as the child's weight not being life-threatening, the judgement of the court may be sought. Sometimes, the fact that professionals and parents are working together to care for the child seems to help eating to recommence and court proceedings can be avoided. The weight chart in Figure 6.6 is from a case seen by the author which demonstrates this phenomenon. The sharp increase in the child's weight correlates with the parents' eventual agreement to seek court approval to enforce nasogastric feeding. Court approval was never actually required.

TACKLING OTHER FORMS OF SELF-DESTRUCTIVE BEHAVIOUR

Some children with eating disorders, particularly multi-impulsive bulimia, may cut themselves. This may be in response to hating their bodies; because of the tranquillising effect of releasing blood; feeling depersonalised and needing to cut themselves to feel pain and in touch with themselves; and/or because experiencing physical pain is more bearable than experiencing psychic pain. It is obviously important to prevent, or at least try to reduce, this form of self-destruction and to give the child a clear message that you care about them, even if they do not. (See Chapter 2 – *Nursing/multi-disciplinary intervention, Maintaining the child's safety*).

INDIVIDUAL WORK

Nurses can play a key role in providing special individual time for young people with eating disorders. Topics may include the following:

Enhancing a healthy body image

Research suggests that patients with anorexia nervosa overestimate their body size (e.g. Bell et al, 1986). Enhancing a more accurate body image must help the anorectic to tolerate weight gain more easily and eventually to maintain a healthy weight. Some exercises, using ideas from a self-directed programme of body image therapy for adults (Cash, 1991), are as follows:

✦ Help the young person to identify when they feel particularly fat. Ask them to complete a self-monitoring diary (Figure 6.8). Perhaps when they are weighed or go swimming, they are made especially conscious of their body size.

✦ Ask the young person to write a list of the body parts they dislike and give each a rating of 1–10, where 1 represents a mild dislike and 10 total disgust. Alternatively, draw around the child on a large piece of paper and ask them to colour in the parts they dislike. The young person creates a key to indicate their strength of feeling.

✦ Teach relaxation skills (see Chapter 4 – *Individual work, Relaxation*), which can enhance contentment in mind and body, as well as being used in desensitisation work, to reduce tension associated with particular events or thinking about particular body parts.

WHAT HAPPENED	WHAT I THOUGHT	WHAT I FELT AND WENT ON TO DO
My key nurse weighed me	She's looking at my bottom and is amazed how large it is.	I felt humiliated and jumped off the scales before she could read them. I covered myself up and refused to stand on the scales again
Susan, Jane and myself having a make-up session	My face is too fat to wear make-up. I look stupid	Said I didn't want to carry on and left Jane and Susan having a good time.

Figure 6.8 Example of a diary to self-monitor body image work.

The child starts to relax and then thinks about the stressor for 15 seconds, followed by further concentration on relaxing. The time spent imagining the stressor is slowly increased to 1 minute.

◆ Desensitisation could be used, employing a full-length mirror: the child looks in the mirror for specified times while practising relaxation.

◆ Use a cognitive approach to challenge the child's beliefs. Using the self-monitoring diary, discuss the young person's interpretation of events and offer alternatives. For example, perhaps she/he thought the nurse was staring at their bottom with disgust, when in fact the nurse was not, but because the child was feeling so low she/he assumed the worst.

◆ Another way to challenge the child's negative self-esteem is to ask them to list the parts of their body that they like. There is a tendency to focus on the 'hated' parts at the expense of the 'liked'. Look at the coloured body outline and compare the area of 'liked' (not coloured) with the 'hated' (coloured) parts. Although the 'liked' parts may cover only a small area, such as the eyes, they may have great significance (we look at a person's eyes when we talk to them).

◆ Using a long mirror, the child, dressed in a swimming costume, describes what she/he sees, incuding size, posture and general appearance, and the nurse reinforces accurate comments.

◆ Encourage the child to use corrective thinking when they are exposed to triggers that spark negative and distorted thoughts. For example, they might look at a magazine, see particularly thin models and think to themselves, 'Why can't I look like that?' Corrective thinking would involve saying 'STOP' to themselves, as soon as this negative and unrealistic thought came into their head. They must then come up with their own counter-argument (e.g. 'I don't need to look like a supermodel to be attractive'). Corrective thinking work could be recorded in a diary and discussed in individual work. Rewards might be given for positive thoughts.

◆ Ask the child to think of a person who is not thin that they admire. Explore what it is about them that they like.

◆ Use desensitisation to confront avoidant behaviours, such as using a towel to cover legs and tummy until reaching the water's edge of a swimming pool.

Acknowledging the healthy side of the child

The idea of an anorectic part and healthy part of the child (see *Weight restoration, Psychodynamic approach to mealtimes* above) can be used visually in individual sessions. The young person could draw each part in whatever shape or form and then write down what each has to offer (Figure 6.9). Alternatively, balancing scales can represent each part of the child, and counters or weights represent the advantages of each. It may be necessary to start this work by asking the child to keep a diary which includes columns for activity, thoughts and feelings, in order to identify the healthy and unhealthy parts. The child should make entries before or after meals and at periods in between.

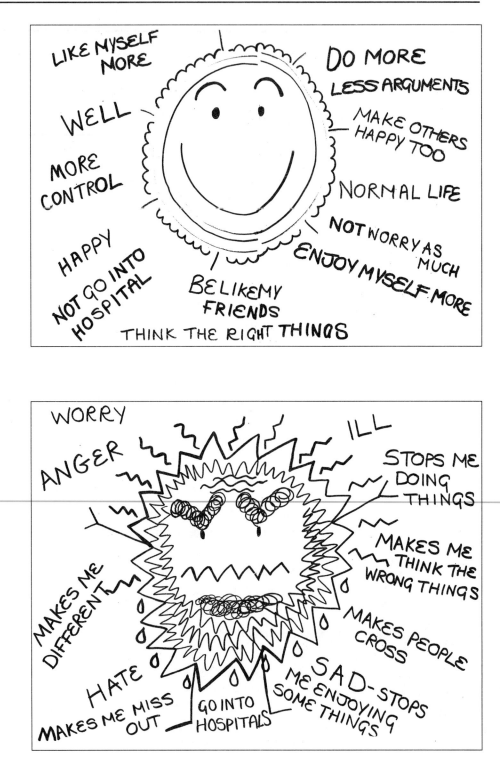

Figure 6.9 One girl's visual image of her anorexia and her healthy side. Reproduced with permission from the artist.

Enhancing self-esteem

Establishing what activities the child is good at, ensuring time is found for them, and giving positive reinforcement is one of the simplest ways to improve self-esteem. As the control of eating is taken away from the child, it is important to find other areas where they do feel in control. For example, organising and decorating their bedroom in whatever way they wish (see chapter 2 - *Individual work, Improving self-esteem*).

'Growing up work'

Conflicts surrounding adolescence are considered central to the development of anorexia nervosa (Crisp, 1983). The struggle for autonomy and identity may seem overwhelming and the adolescent regresses to a safer, 'younger age'. Where there have been adverse sexual experiences, there will obviously be concerns around developing sexuality. 'Growing up work' can help to address such conflicts and concerns (see Chapter 10 – *Individual work, 'Growing up work'*).

Education

The nurse, together with a dietician, should teach the child about healthy eating and the dangers of vomiting and laxative abuse. Helping the young person to identify factors that led to fasting, bingeing or vomiting and laxative abuse may enable coping strategies to be found. For example, eating small frequent meals may reduce the craving to binge.

INDIVIDUAL PSYCHOANALYTICAL PSYCHOTHERAPY

Rather than face anxieties present in interpersonal relations, the child turns to omnipotent control. By not eating and controlling his or her weight, the child can feel strong and less vulnerable. Individual psychotherapy can enable the child to begin to express his or her anxieties, and then start taking some responsibility for ensuring that his or her needs are met. Initially, the child projects all emotional pain on to the therapist, before being able to feel, and later verbalise, her/his own experience. Fasting has become a way of communication and only when another medium is found can the child resume eating (Magagna, 1993).

GROUP WORK AND MILIEU THERAPY

An inability to verbalise feelings and strong denial will result in the anorectic patient using immature defence mechanisms, such as splitting and projective identification (Ehle, 1992). Parents, nurses and other professionals will be played off against one another, after the child has classified each as good or bad. One of the hardest, but probably most therapeutic, positions to be placed in by the child is that of the person they hate. It is important that you are able to demonstrate to the child that they are still respected and cared for. You are in a position to teach the child that it is safe to express their most frightening aggressive feelings. By working together with other nurses and parents to counteract splitting, the child can eventually start to assimilate good and bad. This important group work can take place within the therapeutic milieu of an inpatient unit and/or within group psychotherapy.

Body image therapy in a group setting has the advantage of activating peer support. The perceptions of like-minded individuals are probably more important than those of an adult not acutely concerned with body shape. Possible group exercises include :

◆ A volunteer in the group stands in front of a full-length mirror and comments on her/his size, posture and general appearance. Two allocated 'helpers' then give their opinions, before the discussion is broadened to the whole group. Generally the perceptions of others will be closer to reality.

◆ The exercise above may also be done using pre-recorded filming of the child. Video may be less threatening, as it is slightly removed from the here and now.

◆ Group relaxation may help to couple body awareness with a feeling of ease (see Chapter 4 – *Individual work, Relaxation*).

SOCIAL SKILLS TRAINING

The child's ability to assert her/himself rather than withdraw from conflictual situations seems to be an important factor in determining a positive outcome to treatment. Social skills training can be used to teach assertiveness and improve self-confidence. It is probably most easily organised by nurses on an inpatient psychiatric unit but could be a valuable area for school nurses to embark on. Role-playing non-threatening situations, such as returning faulty goods to a shop, can lead on to more pertinent issues, such as dealing with bullying or complaining to a parent about not being heard. Issues around sexuality can also be addressed in social skills training (see Chapter 10 – *Group work, 'Growing-up work'*).

FAMILY THERAPY

Family therapy has been shown to be effective in treating children and adolescents with anorexia and bulimia nervosa (Russell et al, 1987). Important areas to focus on include enhancing the quality of parenting, improving family communication, and linking relevant aspects of family history that may be maintaining the illness (Lask, 1993). One of the most crucial tasks of the family therapist is to help the parents to work together and take control of the situation, while understanding their child's anxieties about eating. If the child's anxieties about eating control the parents, the child will lose weight.

Complex issues relating to culture may need to be addressed. Timimi and Adams (1996) broadly explore some of the problems faced by British–Asian children and adolescents. The notion of a 'culture clash' between the parents' culture and the adolescent culture to which their children are exposed has been cited as a significant factor in the development of eating disorders. However, professionals must guard against cultural stereotyping, which may lead to an impasse in treatment.

Bushra, a 14-year-old girl, was admitted to the psychiatric unit with anorexia nervosa. Her parents had come to Britain when Bushra was 18 months old. Father had a strong need for his family to retain its cultural identity, to the point where he had said he would die prematurely if his children strayed too far from their cultural roots. Bushra's behaviour clearly challenged this: she cut her hair, refused to speak Punjabi and ceased to wear traditional dress. A white female doctor started family therapy. In sessions, the father appeared bored, edgy or angry. In team meetings, staff (who were all white) discussed cultural issues, which invariably led to culturally stereotypical ideas – difficulties in expressing feelings and a tendency to somatise, subservience of women, and so on. Eventually, the therapist and team felt that father was becoming increasingly isolated within the family and that family therapy was not helpful. Timimi and Adams highlight the possible fantasies behind this unsuccessful intervention. The suspicions within the father, relating to the therapist and institution, stealing the soul from his daughter, and the immediate conclusions drawn by the therapist and team, resulting in the therapist identifying with Bushra and consequently confirming the father's fears. In this instance, cultural stereotyping served only to distance the participants in family therapy.

PARENTAL COUNSELLING

It appears that children with anorexia nervosa fare better if parents work together, rather than against each other. This is the clinical impression of many professionals working in this field. Parental counselling on child management issues seems to be as effective as family therapy.

SCHOOL

Children with anorexia nervosa are generally perceived as successful pupils by their school teachers, being diligent in their work and often high achieving. However, using different measures of success, these young people are frequently observed to be isolated from their peers and miserable (Tate, 1993). The child's denial of illness and obsessional pursuit of perfection result in special educational needs. Finding activities to help raise self-esteem, encouraging peer relationships and diverting the child from compulsive working will be important.

Children with pervasive refusal syndrome will refuse to engage in school activities along with every other area of functioning. Those with food-avoidant emotional disorder may experience school phobia. Both groups of children will require a gradual re-introduction into school.

SELF-HELP

The Eating Disorders Association is a registered charity which has a register of local support groups and publishes a newsletter called *Signpost* for sufferers and their families.

Eating Disorders Association
Sackville Place
44–48 Magdalen Street
Norwich
Norfolk NR3 1JE

A number of self-help books have been published which can be used by the patient alone or with nurse supervision (e.g. Fairburn 1995; Schmidt and Treasure, 1995).

CHILDREN AND ADOLESCENTS EATING EXCESSIVELY

Eating excessively is an important factor in the development of obesity, together with genetic predisposition, metabolic disturbance and environmental influences. There is unlikely to be a single cause of obesity and, indeed, each contributing element can be seen as interlinked. A genetic disposition and some metabolic disturbance or environmental influence may result in increased food intake, and abnormal eating patterns may produce a secondary metabolic derangement (Figure 6.10).

Obesity is an 'abnormal generalised increase in the size of the adipose organ' (Taitz, 1983, p. 1). It is usually diagnosed in any individual whose weight for height exceeds 120%. In children, it is essential that weight is measured against standards for height and age. Tanner–Whitehouse norms are used in Britain. However, diagnosis is somewhat arbitrary, because standard centiles will be shifted upwards with improved living conditions or social class, different ethnic groups probably require different standards, and it is unclear at what point being overweight will cause ill-health. Obesity may cause cardiovascular disease, respiratory, orthopaedic and skin problems, diabetes mellitus and severe psychosocial problems. Given these serious consequences, diagnosis and treatment must surely be imperative. However, focusing on the need for weight loss can result in self-loathing and feelings of failure if dieting is unsuccessful. The advantages and disadvantages of treatment must therefore be considered before embarking on a vigorous attempt to cure obesity.

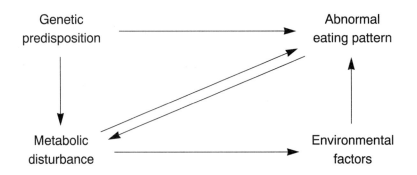

Figure 6.10 Factors that interact in the development of obesity. Reproduced from Taitz, L.S. (1983) *The obese child.* Blackwell Scientific Publications, Oxford, p.32, with permission.

ASSESSMENT – CHILDREN AND ADOLESCENTS EATING EXCESSIVELY

PHYSICAL ASSESSMENT

The diagnosis of obesity can essentially be made by observation during a physical examination. However, measurement of weight, height and skinfold thickness enables the doctor to determine the extent of excess weight and body fat. A child whose weight is 20% or more above the mean for sex and height is considered obese. Skinfold thickness provides a more direct measure of body fat and is a useful adjunct to height and weight, particularly with certain children, such as those who are short and very muscular.

Physical assessment will also include the identification of endocrine or genetic disorders that may be underlying the obesity, although in children these account for less than 10% (Williams et al, 1993), and the establishment of any physical damage caused by the obesity. Obesity will increase the risk of respiratory infection, particularly in infants, because the pressure of excess adipose tissue compromises respiratory function. Some children will develop 'obesity–hypoventilation syndrome' (pickwickian syndrome), although this is a rare complication in young people. However, all obese children are likely to hypoventilate to some degree and suffer hypoxaemia. Some of those with obesity–hypoventilation syndrome will develop upper airway obstruction, as the mechanical effect of obesity in the head and neck produces a backward projection of the tongue, occluding the oropharynx and resulting in periodic apnoea. These respiratory complications may interact with circulatory problems, including hypervolaemia and increased cardiac output. Obese children may have a raised blood cholesterol level and hypertension, both of which are risk factors for developing premature cardiovascular disease. Unlike adults, diabetes mellitus is a rare sequelae of obesity in childhood. However, raised fasting blood glucose and insulin levels are common in adolescents. Pancreatitis, a rare disease of childhood, is more common in obese pubertal girls and may lead to diabetes mellitus and malabsorption. Skin folds in obese children may result in skin infections, such as intertrigo and monilial dermatitis. Striae are common, as elastic fibres are stretched and broken. Finally, orthopaedic problems may result from the weight exerted on joints. Perthes' disease and genu valgum are possible sequelae, and adolescent boys may develop slipped femoral epiphysis with coxa vara (Taitz, 1983; Williams et al, 1993).

INDIVIDUAL ASSESSMENT

Depending on the age of the child, the individual assessment may be done with the parent(s) present or talking to the young person on their own. Areas to be considered should include:

✦ *Diet* It is obviously important to establish the eating habits of the child, including diet content and pattern of intake over 24 hours, the child's knowledge of the nutritional value of food and the cues to eat that the child responds to, such as appetite, boredom, sadness, and so on. It is probably helpful to ask the parent or child to keep a diary of food intake, including a record of the cues to eat. On an inpatient setting, nurses should also complete a food intake chart and observe and record the child's eating behaviour.

✦ *Exercise* The child or parents could be asked to keep a record of physical activity over the course of a week or asked questions regarding physical education at school, outside school activities and interests, mode of transport to school, and so on.

✦ *Cigarette smoking* Due to the increased risk of chest infection and premature development of cardiovascular disease in the obese, it is important to establish whether the young person is smoking and therefore putting themselves in greater danger of developing such complications.

✦ *Self-esteem* Society in the Western world has a very negative view of obesity. Fat people have been characterised as being greedy, lazy, stupid and dirty. Even pre-school children have been shown to dislike others who are obese. There is also evidence that discrimination exists in education and employment (Taitz, 1983; Williams et al, 1993). It is not surprising, therefore, that those who are obese will often have low self-esteem. Children, lacking inhibition, can be particularly cruel to their peers, teasing and excluding them from games. Asking the child what they are good at, who their friends are and whether they ever feel sad, should begin to help establish a picture of their self-image. It is also important to look for signs of depression, as there appears to be an increased incidence amongst obese children (Wallace et al, 1993) (see Chapter 2 – *Introduction* for signs of depression).

✦ *Body image* During adolescence obese individuals are likely to focus on their body size, regarding it as grotesque and loathsome. Some studies suggest that obese individuals overestimate their body size, whereas others suggest that they underestimate their size (Taitz, 1983; Bell et al, 1986). A silhouette chart could be used in a similar way to body image assessment in anorexia nervosa (see *Individual assessment, body-image* above).

INDIVIDUAL PSYCHOTHERAPY ASSESSMENT

An assessment with a psychoanalytical psychotherapist may reveal an underlying meaning or purpose for the development of obesity. In a similar way to anorexia nervosa, aggressive feelings may be turned inwards because the child does not have a method of solving conflicts in inter-personal situations. This results in self-destructive behaviour which, in the case of obesity, means overeating. Alternatively, eating may provide comfort to blot out anxieties or be a substitute for love and affection. This may occur when, as an infant, the feeding relationship between mother and child dominated over other parent–child relationships (Taitz, 1983). Developing a thick layer of fat may also provide protection against a hostile world.

Nesta, aged 13, had been sexually abused by her step-father. He had also shown violence towards Nesta's mother. Her mother was child-like, having had a deprived childhood herself, and looked to Nesta for friendship. During the course of Nesta's admission to the psychiatric unit, it became evident that she sought comfort in food and felt 'safe' behind her layer of fat. The feeling of security that it gave her was not only psychological, but also physical. In her eyes, it made her less attractive and certainly made her a heavy force to be reckoned with.

FAMILY ASSESSMENT

Areas to be considered when meeting the family include:

✦ *Prevalence of obesity* There is a familial tendency in obesity, which is likely because of genetic and environmental factors. An obese child whose parents are both obese is likely to remain so, unless treated. The relationship between social class, ethnic group and obesity is complex. Although low socio-economic class tends to lead to undernutrition, the increased likelihood of bottle feeding in infancy and the early introduction of solids, together with the attitude that fatness correlates with affluence and good health, can lead to an increased prevalence of obesity. Urbanisation is associated with an increase in obesity, due to rising income, changing diet and more sedentary occupations. Immigration from poor rural communities into industrialised cities might therefore be expected to produce an increased prevalence of obesity (Taitz, 1983; Kumanyika, 1993). It is important to establish the family attitudes to eating and body size.

✦ *Nutritional knowledge* Poor parental knowledge about nutrition is linked with the development of obesity in the child (Blank Sherman et al, 1992). A lack of structure to eating patterns and a high intake of 'junk' foods typically contributes to obesity.

✦ *Family functioning* Parental neglect during childhood is related to an increased risk of obesity during young adulthood (Lissau and Sorensen, 1994). Therefore, it is important to observe for signs of neglect, such as poor parental support (either a lack of support or over-protectiveness) and poor hygiene. Viewing obesity as a psychosomatic disorder, it is probably helpful to consider Minuchin's model for the psychosomatogenic family (Minuchin, 1974). The family is characterised by enmeshment, over-protectiveness, rigidity and a lack of conflict resolution. It is easier to eat and seen as potentially less destructive to the family, than dealing with areas of family conflict.

A home visit is always a useful adjunct to meeting the family in a clinic or hospital setting. It will provide clues regarding family lifestyle and functioning (see Appendix A).

SCHOOL ASSESSMENT

Visiting the child's school will provide useful information regarding academic achievement, school attendance and psychosocial adjustment. Teachers will hopefully be aware of any difficulties the obese child is experiencing, for example in physical education or bullying (see Appendix B).

NURSING/MULTI-DISCIPLINARY MANAGEMENT – CHILDREN AND ADOLESCENTS EATING EXCESSIVELY

ESTABLISHMENT OF A HEALTHY WEIGHT

Diet

A high-fibre diet will promote health and help to satisfy appetite. If the child is in a period of rapid growth, such as the young baby or pubertal adolescent, help should be given to maintain weight rather than reduce it. As the child grows in length, they will become slimmer. This gradual weight reduction is preferable. After the second year of life until puberty, and after the adolescent growth spurt, excessive weight gain will require a reduction in energy intake. Limitation of sweets and high-calorie snacks may be all that is necessary. In more serious cases of obesity, a calorie-controlled diet will be required. A diet sheet should be drawn up in consultation with the dietician. A 10-year-old may lose weight on a diet of 1500 kcal, whereas a teenager may lose weight on as much as 2500 kcal. It is better to bring down the energy intake gradually until there is a loss of about 500 g a week (Stark, 1990; Williams et al, 1993). Small, frequent meals may help to satisfy cravings (See Figure 6.11).

Improving nutritional knowledge

Education on healthy eating will obviously need to include parents, as they are likely to buy the family food and do most of the cooking. The dietician should be able to provide useful, easy to read literature and answer any questions the parents or child might have. In a clinic in Belgium, a game is used to teach children just how much 'healthy' food can be eaten compared with 'junk', using sections of pie charts. A similar game has been created by the author (Figure 6.12). Nurses or parents could take children shopping to reinforce what has been learnt. Pazzaglia et al (1993) have highlighted the high incidence of stereotypical food-related behaviour that seems to occur in films, such as healthier diets being eaten by those of higher socio-economic class and fat people eating large quantities of unhealthy food. Adolescents may enjoy discussing the content and style of food scenes in films.

Exercise

Weight reduction is usually most successful when diet is combined with exercise. Calorie restriction reduces the basal metabolic rate, making it harder actually to lose weight, and can produce a loss of lean body mass when there is limited physical activity. Exercise also has the added benefit of reducing appetite (Williams et al, 1993; Beumont et al, 1994). It is important to find ways of exercising that the child will enjoy. Some obese children may be embarrassed going to busy public swimming pools, but it may be possible to find a time when there are fewer people around. It is also a good idea to find ways of increasing the amount of physical activity that the child can assimilate into their normal day routine, such as walking to school instead of catching the bus, encouraging them to play outside after school instead of watching television, and so on. Children

---

Figure 6.11 Example of a diet sheet to produce weight loss.

On waking
A glass of water

Breakfast
A bowl of cereal with semi-skimmed milk
A slice of toast with low-fat spread and sugar-free fruit spread
A glass of fresh orange juice

Mid-morning
A glass of cordial
A piece of fruit

Lunch
A portion of lean meat or a low-fat vegetarian alternative
A portion of potato, rice or pasta (no added fat)
A portion of vegetable
A piece of fruit or a very low-fat yogurt
A glass of water

Mid-afternoon
A glass of cordial
A piece of fruit

Supper
As lunch

---

who are severely overweight need to have their level of exercise increased gradually, so that their circulatory and respiratory systems are not put under too great a strain.

Finding alternatives for comfort

Many obese individuals eat to relieve sadness, anger or boredom. Giving food on these occasions reinforces this behaviour. We need to help children identify when they need comfort and teach them to find alternative ways to receive it. Initially, this will require the nurse to be alert to the signs of sadness, anger or boredom, to comment on this observation to the child and find ways of helping the child gain some relief. Talking with the child, putting an arm around them, providing the opportunity for an 'angry time' (a special time and place to vent angry feelings) are possible alternatives to eating (see Chapter 3 – *Individual work,* possible channels for venting angry feelings).

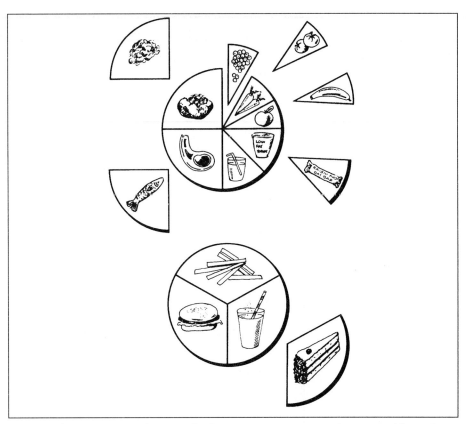

Figure 6.12 Game to make a meal. The segments correspond very roughly to the calorific value of the food; less healthy foods taking up a third of a meal and healthy meals accomodating a source of protein and carbohydrate, some low fat food/drinks and plenty of fruit and vegetables.

Behavioural approaches

There is a danger in rewarding weight loss, because the child is likely to experience periods of 'failure' (no weight loss or weight gain) and, because self-esteem is likely to be low already, their self-image could be damaged further. However, praising the child when they have achieved some weight loss, but not making a big issue when, one week, there is no loss or a slight gain, will probably boost motivation. Buying new clothes as weight is lost may be a good incentive for the fashion-conscious teenager. Incentive charts are best used for non-eating activities, such as exercise (see Chapter 7 – *Points to remember when using incentive charts and rewards*).

Cognitive approaches

Cognitive work may help the young person to feel more in control of their eating behaviour and can be an enjoyable form of individual work. The child might be asked to imagine a difficult food-related situation, such as walking into a newsagent's shop and being faced with a wall of tempting sweets. Teaching the young person to use 'thought-stopping' and relaxation may be helpful. The child, when faced with the sweets in their imagination, says 'STOP' to themselves, or has some other special word that is individual to them, and imagines removing themselves from the tempting situation. Relaxation techniques may be taught to facilitate this process (see Chapter 4 –*Individual work, Relaxation*). At a later stage, this work could be put into practice.

Self-help groups

Groups such as Weight-watchers, which are run all over the country, can provide invaluable support, particularly in helping weight loss to be maintained.

INDIVIDUAL WORK

In addition to health education and cognitive work, the nurse can play an important part in helping to raise the child's self-esteem (see Chapter 2 – *Individual work, Improving self-esteem*). Additional exercises specific to the obese child include:

◆ Reframing situations that the child brings to you, such as the time another child told them to go away – perhaps that other child just wanted to be alone.

◆ Role-play bullying situations to help the young person learn coping strategies.

◆ Some body image work used for children refusing to eat (see above – *Middle childhood to teens*) could also be used for the obese child.

◆ Helping the young person to find people who he or she can turn to when tempted to turn to food.

INDIVIDUAL PSYCHOANALYTICAL PSYCHOTHERAPY

Unfortunately, there is little evidence to support the effectiveness of individual psychoanalytic psychotherapy in the treatment of obesity. However, psychotherapy may be able to help the child to find alternative ways of dealing with anxieties, rather than turning to food. An assessment by a psychotherapist should establish whether a particular child is able to make effective use of psychotherapy.

GROUP WORK

Group work on an outpatient or inpatient basis can incorporate goals related to weight loss and improving self-esteem. Blank Sherman and co-workers (1992) described a series of nine group sessions with schoolchildren, which covered topics related to health and self-esteem. Boys and girls were separated to limit embarrassment. Each session involved three main components: a compliment activity, the main topic and a physical activity. Perhaps an additional component could be finishing the group with relaxation and massage. Massage can relieve tension and help the child to feel better about their body. The hands or feet could be massaged with a pleasant foot lotion or shoulders massaged through light clothing. Staff offering massage must accept that some children may not feel comfortable with this physical contact and should not persuade a child otherwise. Possibly as their confidence and self-esteem improves, they may feel differently.

FAMILY THERAPY

Flodmark and colleagues (1993) have demonstrated the effectiveness of family therapy in the treatment of obesity. The approach to family therapy used in this study was based on Minuchin's proposal of how to treat psychosomatic families and de Shazer's brief solution-based therapy. Interventions focused on family structure, addressing confusions in family hierarchy, blurring of boundaries, the existence of rigid or pathological coalitions, and helping the family to find solutions using their present strengths. This solution-based approach seemed to facilitate change, perhaps because it reduced the family's feelings of guilt, by not dwelling on past or present 'failures'.

SCHOOL

As with all children who are experiencing psychosocial problems, it is important to consider whether their schooling is appropriate. A child who is severely incapacitated by obesity may benefit from being in a school that can provide for their special needs. A vast school where there are many staircases or considerable distances to walk between classes is likely to put the severely obese child under immense physical strain and lay them open to ridicule. Understandably school refusal is likely to ensue.

CONCLUSION

The act of eating has enormous cultural and emotional significance. Therefore, it is perhaps not surprising that mental health problems may present themselves primarily as problems concerned with eating.

Essentially, the young child who has problems with eating is likely to respond to a straightforward behavioural approach. Parental training and support will be an integral part of this treatment. Where family dynamics are contributing to the child's eating behaviour, family therapy may be appropriate and if the mother is suffering post-natal depression, she may benefit from individual therapy.

Older children and adolescents who present with anorexia nervosa and related eating disorders require a more psychodynamic approach. The aetiology is likely to be complex and the problem more persistent. An eclectic multi-disciplinary approach will be essential.

One of the key points for the nurse to remember is that these children are so desperate to control their weight, they will go to great lengths, often secretly, to avoid food or expel it from their bodies. Nursing staff must assume that children with anorexia nervosa and related disorders will induce vomiting, take laxatives, exercise fanatically, and hide or discard food. By doing so, nurses can take the appropriate action to ensure that the child is well cared for. It is also important to remember that this secretive behaviour is a part of the illness, rather than part of a naturally devious personality.

A further aspect of nursing these children that can be difficult is their tendency to split staff, perhaps seeing one of their key nurses as 'bad' and the other as 'good'. It is important to understand that splitting is a defence mechanism and not actually a personal show of admiration or attack on the staff concerned. The young person feels confused by the mixed feelings that they quite naturally hold for their parents and/or significant others, and manages this by project-ing 'good' and 'bad' feelings on to different people. They are quite likely to see one parent as 'good' and the other as 'bad'. The 'bad' feelings are the ones that cause the child most concern, and so they tend to be projected on to someone who the child believes can 'hold' them, some-one who will not crumble. It is important that the nurse who is being subjected to the child's anger and feelings of hatred can demonstrate that they can remain strong. In this way, the young person can learn that it is all right to have and express negative feelings; they will not destroy the subject to whom they are felt. Raising the young person's self-esteem will be crucial if weight restoration is to be maintained. The child must feel that they are worth taking notice of and find alternative ways of communicating their distress.

In working with obesity, the nurse must be aware of her or his own misconceptions and prejudices concerning fatness. The child is likely to have poor self-esteem and the nurse will be in a better position to help, having previously discussed and worked through her or his own attitudes and feelings in clinical supervision.

Generally, a healthy diet and exercise is all that is required to help a growing young person to lose weight. It is necessary to start with a low level of exercise, perhaps taking the child for short walks, to safeguard their health.

Just as children who are trying to lose weight will go to great lengths to achieve their goal secretly, the obese child may secretly help themselves to food and eat in private. Food has become an important crutch and this behaviour, which could be seen as unpleasantly devious, is a part of the child's problem. A firm, but understanding, stance should be taken.

REFERENCES

American Psychiatric Association (1992) *Practice Guideline for Eating Disorders*. Washington, DC: American Psychiatric Press.

Bell C, Kirkpatrick SW and Rinn RC (1986) Body image of anorexic, obese and normal females. *Journal of Clinical Psychology* **42(3)**: 431–439.

Berwick DM, Levy JC and Kleinerman R (1982) Failure to thrive: diagnostic yield of hospitalisation. *Archives of Disease in Childhood* **57**: 347–351.

Beumont PJV, Arthur B, Russell JD and Touyz SW (1994) Excessive physical activity in diet disorder patients: proposals for a supervised exercise programme. *International Journal of Eating Disorders* **15(1)**: 21–36.

Bhadrinath BR (1990) Anorexia nervosa in adolescents of Asian extraction. *British Journal of Psychiatry* **156**: 565–568.

Blank Sherman J, Alexander MA, Gomez D, Miyong K and Marole P (1992) Intervention program for obese school children. *Journal of Community Health Nursing*. **9(3)**: 183–190.

Browning CH (1977) Anorexia nervosa: complications of somatic therapy. *Comprehensive Psychiatry* **18**: 399–403.

Cahill, C (1994) Implementing an inpatient eating disorders program. *Perspectives in Psychiatric Care* **30**: 26–30.

Cash TF (1991) *Body-image Therapy – A Program for Self-directed Change*. New York: Guilford Publications.

Chatoor I and Egan J (1983) Non-organic failure to thrive and dwarfism due to food refusal: a separation disorder. *Journal of the American Academy of Child Psychiatry* **22(3)**: 294–301.

Chatoor I, Conley C and Dickson L (1988) Food refusal after an incident of choking: a post-traumatic eating disorder. *Journal* of the American Academy of Child and Adolescent Psychiatry **27(1)**: 105–110.

Crisp AH (1983) Anorexia nervosa. British Medical Journal **287**: 855–858.

Douglas J (1989) Eating and feeding difficulties. In *Behaviour Problems in Young Children*, pp 67–87. London: Tavistock/Routledge.

Ehle G (1992) Experiences with 'planned' dynamic group psychotherapy of patients with anorexia nervosa. *Group Analysis* **25**: 43–53.

Fairburn C (1995) *Overcoming Binge Eating*. New York: Guilford Press.

Flodmark C–E, Ohlsson T, Ryden O. and Sveger T (1993) Prevention of progression to severe obesity in a group of obese school children treated with family therapy. *Pediatrics* **91(5)**: 880–883.

Fosson A and Wilson J (1987) Family interactions surrounding feedings of infants with non-organic failure to thrive. *Clinical Pediatrics* **26**: 518–523.

Fosson A, Knibbs J, Bryant-Waugh and Lask B (1987) Early onset anorexia nervosa. *Archives of Disease in Childhood* **62**: 114–118.

Frampton I and Wilkinson A (1997) W4H, Great Ormond Street Hospital for Children NHS Trust, London.

Gilbert S (1986) Cultural aspects of eating and body weight. In *Pathology of Eating*, pp 3–10. London: Routledge and Kegan Paul.

Graham P (1991) Feeding and eating disorders. In *Child Psychiatry: A Developmental Approach*, 2nd edn, pp 73–84. Oxford: Oxford University Press

Green WH, Campbell M and David R (1984) Psychosocial dwarfism: a review of the evidence. *Journal of the American Academy of Child Psychiatry* **23(1)**: 39–48.

Hall RCW, Tice L, Beresford TP, Wooley B and Klassen Hall A (1989) Sexual abuse in patients with anorexia nervosa and bulimia. *Psychosomatics* **30(1)**: 73–79.

Hampton D (1993) Tackling feeding problems: a community-based approach. *Health Visitor* **66(11)**: 407–408.

Higgs JF, Goodyer IM and Birch J (1989) Anorexia nervosa and food avoidance emotional disorder. *Archives of Disease in Childhood* **64**: 346–351.

Holden NL and Robinson PH (1988) Anorexia nervosa and bulimia in British blacks. *British Journal of Psychiatry* **152**: 544–549.

Homer C and Ludwig S (1981) Categorization of etiology of

failure to thrive. *American Journal of Diseases in Childhood* **135**: 848–851.

Klein MJ (1990) The home health nurse clinician's role in the prevention of non-organic failure to thrive. *Journal of Pediatric Nursing* **5(2)**: 129–135.

Kumanyika S (1993) Ethnicity and obesity development in children. *Annals of the New York Academy of Sciences* **699**: 81–92.

Lask B (1993) Family therapy. In *Childhood Anorexia Nervosa and Related Eating Disorders*, pp 211–220. Hove: Lawrence Erlbaum Associates.

Lask B and Bryant-Waugh, R. (1993) *Childhood Onset Anorexia Nervosa and Related Eating Disorders*. Hove: Lawrence Erlbaum Associates.

Lask B, Britten C, Kroll L, Magagna J and Tranter M (1991) Children with pervasive refusal. *Archives of Disease in Childhood* **66**: 866–869.

Lissau I and Sorensen TIA (1994) Parental neglect during childhood and increased risk of obesity in young adulthood. *Lancet* **343**: 324–327.

Magagna J (1993) Individual psychodynamic psychotherapy. In *Childhood Anorexia Nervosa and Related Eating Disorders*, pp 191–208. Hove: Lawrence Erlbaum Associates.

Minuchin S (1974) The psychosomatogenic family model. In *Families and Family Therapy*, pp 241–254. London: Tavistock Publications.

Minuchin S Rosman B and Baker L (1978) *Psychosomatic Families: Anorexia Nervosa in Context*. Cambridge, Massachusetts: Harvard University Press.

Nunn P and Thompson SL (1996) The pervasive refusal syndrome: learned helplessness and hopelessness. *Clinical Journal of Child Psychology and Psychiatry* **1(1)**: 121–132.

Oates RM, Peacock A and Forrest D (1985) Long-term effects of non-organic failure to thrive. Pediatrics **75**: 36–40.

Pazzaglia SG, Williams J and Achterberg C (1993) Food and nutrition messages in film. *Annals New York Academy of Sciences* **699**: 295–297.

Ravelli AM, Helps B, Devane S, Lask BD and Milla PJ (1993) Normal gastric antral myoelectrical activity in early onset anorexia nervosa. *Archives of Disease in Childhood* **69**: 342–346.

Robb ND, Smith BGN and Geidrys-Leeper E (1995) The distribution of erosion in the dentitions of patients with eating disorders. *British Dental Journal* **178**: 171–175.

Russell GFM, Szmukler GI, Dare C and Eisler I (1987) An

evaluation of family therapy in anorexia nervosa and bulimia nervosa. *Archives of General Psychiatry* **44**: 1047–1056.

Rutter M (1967) A children's behavioural questionnaire for completion by teachers – preliminary findings. *Journal of Child Psychology and Psychiatry* **8**: 1–11.

Sanders MR, Patel RK, Le Grice B and Shepherd RW (1993) Children with persistent feeding difficulties: An observational analysis of the feeding interactions of problem and non-problem eaters *Health Psychology* **12(1)**: 64–73.

Skuse D (1985) Non-organic failure to thrive: a reappraisal. *Archives of Disease in Childhood* **60**: 173–178.

Skuse DH (1989) Emotional abuse and delay in growth. *British Medical Journal* **299**: 113–115.

Schmidt U and Treasure J (1995) *Getting Better Bit(e) by Bit(e)*. Hove: Lawrence Erlbaum Associates.

Stark, O (1990) Obesity in childhood. *Maternal and Child Health* **15(10)**: 290–293.

Stein A, Woolley H, Cooper SD and Fairburn CG (1994) An observational study of mothers with eating disorders and their infants. *Journal of Child Psychology and Psychiatry* **35(4)**: 733–748.

Taitz LS (1983) *The Obese Child*. Oxford: Blackwell Scientific Publications.

Tate A (1993) Schooling. In Lask B and Bryant-Waugh R (eds) *Childhood Anorexia Nervosa and Related Eating Disorders*, pp 233–248. Hove: Lawrence Erlbaum Associates.

Timimi S and Adams R (1996) Eating disorders in British–Asian children and adolescents. *Clinical Child Psychology and Psychiatry* **1(3)**: 441–456.

Tranter M (1993) Assessment. In Lask B and Bryant-Waugh R (eds) *Childhood Onset Anorexia Nervosa and Related Eating Disorders*, pp 109–126. Hove: Lawrence Erlbaum Associates.

Wallace WJ, Sheslow D and Hassink S (1993) Obesity in children: a risk for depression. *Annals of the New York Academy of Sciences* **699**: 301–303.

Williams CL, Bollello M and Carter BJ (1993) Treatment of childhood obesity in pediatric practice. *Annals of the New York Academy of Sciences* **699**: 207–219.

Wolke D and Skuse D (1992) The management of infant feeding problems. In Cooper PJ and Stein A (eds) *Feeding Problems and Eating Disorders in Children and Adolescents*, pp 27–59. Reading: Harwood Academic Publishers.

Woolston JL (1983) Eating disorders in infancy and early childhood. *Journal of the American Academy of Child Psychiatry* **22(2)**: 114–212.

Yellowlees PM, Roe M, Walker MK and Ben-tovim DI (1988) Abnormal perception of food size in anorexia nervosa. *British Medical Journal* **296**: 1689–1690.

7 PROBLEMS WITH ELIMINATION

INTRODUCTION

Problems with elimination, such as wetting (enuresis) and soiling (encopresis), can have a tremendous impact on the child and family. The child is likely to have a low self-esteem and feel isolated from peers, avoiding certain activities and quite possibly being teased. At home, the parents may develop a negative attitude towards the child but, at the same time, feel responsible and guilty. Their loss of confidence in parenting skills may be exacerbated by outside pressure, from the extended family or school, to stop the child wetting or soiling. There is the practical and financial burden of washing or replacing clothes and linen, and a constant battle to remove unpleasant odours from the home. Tensions are likely to rise in the family, and the child suffers a further blow to self-esteem. Some children may develop behavioural problems (Richman et al, 1982) and some may become the victim of abuse (Pratten and Sluckin, 1985). For these reasons it is imperative that the problem is recognised and treatment offered. Emotional factors may play a part in the aetiology of enuresis and encopresis, and will certainly be a cause for concern once the problem has arisen. Nurses working in hospital or the community, particularly school nurses, have an important role to play in identifying children with enuresis or encopresis and offering appropriate help.

ENURESIS

In the first months of life the bladder empties automatically by reflex and is described as being 'unstable' because the detrusor muscle lining is constantly contracting and relaxing. Gradually these contractions are unconsciously inhibited, allowing the bladder to accommodate an increased volume of urine. Between the age of 1 and 2 years, stretch receptors in the bladder wall start to convey sensory impulses to the brain and the child becomes aware of a full bladder for the first time. At about the age of 3, the child is able consciously to hold on to urine, by tensing muscles in the pelvic floor, and by 4 years can initiate micturition by contracting the detrusor and abdominal muscles and relaxing the external sphincter and perineal muscles.

Enuresis is said to occur when there is **'involuntary discharge of urine by day or night or by both, in a child aged 5 years or older, in the absence of congenital or acquired defects of the nervous system or urinary tract'** (Forsythe and Butler, 1989). The terms 'diurnal' and 'nocturnal' enuresis are used to refer to day-time and night-time wetting, respectively; enuresis is said to be 'primary' where the child has never acquired continence and 'secondary' where there has been a loss of control after a period of continence for at least 12 months, beyond the age of 3 years.

Rutter et al (1973) found that 15% of boys and 12% of girls aged 7 years wet the bed *less than* once a week and that 7% of boys and 3% of girls were wet *at least* once a week. The differences in frequency of wetting amongst the same age group is significant because it influences the proportion of children who are likely to be referred for help. At 14 years of age, 2% of boys and 1% of girls wet the bed less than once a week and 1% of boys and 0.5% of girls were wet at least once a week. Research by Rutter and colleagues therefore suggests that twice as many boys than girls experience nocturnal enuresis. However, in a study by Foxman et al (1986), looking at 5–13 year olds, similar prevalence rates were found amongst boys and girls who wet the bed at least once a week (7% of boys and 6% of girls). Nevertheless, in the group of children who wet the bed at least once in a 3-month period, more boys had problems than girls (16% of boys and 12 % of girls). All studies indicate a higher prevalence of diurnal enuresis amongst girls than amongst boys. Day-time wetting is less common, with only 1–1.1% of girls and 0.3–0.8% of boys aged 4–7 years wetting regularly during the day (Fielding, 1988).

There are many factors that may contribute to the development of enuresis:

◆ Family history of enuresis

◆ Maturational delay

◆ Organic pathology

◆ Poor toilet training

◆ Stressful life events

◆ Emotional disturbance

◆ Family discord

◆ Urinary tract infections

◆ Small functional bladder capacity

◆ Sleep apnoea

◆ Constipation

◆ Abnormal discharge of anti-diuretic hormone

◆ Diet

ASSESSMENT – ENURESIS

The aim of assessment is to identify possible contributing factors to the development of enuresis and to establish a treatment plan which best suits the individual child and family. Meeting with the child and parents and organising a simple medical examination may be all that is required to achieve these aims. However, sometimes it will become apparent that a more in-depth assessment is required. Therefore, it may be appropriate to use all or only part of the following assessment framework.

INTERVIEWING THE PARENTS

Useful areas to cover have been compiled using ideas from questionnaires devised by Blackwell (1989a) and Butler (1987), together with the incorporation of enuresis research findings and clinical experience.

Enuresis and toiletting

◆ Is the child wet in the day and/or at night?

◆ How often is the child wet?

◆ Has the child ever been dry?

> If so, for how long? (i.e. Is the enuresis primary or secondary?)

◆ How independent is the child with regard to toiletting and coping with wet episodes?

> Can the child take him/herself to the toilet?
> Can the child sit him/herself on the toilet unaided?
> Can the child undress and dress him/herself?
> Can the child clean him/herself after going to the toilet?
> What does the child do if they are wet?

◆ How frequently does the child need to go to the toilet? (i.e. How great is their bladder capacity?). Approximately 85% of children have a reduced bladder capacity, which is probably linked to maturational delay (Gandhi, 1994).

◆ Is the child able to 'hold on' or do they have to rush to the toilet? (i.e. Does the child suffer from 'urgency'?). Urgency is sometimes associated with enuresis and refers to the sudden urge to pass urine.

◆ Has anyone else in the family ever suffered from enuresis?

> Mother
> Father
> Sibling(s)
> Bakwin (1971) found that 70% of all night-wetting children had a family history of nocturnal enuresis.

◆ Does the child have any fears associated with the toilet?

Stressful life events

Stressful events that occur during the period when bladder control is usually acquired, that is between the ages of 1 and 4 years, may disrupt this area of development and lead to primary enuresis. Stressful experiences later in life may cause secondary enuresis.

◆ Has the child experienced any stressful events recently or during toilet training? Such as:

> A change of school
> Birth of a new sibling
> Admission to hospital
> Moving home
> Separation from mother
> Death or divorce in family
> Bullying at school

Developmental milestones

◆ When did the child reach other developmental milestones? (i.e. Are they generally a late developer?) Such as:

> When did the child walk?
> Start talking?

Emotional disturbance

There is evidence to suggest that emotional disturbance among enuretic children is 10–15% higher than in non-enuretic children (Schaefer, 1979). This is particularly true of girls and of children who have diurnal enuresis, but there is no specific emotional disorder associated. Enuretic girls are more deviant than non-enuretic girls, but the relationship between enuresis and behavioural problems in boys is less pervasive (Rutter et al, 1973). It is not clear whether emotional disturbance causes enuresis, is a consequence of wetting, or simply co-exists because of similar causative factors.

◆ Do the parents have any other concerns about the child? Such as :

Behavioural problems

Sleeping difficulties

Does the child appear sad or depressed?

Worrying and anxious?

Constipation

Chronic constipation may contribute to the development of enuresis, by causing pressure on the bladder leading to 'frequency' (Blackwell, 1989a). O'Reagan et al (1986) indicated that constipation is a commonly unrecognised cause of enuresis.

Home circumstances

Unsatisfactory housing may play a part in the aetiology of enuresis, through the stress it places on the family and/or a lack of adequate toilet facilities, and may affect the success of treatment. Simple factors in lifestyle can also be important in the cause and effectiveness of treatment.

◆ Do the parents feel happy where they live /that their housing is adequate?

◆ Does the child share a room or bed?

If there are bunk beds, is the child on the top or bottom?

◆ Does the child have easy access to the toilet?

Is there a light on at night?

Is there a footstool for the child to reach the toilet, or a potty available?

◆ What facilities does the family have to wash clothes/linen?

◆ Is there a problem with the smell of urine?

Measures used to overcome the problem

◆ Has there been any professional help?

If so, was any of it successful?

◆ Have the parents taken any measures themselves? Such as:

Restricting fluids

Using pads or nappies

Lifting (for nocturnal enuresis)

Rewards or punishments

Lifting (taking the child to the toilet at intervals during the night) and restricting fluids were the most widely used methods by mothers, in a study on maternal views of nocturnal enuresis by Butler and Brewin (1986).

Effect of enuresis on the child

✦ Has it stopped him/her from staying overnight with friends or participating in certain activities, such as school trips?

✦ Does the child seem upset when he/she is wet?

✦ Has the child become more withdrawn or lacking in self-confidence?

In the study by Foxman et al (1986), more than half the children with enuresis were perceived as being distressed by their wetting, one-third a 'great deal'.

Parents' attitudes to enuresis

✦ How concerned are the parents about the wetting? Two-thirds of parents in the study by Foxman et al (1986) were worried about their child's wetting.

✦ What do the parents consider is the cause for the enuresis?

The child is a deep sleeper (where enuresis is nocturnal).

The child is not bothered about being dry.

There is a developmental reason or organic cause.

The child is a 'worrier'.

The child drinks too much.

These beliefs have all been found amongst mothers of enuretic children, with deep sleep being the most firmly held view (Butler and Brewin, 1986). However, there is no evidence that deep sleep causes enuresis and, indeed, wetting can occur at any stage of sleep (Mikkelsen and Rapaport, 1980).

✦ How has the problem affected the parents? For example:

Do they feel irritated or angry with the child?

How do they feel about taking the child out? (They may find it difficult practically and/or embarrassing.)

What is it like coping with the washing of clothes/linen?

Diet

Some food and drinks contain substances that have a diuretic effect and may contribute to enuresis (Blackwell, 1989a). Egger et al (1992) have identified an extensive list of foods that may provoke enuresis, including carbonated drinks, milk products, chocolate and citrus fruits.

♦ Have the parents noticed whether any foods or drinks are associated with their child's wetting?

♦ Does the child eat a lot of chocolate or drink tea, coffee or fizzy drinks in excess?

BASELINE RECORDING

This should be done by parents, or nursing staff if the child is hospitalised, involving the child. An older child or teenager may wish to make their own recording but, from clinical experience, young people often appreciate parental/adult help and support. It may be necessary to ask a teacher or welfare assistant to complete, or supervise the completion of, a diurnal enuresis chart if the child is at school. A baseline recording should be made for 1–2 weeks.

Drawing up an assessment chart

The chart should be drawn up to fit the individual child:

♦ Recording of diurnal enuresis will involve the child going to the toilet at regular intervals in the day to assess the extent of wetting. It is helpful to fit these times around the child's normal routine (Figure 7.1).

♦ A child who is experiencing 'frequency' and 'urgency' will need to go to the toilet more regularly, perhaps hourly (Figure 7.2).

♦ Night-time wetting is simply recorded in the morning. The child should not be 'lifted' during the assessment (Figure 7.3).

MEDICAL HISTORY AND EXAMINATION

It is important to exclude any physical cause for enuresis. These include urinary tract infections, congenital abnormalities such as hypospadias, obstructive uropathy and defects of the neurological system. Urinary tract infections (UTIs) are fairly common: 5% of girls and 2.5% of boys will suffer from a UTI at some time. However, it is generally thought that enuresis causes UTIs rather than vice versa. Organic pathology affecting micturition is rare (Blackwell, 1989a).

♦ The child should be asked whether he/she is experiencing any symptoms that would suggest a UTI, such as dysuria.

♦ A mid-stream urine specimen should also be sent to the laboratory to exclude infection.

♦ A doctor must take a medical history from the parents and examine the child. If there are signs of organic pathology, further investigations will be organised. Parents may report that the child has irregular breathing or snores at night, suggesting sleep apnoea. Weider and Hauri (1985) have demonstrated a link between sleep apnoea, caused by obstruction of the airway by tonsils or adenoids, and nocturnal enuresis.

	On Waking	After break-fast	Before first lesson at school	Break-time	Before lunch	Before after-noon lessons	Before leaving school	Before tea	After tea	Before bed	Other times when Susan asks to go to the toilet (indicate time)		
Monday	WET	DRY	WET	WET	DRY	DRY	WET	DRY	DRY	DRY	8.00 P.M WET		
Tuesday	WET	WET	WET	DRY	DRY								
Wednesday													
Thursday													
Friday													
Saturday													
Sunday													

Write 'wet' or 'dry' as appropriate

Figure 7.1 Example of a baseline record chart for diurnal enuresis.

	7.00 a.m.	8.00	9.00	10.00	11.00	12.00	1.00 p.m.	2.00	3.00	4.00	5.00	6.00	7.00	8.00	9.00
Monday	WET	DRY	DRY	WET	WET	DRY	WET								
Tuesday															
Wednesday															
Thursday															
Friday															
Saturday															
Sunday															

Write 'wet' or 'dry' as appropriate

Figure 7.2 Baseline record chart for a child experiencing 'frequency' and 'urgency'.

	Monday	Tuesday	Wednesday	Thursday	Friday	Saturday	Sunday
DRY	✓			✓			
WET		✓	✓				

Tick in the morning as appropriate

Figure 7.3 Baseline record for nocturnal enuresis.

INTERVIEWING THE CHILD

The following ideas for questions have been taken from Butler (1987):

◆ Why does the child think he/she is meeting you?

◆ Who is most worried about the child's wetting?

Children may find it easier to express their feelings through drawing. Suggestions for pictures could include:

◆ A picture of him/herself waking up with a *wet* bed (nocturnal enuresis).

◆ A picture of him/herself waking up with a *dry* bed (nocturnal enuresis).

◆ A picture of him/herself discovering that he/she is *wet* during the day (diurnal enuresis).

◆ A picture of him/herself discovering that he/she is *dry* during the day (diurnal enuresis).

Notice the emotions that are portrayed and whether the child draws him/herself alone or involves others in the picture (Figure 7.4).

◆ Ask the child to name three bad things about wetting

◆ One good thing about wetting

◆ Three good things about being dry

◆ One bad thing about being dry

Some children see wetting as interfering with many aspects of their life. Enuresis may prevent a child from staying the night at a friend's house or even going out with peers. It may result in uncomfortable and embarrassing rashes between the legs and can mean the young person spends much of their time washing. Wetting might make parents angry or upset and the child is likely to be aware of the burden 'their problem' is putting on the family. However, some children may feel a sense of comfort from wetting, perhaps because of the additional care they receive from parents. It is helpful at this stage to encourage the child to think of the positive consequences of being dry in order to facilitate treatment.

◆ How do the different family members react to the child wetting?

    Mother

    Father

    Sibling(s)

In some families, enuresis is considered an intrinsic part of growing up. Parents may be unaware of the distress that the child is experiencing.

◆ Who knows about the wetting? Many children will try to keep it a secret from friends.

◆ Why does the child think he/she is wet?

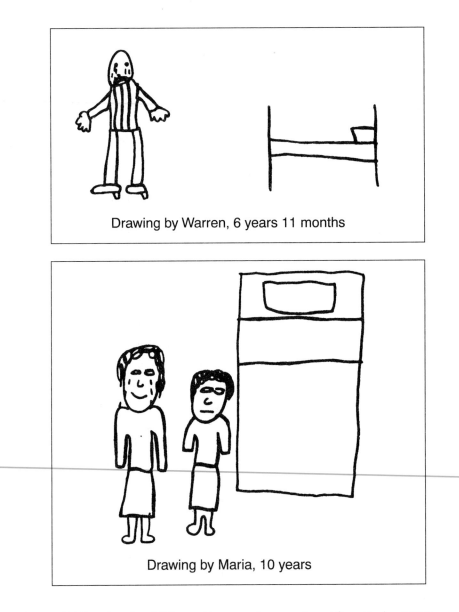

Drawing by Warren, 6 years 11 months

Drawing by Maria, 10 years

Figure 7.4 Drawings by children with enuresis. reproduced from Butler (1983) Nocturnal Enuresis – Psychological Perspectives, with permission from Wright, London.

◆ What attempts has the child made to stop the wetting?

Has anything helped?

Some children may find it very difficult to talk about their enuresis. A useful way to communicate with young children is with puppets. The nurse's puppet is then asking the child's puppet about their wetting. Older children or adolescents may find it reassuring to know how many other young people are suffering from incontinence.

INDIVIDUAL PSYCHOTHERAPY ASSESSMENT

There are various psychodynamic theories suggesting that enuresis is a symptom of an underlying disturbance, but little concrete evidence to support them. However, where there is a concern regarding the emotional state of the child or where enuresis is part of a wider mental health problem, an assessment with a psychoanalytical psychotherapist may reveal underlying conflicts within the child's psyche. Psychodynamic theories include:

✦ The child has *aggressive* feelings towards the parent(s) which he/she feels unable to express overtly (Fenichel, 1945).

✦ The child remains at, or *regresses* to, an earlier stage in development, in order to maintain the safe and secure feelings of infancy (Winnicott, 1953).

✦ The child's anxieties and conflicts are not 'contained internally', so they emerge externally as somatic symptoms such as wetting and constipation.

✦ The child *suppresses* a sexual drive, perhaps an older child returning to enuresis as a form of infantile satisfaction and suppressing a desire to masturbate.

FAMILY ASSESSMENT

If the initial interview with one or both parents suggests family discord, or if the child's enuresis is part of a more pervasive emotional problem, it will be important to arrange a family assessment with a family therapist. Issues that may be important include:

✦ Marital problems

✦ Mother–child separation issues, particularly during the 'sensitive period' for bladder control development

✦ Sometimes, enuresis may follow sexual abuse, but in such cases there will be other indicators that elicit concern

HOME VISIT

It may be helpful to visit the child's home, in order to assess the conditions for treatment and to help engage the child and family. Taking note of where the child sleeps, toilet facilities, and washing and drying facilities will be important (see Appendix A – *Home visit*).

SCHOOL VISIT

A school visit will give you a clearer picture of school toilet facilities and make it easier to explain to teachers or welfare assistants how they can help assess the extent of the child's wetting (see Appendix B – *School visit*).

NURSING/MULTI-DISCIPLINARY INTERVENTION – ENURESIS

Following a thorough assessment, a decision regarding therapeutic intervention can be made, which in some cases may be to do very little. If the child is slow in developing bladder control, but this has also been the case in other areas of development, or if a child has recently experienced an acute episode of stress, such as admission to hospital, it is probably advisable not to intervene actively, but to wait and review progress. Where the child is experiencing diurnal and nocturnal enuresis, or other health problems, it is usually better to tackle one area at a time. For example, if the child is obese and suffering from nocturnal enuresis, it may be too much to subject the child to a reducing diet with incentives to lose weight and a behaviour programme to overcome wetting. If there is a decision to treat the enuresis actively, a combination of therapeutic approaches can be planned, based on information derived from assessment.

INCENTIVE CHARTS AND REWARDS

A behaviour programme involving incentive charts and rewards can be effective for both diurnal and nocturnal enuresis. Positively reinforcing dry pants or a dry bed can reduce wetting, not because the child is deliberately wet but because, over a period of time, a change of behaviour is brought about by **operant conditioning**. Incentive charts or rewards can be used on their own or in conjunction with an enuresis alarm.

Points to remember when using incentive charts and rewards

◆ *Type of reward* The decision whether to use an incentive chart or to reward the child in some other way can be made from your knowledge of the child. Older children may prefer to record their progress in a diary and be given rewards, such as staying up later in the evening or having extra pocket money. Incentive charts can also incorporate extra rewards or treats after a certain number of dry episodes, although for some children a special chart is sufficient reward. All rewards must be accompanied by praise and positive attention.

◆ *Incentive charts* Using imagination is the key to producing a truly individual chart. It is a good idea to think of a theme that is appropriate for the child, such as football, and involve him/her in its creation. If possible, have the parents and child create the chart. There is no end to the possibilities of incentive charts; they may involve colouring in, sticking on stars, joining up dots or moving objects (see Plate 6 which appears in the unfolioed section between p56 and 57 and Figure 7.5).

Rebecca, aged 13, who had a problem of diurnal enuresis with frequency, devised a complicated weekly chart on her personal computer, incorporating symbols to represent when she was very wet, wet and damp. The key to her chart was kept in the computer and so, apart from herself, only her mother and I, as therapist, could interpret it. This meant that her progress could be kept private from her brother or friends who might pick up a chart.

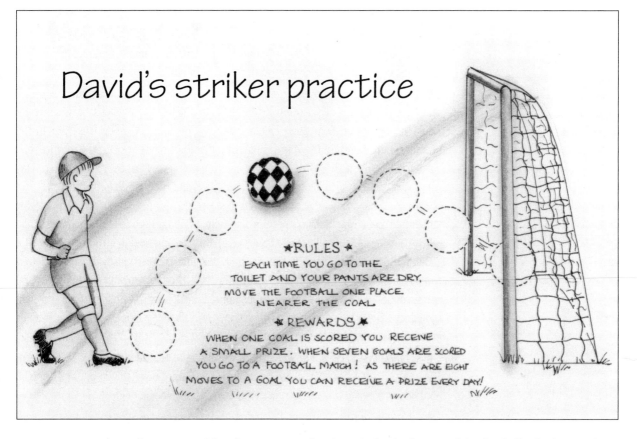

Figure 7.5 David's striker practice. The chart is covered with sticky back plastic and the football, which is card, is held in place with bluetac®.

◆ *Rewards must be achievable* To foster the child's confidence in the programme and to maintain their interest, rewards must be attainable instantly. If a child is wetting their pants at least four times in the day, the behaviour programme should involve at least six visits to the toilet, in order to ensure some visits when the child will be dry and therefore rewarded. With nocturnal enuresis, a reward should be given each morning that the child has been dry. Larger rewards may accompany a number of dry nights.

◆ *Immediacy of rewards* As soon as the child and parent/supervising adult have identified that pants are dry, the reward should be given.

◆ *Consistency of the programme* Continuity and consistency are essential for a behaviour programme to work. This will need particular consideration if more than one adult is involved in supervision, for example on a busy paediatric ward.

◆ *Encouraging visits to the toilet* As well as encouraging dryness, it is important to encourage the child to visit the toilet regularly and attempt to pass urine (see below –

Overcoming fears of the toilet). As well as going at specified times during the day (if diurnal enuresis) and before bed, the child must obviously go to the toilet when they sense a full bladder. It may be an additional help to the programme if passing urine in the toilet or recognising the need to go to the toilet is rewarded.

◆ *Supervision by a parent or adult is essential* Where the child has diurnal enuresis, the adult should generally accompany the child into the toilet to assess visably whether the child is dry or wet. Sometimes children will say they are dry, when it is clear to the contrary, either because they have got accustomed to being wet or because they feel bad about it. The adult should then ask the child to feel his/her pants to check again. This approach will help the child to recognise being wet and reassure them that there will not be a punishment, but some help offered to wash and change. A teenager who is highly motivated to become dry may not need accompanying into the toilet, but could change their pants regardless of being dry or wet and have them checked by an adult outside. The adult must be able to check in some way, so that the reward be justly earned and given immediately after going to the toilet. (If the child cheats, they will not gain from the programme!) Similarly, with nocturnal enuresis, the adult or parent should ask the child whether their bed is dry or wet and then check with them. Again, help should be given to wash, dress and change the bed linen.

◆ *Managing wet clothes/linen* Some provision should be made for wet clothes or linen, perhaps a plastic bag to take to school or a bucket at home. Children should not be involved in washing clothes/linen, as being wet is punishment enough.

◆ *A supply of dry clothes/linen* There must be a ready supply of dry clothes and bed linen, so that the child starts to recognise and enjoy feeling fresh and dry. Where this is difficult for parents, social services may be able to assist with the cost.

◆ *Progress record* A reward system must include a regular review of progress. A progress chart should be kept by the supervising adult, similar to the assessment chart used (see Figures 7.1–7.3). The professional coordinating the child's treatment, such as the school nurse, should meet with the parent(s) and child at least fortnightly to review progress. If there is no progress after 3 weeks, the programme may need to be adjusted, or an alternative treatment offered. A system that is not working will reduce the child's self-esteem still further.

ENURESIS ALARMS

The alarm system consists of a sensor connected to an alarm box. When the sensor is wet, an electrical circuit is completed and the alarm sounds. Two basic varieties are available: (1) the 'mini-alarm', which can be used for diurnal or nocturnal enuresis, has a sensor that is small enough to fit into the paper layers of a pant liner and a small alarm box which attaches to clothes or pyjamas (Figure 7.6); and (2) the 'bell and pad', which can be used only at night, has a large flat sensor which goes under a sheet and an alarm box which is placed next to the bed (Figure 7.7). It is unusual to use an alarm during the day for the obvious reason of causing the child

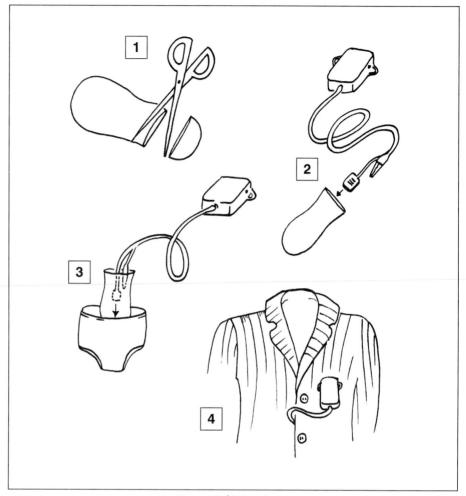

Figure 7.6 Mini-alarm.

embarrassment. 'Alarms' do exist that produce vibration rather than sound, and have been devised for those who are hard of hearing, but could possibly be used during the day.

The enuresis alarm changes behaviour by **operant** and/or **classical conditioning**. The shock or startle of the alarm causes muscular tightening in the pelvic floor which stops the flow of urine until the toilet can be reached. The child may learn to associate the sound of the alarm with a full bladder and gradually becomes aware of the need to micturate before the alarm sounds; a 'conditioned stimulus', that is the alarm, becomes associated with an 'unconditional' one, the full bladder (classical conditioning). Alternatively, or additionally, the child may learn to go to the toilet to avoid the unpleasant sound and be rewarded for dryness (operant conditioning).

Enuresis alarms should be used only if parents can provide the necessary support, which will involve getting up at night in the case of nocturnal enuresis. It is unsuitable for some children, as they may be frightened by the alarm, and cannot be used where children share a bed. Re-organisation of sleeping arrangements at home may overcome some obstacles.

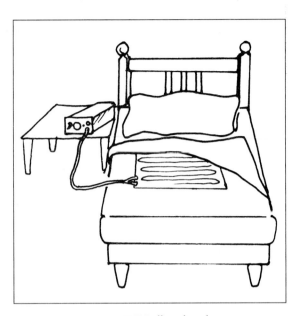

Figure 7.7 Bell and pad.

Points to remember when using an alarm

✦ *Incentive charts or rewards must be used in conjunction with an alarm* A programme involving an incentive chart or another reward system should be set up as above.

✦ *Setting up the alarm* The parent or supervising adult should assist the child in setting up the alarm each time. It is important to ensure that the sensor is thoroughly dry and that the alarm is switched on. Some children and parents may be concerned that the sensor could cause an electric shock; they can be reassured to the contrary. It is helpful to demonstrate the alarm using tap water and allow the child to practise switching it off when it sounds.

✦ *Encouraging visits to the toilet and responding to the alarm* The child should be rewarded for going to the toilet when the alarm sounds, when sensing a full bladder and at specified programme times. Rewarding the child's positive response to the alarm will mean that he/she is having a reward when wet, but initially this may be helpful in establishing the alarm programme. It takes a great deal of motivation to get up in the middle of the night, and this must be recognised in some way.

✦ *Parental or adult supervision* As well as providing the supervision and support required for the reward system (see above), where there is nocturnal enuresis parents will need to get up in the night to help the child wash, change the sheets and re-set the alarm. If the alarm does not wake the parents in another room, a baby call system could be used or the child asked to wake parents. It is very important that the child does not have to cope with getting up at night alone.

✦ *Review progress* Progress should be monitored fortnightly in the same way as reviewing the reward system, but the record chart must also include how frequently the alarm sounds. If the alarm is effective, wetting should stop in 5–10 weeks.

Success rates using alarms for nocturnal enuresis vary from 60% to 80% (Forsythe and Butler, 1989), although some 30–50% of these will relapse, usually within 6 months to 1 year. There have been fewer studies evaluating the effectiveness of alarms with diurnal enuresis.

> Leo, aged 10, had never achieved continence at night. His mother brought him to the clinic, determined to help him overcome the problem. Leo wanted to be able to stay with friends but felt embarrassed. A behaviour programme using an enuretic alarm was set up. Leo's parents took it in turns to get up with Leo at night. In 4 weeks Leo was dry.

> Sam, aged 9, also had primary enuresis. His family lived in poor housing conditions. Sam shared a bedroom with his two brothers, although his younger brother was currently sleeping with the parents, because he was having frequent asthmatic attacks. Sam's older brother was studying for his school exams. The father had heard about enuresis alarms and wanted Sam to try using one. Perhaps predictably, the alarm was not a success. The parents expected Sam to get up on his own at night, because they were preoccupied with caring for his younger brother, and the older brother resented being woken by the alarm.

BLADDER TRAINING

Bladder training may be particularly helpful for children with 'urgency' and 'frequency', but can give any child a greater sense of control in their treatment. Children under 7 years of age may find the techniques difficult to grasp. Holding practice and retention control training have been shown to increase bladder capacity (Harris and Purohit, 1977).

Holding practice and toiletting twice in quick succession

Holding practice is useful for children suffering from diurnal enuresis. If the assessment has revealed that the child is wet most of the specified times in the day and seems to be wet again about 10 minutes after having visited the toilet, holding practice and visiting the toilet twice in quick succession may be helpful (Blackwell, 1989a).

✦ Initially the child should be asked to visit the toilet every hour and to 'hold on' in between. When a week of dryness has been achieved, the length of holding time is increased, perhaps by just 10 minutes.

✦ The 'holding time' should gradually be increased by 20, 40 and then 60 minutes as dryness is achieved each subsequent week, until toilet times can be fitted around the child's daily routine.

◆ This approach should be reinforced positively with an incentive chart or another reward system.

◆ If the child seems to experience a small amount of wetting soon after visiting the toilet, it may be helpful if they void urine twice in succession, perhaps one minute apart.

Retention control training

Retention control exercises are useful for children with diurnal and nocturnal enuresis, those suffering 'urgency' and 'frequency', and children who appear unaware of the need to micturate (Blackwell, 1989a).

◆ Once a day, perhaps straight after school, the child drinks a large volume of fluid (between 500 ml and 1 litre, depending on the child's size).

◆ The child is asked not to void urine, but to 'hold on' for a specified time (1–5 minutes). The time must be managable for the child,

◆ When the timer rings, the child goes to the toilet.

◆ After the child has succeeded in staying dry on three consecutive occasions, the time interval is increased by 1 minute.

◆ It is important that the supervising adult stays with the child throughout, giving encouragement and praise.

Pelvic floor exercises

Pelvic floor exercises can help 'urgency'. However, they may be difficult for a young child.

◆ The child slowly contracts the pelvic floor muscles, starting from the back and slowly moving to the front. Ask the child to pull up their back passage, as if trying to stop their bowels from opening, and then to include the front passage, as if holding on to urine. Ask the child to imagine they have diarrhoea and a desperate urge to pass water, but need to hold on until they reach the toilet. The exercise should be repeated five times.

◆ Repeat the above exercise but with a fast staccato action. Repeat ten times.

◆ Lying on the floor with knees raised, feet on the floor and slightly apart, the child pulls in the stomach muscles so that the arch of the lower back touches the floor. This position is held for a count of 10 and then slowly released.

INDIVIDUAL WORK

Improving self-esteem

Basic education concerning the urinary system and the prevalence of enuresis may help the child to feel more in control and less embarrassed about their problem. A simple diagram can illustrate the internal and external sphincters and perineal muscles (Figure 7.8).

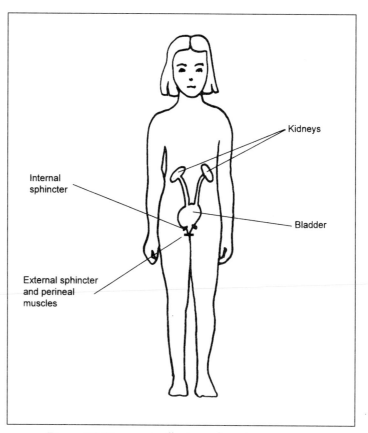

Internal
sphincter

External sphincter
and perineal
muscles

Kidneys

Bladder

Figure 7.8 Diagram to illustrate the urinary system.

Drawing a graph to show the child's progress (Figure 7.9) can boost their confidence in being able to become dry, as their achievement is clearly visible (Blackwell, 1989a).

The child's self-image is likely to be poor and they are likely to be experiencing teasing from peers. There are a number of exercises the nurse can do to help improve self-esteem and confidence (see Chapter 2 – *Individual work, Improving self-esteem*).

Overcoming fears of the toilet

As well as taking time to listen to the child's fears concerning the toilet, a number of practical steps may be taken to overcome them. The child may find it helpful if a light is left on at night for visits to the bathroom, a footstool may be needed for a small child to feel secure sitting on the toilet, or the child may need to be accompanied to the bathroom for a period of time. School toilets are often a distance from the classroom and sometimes in an outside building. Children may have been bullied in the toilets or may just find them cold and uninviting. Liaison with the head teacher may enable such obstacles to be overcome.

If these simple measures do not help to overcome the child's fears, a desensitisation pro-gramme, involving a clinical psychologist, may be necessary. This will involve the child mastering a hierarchy of small steps towards sitting happily on the toilet. The first step might involve

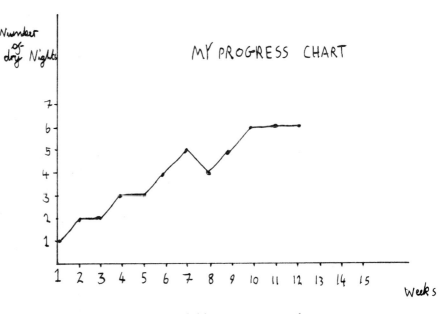

Figure 7.9 A child's own progress chart.

looking at a picture of a toilet, with the aid of relaxation techniques (see Chapter 4 – *Individual work, Desensitisation*).

INDIVIDUAL PSYCHOANALYTICAL PSYCHOTHERAPY

The psychotherapist will advise the multi-disciplinary team on whether she/he considers that individual psychotherapy would be beneficial. There is little evidence that psychotherapy does reduce wetting, although Novick (1966) reported that 20% of 45 children became dry with psychotherapy, essentially aimed at reducing the child's sense of guilt and reducing punitive measures used by the mother.

FAMILY THERAPY

The multi-disciplinary team will need to decide whether family therapy is indicated. Assessment may have revealed family discord which, even if unrelated to the child's enuresis, is likely to influence the effectiveness of treatment.

HYPNOSIS

Hypnosis and self-hypnosis can be effective in treating enuresis. In a study by Banerjee and co-workers (1993), a 72% success rate was demonstrated with nocturnal enuresis after 3 months of hypnosis, and a 68% success rate at the 9-month follow-up, during which time the children had been practising self-hypnosis. In comparison, children treated with imipramine initially demonstrated similar results (76% success rate), but at 9 months' follow-up only 24% were still dry. A therapist qualified in hypnosis must be involved in treatment. If the child has a key nurse involved in their care, she/he could accompany the child in the hypnosis session and then encourage and support the child in self-hypnosis. During the relaxed state of hypnosis, the child is given suggestions of self-control and improved self-image, and may be taken through some guided imagery involving the experience of a full bladder and going to the toilet. The child can be taught how to hypnotise him/herself and instructed to practise daily or twice daily (Waxman, 1991).

DIET

The child's diet helps prevent constipation (see below – *Constipation and encopresis*) and in which foods known to have diuretic properties are taken in moderation.

MEDICATION

Medication may be useful on a short-term basis, perhaps to increase the likelihood of dryness over a holiday period, or to improve the efficacy of a behavioural programme. Two main types of drug may be prescribed: one reduces the amount of urine produced by the kidneys and the other probably increases functional bladder capacity.

Desmopressin, a synthetic analogue of anti-diuretic hormone (ADH), used in doses of 20–40 μg, can reduce urine production for 5–9 hours. It comes in the form of a nasal spray (Desmospray) or alternatively as tablets. There are no known side-effects, although if the dose is too high fluid retention may occur. If the child has damaged nasal mucosa, perhaps from a cold, or a faulty technique is being used in administration, Desmospray will be ineffective (Klauber, 1989; Lyon, 1991). Bradbury and Meadow (1995) have demonstrated the effectiveness of combining the use of an enuresis alarm with desmopressin. They suggest that this approach is particularly useful when enuresis is severe, the child has behavioural problems and/or there are family problems. Behavioural and family problems can reduce the amount of support the child is likely to get and reduce the motivation of both child and parents. Medication may boost their confidence and enthusiasm for a treatment programme.

Trycyclic antidepressants, imipramine or amitriptyline, are thought to reduce bladder instability and increase functional bladder capacity. They can be used for diurnal or nocturnal enuresis. Fritz and colleagues (1994) demonstrated a 73% success rate using imipramine at a dose of 2.5 mg kg^{-1} and reported that side-effects were rare. Possible side-effects with tricyclic antidepressants include irritability, loss of appetite, headaches, loss of concentration and constipation. Amitriptyline is prescribed in a dose of 10–50 mg depending on the weight of the child.

> Atalanta, aged 9, was wet most nights and had never achieved continence. Her mother was busy working from home and her father was often away on business. Atalanta's mother was exasperated with the endless need to wash bedlinen and pessimistic about her daughter ever being dry. Desmospray gave a reprieve in the wetting, which both boosted Atalanta's self-esteem and gave hope to her mother, which in turn enabled a behaviour programme with an incentive chart to be established.

It is important that constipation, which may contribute to the aetiology of enuresis, is treated. This may simply require a change in diet, but may, in more severe cases, need medication. O'Reagan et al (1986) found that treatment of constipation led to a resolution of enuresis.

LIFTING

'Lifting' can be used on a short-term basis for holidays or to boost a child's confidence and motivation to overcome enuresis, because he or she will have the pleasant experience of waking in a dry bed in the morning. The child may be woken every 1–4 hours, depending on how frequently they are wet in the night. If this method is to be used on holiday, a trial should first be done at home to establish the required frequency of visits to the toilet. Long-term use of lifting is not advisable because it can result in the child wetting at the time they were normally lifted and does not teach the child how to recognise a full bladder.

NATIONAL SUPPORT GROUP

The Enuresis Resource and Information Centre produces a newsletter for parents and children entitled *ERIC says...*

ERIC
65 St Michael's Hill
Bristol BS2 8DZ

CONSTIPATION AND ENCOPRESIS

In the infant defaecation occurs by reflex. As the rectum fills, nerve endings are stimulated and the internal and external anal sphincters relax. However, once the nervous system is fully developed, the external sphincter comes under voluntary control so that the child is able to delay defaecation until it is convenient. This usually occurs by the age of 3 years.

Encopresis refers to the passing of faeces in an inappropriate place, in the absence of organic pathology (Blackwell, 1989b). Encopresis is described as being primary or secondary, depending on whether the child has ever gained bowel control. If the child has achieved control for at least 6 months before showing signs of encopresis, the problem is said to be secondary. This is true of 50–60% of children who are soiling (Fritz and Armbrust, 1982).

Encopresis may also be divided into retentive and non-retentive. If faeces accumulate excessively in the colon and rectum, that is the child becomes constipated, the intestinal wall dilates and liquid faeces from above may leak around the fixed mass, resulting in soiling (Figure 7.10). Retentive encopresis refers to soiling that is associated with constipation. If there is no evidence of constipation, encopresis is said to be non-retentive.

Bellman (1966) reported that the prevalence rate of encopresis in Sweden was 8.1% at age 3 years, 2.8% at 4 years and 2.2% at 5 years. In the Isle of Wight, Rutter and co-workers (1973) reported rates of 1.2% at age 10–12 years in boys and 0.3% in girls of this age. Encopresis is reported as being four to five times more common in boys (Fritz and Armbrust, 1982).

Factors that may contribute to the development of constipation and retentive encopresis include:

◆ Illness

◆ Anal fissures, resulting in a fear of defaecation because of the pain it causes

◆ Chronic use of laxatives

◆ Parental over-concern with bowel regularity and cleanliness

◆ The child is pre-occupied with other activities, so that feelings of urgency to empty the bowels are ignored

◆ A diet containing inadequate quantities of fibre and fluid

◆ Lack of exercise

◆ Emotional disturbance

◆ Stressful life events

◆ Family discord

Factors that may contribute to non-retentive encopresis include:

◆ Poor toilet training

◆ Developmental delay

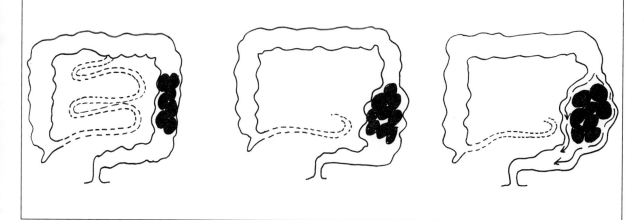

Figure 7.10 Diagram to illustrate constipation with overflow.

◆ Intellectual impairment

◆ Emotional disturbance

◆ Stressful life events

◆ Family discord

ASSESSMENT – CONSTIPATION AND ENCOPRESIS

The aim of assessment is to identify possible causative factors and establish the best form of treatment. Many aspects of the assessment for enuresis can be adapted for encopresis.

INTERVIEWING THE PARENTS

Parents often feel to blame for their child's toileting problems and it is easy for professionals to exacerbate these feelings of guilt by focusing on their possible role in causation. White (1984) believes that a small accidental trigger sets off a snowballing effect, which results in the problem amplifying to a size that is disproportionate to the initial trigger. The initial trigger may never be known, as so many other factors have come into play. White believes it is helpful to externalise the encopresis and to see it as the enemy, affecting everyone in the family. It is one of the by-products of the avalanche. This approach apportions no blame and can enable a therapeutic relationship to develop between professionals and parents having to cope with encopresis.

Useful areas to cover when interviewing the parents are described below.

Encopresis and toiletting

◆ When does the child soil? (Nocturnal encopresis is rare and is often associated with organic pathology.)

◆ How often does the child soil?

◆ Was there a period when he/she did not soil?

If so, for how long? (i.e. Is the encopresis secondary?)

◆ Does the child also wet him/herself? Some 25% of children with encopresis also have enuresis (Fritz and Armbrust, 1982).

◆ How independent is the child with regard to toileting and coping with episodes of soiling?

Can the child take him/herself to the toilet?

How frequently does the child go to the toilet?

Do the parents feel that sometimes the child becomes preoccupied with more interesting activities and puts off going to the toilet?

Can the child sit on the toilet unaided?

Do their feet touch the ground or does the family possess a footstool? (If the child's feet are suspended in the air, it may be difficult to defaecate.)

Are the parents aware of any problems with constipation and, if so, has any medication been used?

Does the child experience any pain on defaecation?

Does the child appear frightened to go to the toilet?

Can the child undress/dress themselves when going to the toilet?

Can the child clean themselves after going to the toilet?

What does the child do when their pants are soiled? (Do they hide the soiled pants?)

Stressful life events

Stressful life events can contribute to primary encopresis if they occur during the period when bowel control is usually achieved and to secondary encopresis later in life.

◆ Has the child experienced any stressful events recently or during toilet training? (see above – *Enuresis assessment, Stressful life events*).

Developmental milestones

See above – *Enuresis assessment, Developmental milestones.*

Emotional disturbance

Emotional and behavioural problems are more commonly associated with encopresis than enuresis.

◆ Do the parents have any concerns regarding the child's behaviour?

◆ Is the child experiencing any problems at school?

◆ Does the child seem particularly sad, worried or angry?

◆ Is the child having difficulties sleeping?

Home circumstances

Similar to enuresis, poor living conditions may play a part in the development of encopresis, because of the stress placed on the family, and/or the maintenance of the problem, owing to the burden of extra washing and having to cope with an unpleasant odour.

◆ Do the parents feel happy where they live/ that their housing is adequate?

◆ What toilet facilities does the family have?

◆ What washing facilities does the family have for clothes and themselves?

◆ Is there a problem with odour?

Measures that have been taken to overcome the problem

◆ Has there been any professional help?

If so, was any of it successful?

◆ Have the parents taken any measures themselves?

Used any rewards or punishments?

Effect of encopresis on the child

See above – *Enuresis assessment, Effect of enuresis on the child.*

The parents' attitudes to encopresis

Some parents may believe the child is being naughty or is out to upset them, but most will feel guilty.

◆ What do you feel has caused this problem? If White's (1984) ideas (see above) on the development of encopresis have not been discussed already, this may be a useful opportunity. The nurse can identify evidence that demonstrates how soiling is beyond anyone's control.

◆ How has encopresis affected the family?

Do the parents, or siblings of the affected child, get angry when the child soils?

How do they cope with the washing and odour?

Is it difficult taking the child out in case he/she soils?

Diet

◆ Does the child eat sufficient fruit and vegetables (at least five portions a day)?

◆ Does the child drink adequately (at least eight glasses a day)?

Exercise

◆ Does the child exercise regularly?

BASELINE RECORDING

See above – *Enuresis assessment.* Assessment charts similar to those in Figures 7.1 and 7.3 should be used. If the child is soiled at each visit to the toilet, increase the number of visits, but ensure that the child wipes him/herself thoroughly each time so that staining of pants does not get confused with soiling. Parents should record the frequency and consistency of bowel motions passed in the toilet or pants.

MEDICAL HISTORY AND EXAMINATION

A doctor must take a medical history and examine the child to exclude organic pathology that would result in soiling (Hirschsprung's disease, congenital hypothyroidism or anorectal anomalies). It is also important to establish whether the child is experiencing abdominal pain, has developed anal fissures and/or is constipated. Plain radiography of the abdomen may be necessary.

INTERVIEWING THE CHILD

See above – *Enuresis assessment, Interviewing the child.*

INDIVIDUAL PSYCHOTHERAPY ASSESSMENT

When there is concern that emotional disturbance is playing an important role in the aetiology of encopresis, or that soiling is only part of a much wider mental health problem, an assessment by a psychotherapist may be enlightening. Psychodynamic theories regarding encopresis include:

◆ Due to an acute episode of stress, the child *regresses* to an earlier and more dependent stage of development.

◆ Due to coercive toilet training, the child *aggressively* rebels, either refusing to defaecate, resulting in retentive encopresis, or passing motions in inappropriate places and so exhibiting non-retentive encopresis (Barker, 1983).

FAMILY ASSESSMENT

Similar family dynamics may contribute to the development of encopresis as contribute to enuresis (see above – *Enuresis assessment, Family assessment*).

HOME AND SCHOOL VISIT

See above – *Enuresis assessment, Home visit, School visit*).

NURSING/MULTI-DISCIPLINARY INTERVENTION – CONSTIPATION AND ENCOPRESIS

RELIEVE CONSTIPATION

Medication

Treatment to alleviate constipation is essential to ensure the success of other nursing/multi-disciplinary interventions. Nolan et al (1991) compared behaviour modification, aimed at reducing encopresis, with behaviour modification plus laxative treatment. The children all had evidence of stool on abdominal radiography, but were not seriously impacted. Treatment included initial clearance with Microlax enemas (containing sodium citrate) and bisacodyl suppositories and tablets, followed by Agarol (a liquid paraffin cocktail), senna granules and/or bisacodyl tablets. Doses were adjusted to ensure daily defaecation. At the 12-month follow-up, 51% of those having laxative and behaviour therapy and 36% of those receiving behaviour therapy alone had achieved remission. It is important to balance the medical benefits of rectal treatment with the psychological trauma it may cause. Children who are suspected of having been sexually abused should not endure this form of treatment if at all possible. From clinical experience, oral laxatives of adequate strength and dose can aid successful treatment of encopresis.

Diet

A diet high in fibre (five portions daily) with adequate fluids (eight glasses daily) can promote bowel regularity. Large amounts of dairy produce or fatty meat can have a binding effect.

Exercise

Regular exercise will promote bowel movements.

INCENTIVE CHARTS AND REWARDS

Behaviour programmes for encopresis should be aimed at reinforcing defaecation in the toilet. They should *not* reinforce clean pants, as this can encourage children to retain faeces and so become constipated. The frequency of visits to the toilet should be greater than the frequency of soiling, established in the assessment, so that the child experiences clean episodes. Food entering the stomach stimulates strong waves of peristalsis in the tranverse colon, which move its contents into the descending and pelvic colon. This is called the gastrocolic reflex and is at its strongest about 20 minutes after eating. Arranging toilet times after meals or drinks is therefore not only practically more convenient and easier for the child to remember, but can also facilitate defaecation. The child should sit on the toilet for long enough to defaecate but not for so long that it becomes boring or punitive (between 1 and 5 minutes). A reward should be given for sitting on the toilet, and an extra reward for passing a motion.

Points to remember when using incentive charts and rewards

Adapt the guidelines above (see *Enuresis*). Themes for incentive charts could follow the child's fantasy character to fight 'sneaky poo' (see below – *Family therapy* and see Plate 7 which appears in the unfolioed section between p56 and 57).

FAMILY THERAPY

Assessment may have revealed important issues, which should be taken up in family therapy. Where there are indicators of family discord, a qualified family therapist must be involved, but a nurse without such qualification can provide valuable family support. The ideas of White (1984) (see above – *Interviewing the parents*) can be used to help the whole family fight against the 'enemy', which White calls 'sneaky poo'. Discussion with the family should facilitate the development of tactics that can be used to win the battle. Where will they gather their strength from? Perhaps the child has a hero he or she can call upon, such as Superman. The parents will need to find ways of supporting each other. If the encopresis is externalised, *it* can be chastised and not the child.

INDIVIDUAL WORK

Improving self-esteem

Education regarding the digestive system and maintaining a healthy diet can help to give the young person a sense of control. A simple diagram can be used to illustrate the path that food takes through the body (Figure 7.11) and what can happen with constipation (see Figure 7.10). Teaching specific exercises for the abdomen may help bowel regularity and also give the child a sense of mastery (Figure 7.12).

A graph can demonstrate visually the child's progress, similar to that used for enuresis (see Figure 7.9) and exercises carried out to raise the young person's self-confidence (see Chapter 2 – *Individual work, Improving self-esteem*). Role play could also be used to help the child to develop strategies to cope with bullying.

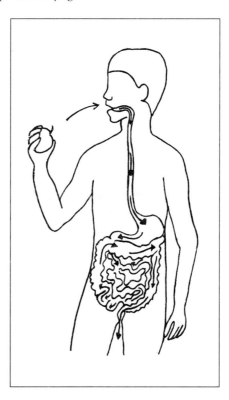

Figure 7.11 Diagram to illustrate the digestive system.

Overcoming fears of the toilet

It is not unusual for children who have been constipated and/or have developed anal fissures to be frightened of passing motions, because of the pain caused. In these situations, it is essential to relieve constipation and perhaps use a topical cream to aid healing and reduce pain. Other measures to overcome fears of the toilet are described above (see *Individual work* for the child with enuresis).

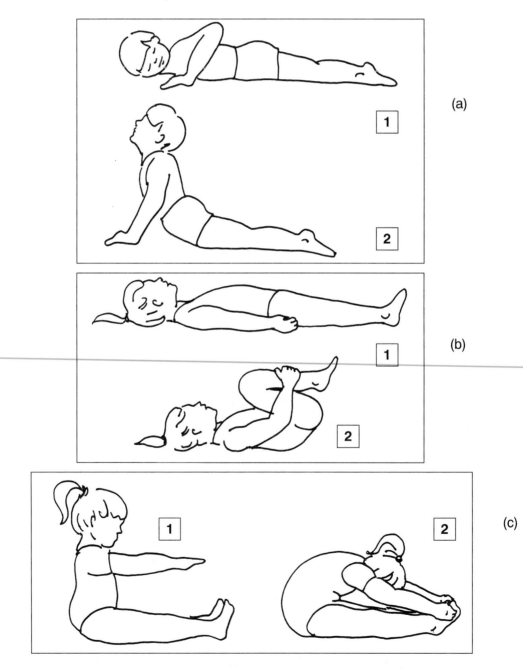

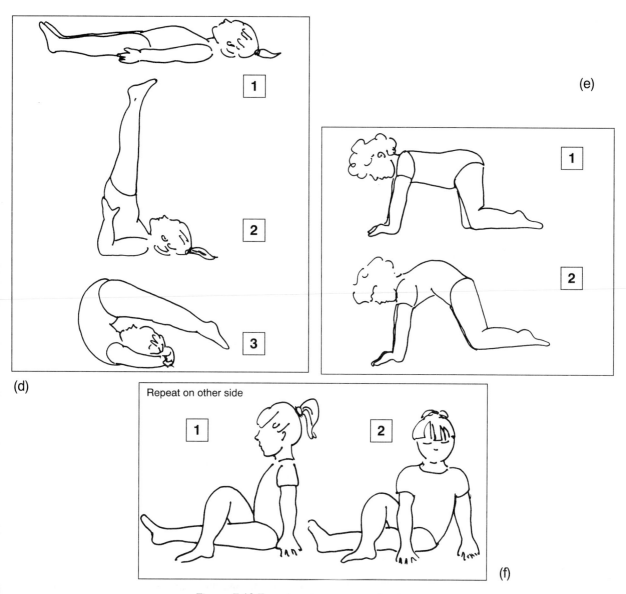

Figure 7.12 Exercises to ease constipation.

Expressing feelings openly

Helping the child to express their feelings openly may help those who are using soiling as a form of protest (see Chapter 5 – *Individual work*).

Individual psychoanalytical psychotherapy

When emotional disturbance is clearly evident, psychotherapy may be indicated.

National support group

ERIC (see *National support group* for enuresis) also provides information for professionals and parents regarding encopresis.

CONCLUSION

Enuresis, and encopresis to a lesser extent, are relatively common childhood problems, but ones that can cause considerable distress for the child and family. Nurses, particularly those working in the community, can play a vital role identifying the problem and initiating treatment.

A thorough assessment is essential if treatment is to be successful. Implementing a behaviour programme without first establishing vital information is likely to result in failure. For example, an enuresis alarm is unlikely to be successful unless the child and parents are highly motivated to follow the programme and there are no practical obstacles, such as the child sharing a bed.

As wetting and soiling can become a highly charged issue within a family, often with the identified child being blamed, it can be helpful to externalise the problem. The family can then unite to fight the problem rather than the identified child.

REFERENCES

Bakwin H (1971) Enuresis in twins. *American Journal of Diseases in Childhood* **121**: 222–225.

Banerjee S, Srivastav A and Palan BM (1993) Hypnosis and self-hypnosis in the management of nocturnal enuresis: a comparative study with imipramine therapy. *American Journal of Clinical Hypnosis* **36(2)**: 113–119.

Barker P (1983) Enuresis, encopresis and hyperkinetic syndrome. In *Basic Child Psychiatry*, pp 127–134. London: Granada.

Bellman M (1966) Studies on encopresis. *Acta Paediatrica Scandinavica. Supplement* **70**: 1+.

Blackwell C (1989a) *A Guide to Enuresis: A Guide to the Treatment of Enuresis for Professionals*. Bristol: Enuresis Resource and Information Centre.

Blackwell C (1989b) *A Guide to Encopresis: A Guide to the Treatment of Encopresis*. Morpeth: Northumberland Health Authority.

Bradbury MG and Meadow SR (1995) Combined treatment with enuresis alarm and desmopressin for nocturnal enuresis. *Acta Paediatrica* **84**: 1014–1018.

Butler RJ (1987) *Nocturnal Enuresis – Psychological Perspectives*. Bristol: Wright.

Butler RJ and Brewin CR (1986) Maternal views of nocturnal enuresis. *Health Visitor* **59**: 207–209.

Egger J, Carter CH, Soothill JF and Wilson J (1992) Effect of diet treatment on enuresis in children with migraine or hyperkinesis behaviour. *Clinical Pediatrics* **31(5)**: 302–307.

Fenichel DM (1945) *The Psychoanalytic Theory of Neurosis*. New York: Norton.

Fielding DM (1988) General information. In Blackwell C (ed.) *A Guide to Enuresis – A Guide to the Treatment of Enuresis for Professionals*, pp 7–11. Bristol: Enuresis Resource and Information Centre.

Forsythe WI and Butler RJ (1989) Fifty years of enuretic alarms: a review of the literature. *Archives of Disease in Childhood* **59**: 748–753.

Foxman B, Valdez B and Brook RH (1986) Childhood enuresis: prevalence, perceived impact and prescribed treatments. *Pediatrics* **77(4)**: 482–487.

Fritz GK and Armbrust J (1982) Enuresis and encopresis. *Psychiatric Clinics of North America* **5(2)**: 283–296.

Fritz GM, Rockney RM and Yeung AS (1994) Plasma levels and efficacy of imipramine treatment for enuresis. *Journal of the American Academy of Child and Adolescent Psychiatry* **33(1)**: 60–64.

Gandhi KK (1994) Diagnosis and management of nocturnal enuresis. *Current Opinion in Pediatrics* **6**: 194–197.

Harris LS and Purohit AP (1977) Bladder training and enuresis; a controlled trial. *Behaviour Research and Therapy* **15**: 485–490.

Klauber GT (1989) Clinical efficacy and safety of desmopressin in the treatment of nocturnal enuresis. *Journal of Pediatrics* **114 (supplement)**: 719–722.

Lyon A (1991) The use of desmopressin in the management of nocturnal enuresis. *Maternal and Child Health* **16**: 170–172.

Mikkelsen EJ and Rapaport JL (1980) Enuresis: psychopathology sleep stage and drug response. *Urologic Clinics of North America* **7**: 361–377.

Nolan T, Debelle G, Oberklaid F and Coffey C (1991) Randomised trial of laxatives treatment of childhood encopresis. *Lancet* **388**: 523–527.

Novick J (1966) Symptomatic treatment of acquired and persistent enuresis. *Journal of Abnormal Psychology* **77**: 363–368.

O'Reagan S, Yazbeck S, Hamberger B and Schick E (1986) Constipation, a commonly unrecognised cause of enuresis. *American Journal of Diseases of Children* **140(3)**: 260–261.

Pratten AR and Sluckin A (1985) Child abuse and encopresis. *Midwife, Health Visitor & Community Nurse* **21**: 400–404.

Richman N, Stevenson J and Graham P (1982) *Pre-school to School: A Behavioural Study*. London: Academic Press.

Rutter M, Yule W and Graham P (1973) Enuresis and behavioural deviance: some epidemiological considerations. In Kolvin I, Mackeith R, Meadow SR (eds) *Bladder control and enuresis*. Clinics in Developmental Medicine No. 5 48/49 pp. 137–147. London: Heinemann/Spastics International Medical Publications.

Schaefer CE (1979) *Childhood Encopresis and Enuresis: Causes and Theory*. New York: Van Nostrand Reinhold.

Waxman D (1991) Use of medical hypnosis in childhood asthma and enuresis. Maternal and Child Health **16(5)**: 189–192, 194–196.

Weider DJ and Hauri PJ (1985) Nocturnal enuresis in children with upper airway obstruction. *Journal of Pediatric Otorhinolaryngology* **9(2)**: 173–182.

White W (1984) Pseudo-encopresis: from avalanche to victory, from vicious to virtuous cycles. In *Selected Papers*, pp 115–124. Dulwich Centre Review.

Winnicott DW (1953) Transitional objects and transitional phenomena. *International Journal of Psychoanalysis* **34**: 89–97.

8 PROBLEMS WITH SLEEPING

INTRODUCTION

The parents of a child who is having problems sleeping are likely to be drained of all energy and to be doubting their own parenting abilities. Fatigue and irritability can lead to marital discord and, in extreme situations, child abuse (Bartlett et al, 1992). In a study by Chavin and Tinson (1980), looking at the effects of sleeping problems on families, 37% of parents thought that the sleeping problem caused serious arguments, 8% admitted administering severe abuse to their child and 2% considered that it had been directly responsible for their marital break-up. Maternal fatigue is thought to be one of the contributory factors causing postnatal depression and sometimes may actually be the primary problem. The characteristics of sleep deprivation are very similar to those of postnatal depression: anxiety, irritability, apathy and aggression, which can result in misdiagnosis and inappropriate treatment (Errante, 1985). The child's lack of sleep is likely to affect their day-time mood and behaviour, perhaps resulting in more frequent tantrums, interfering with feeding, affecting school performance in older children and adolescents, and so on. Certain sleeping problems, such as sleep-walking, also present their own safety hazards and parents may be unable to sleep themselves for fear of the child hurting him or herself. Professionals must therefore be aware and alert to the ramifications of sleep problems, both for the parents and child. Sleep disorders in adolescence are often associated with psychopathology, particularly depression and anxiety. Therefore, the nurse should always consider the possibility of sleeping problems when a child's mental health is clearly jeopardised. It is unclear whether sleep deprivation plays a causal role in adolescent emotional and behavioural problems and/or whether sleep problems are precipitated by psychopathology (Morrison et al, 1992).

Sleeping problems, such as difficulties falling asleep and frequent waking during the night, are common in healthy pre-school children. Research suggests that 15–35% of toddlers and 10–15% of pre-school children wake at least once most nights, that 50% of pre-schoolers resist going to bed and that 4–15% of toddlers and pre-school children take longer than 1 hour to fall asleep once in bed (Wolke et al, 1995). A significant number of adolescents experience sleeping difficulties. Morrison and colleagues (1992) found that 35% of 15 year olds reported problems, 25% feeling in need of more sleep and 10% experiencing difficulties falling asleep.

To understand how sleeping problems arise and how to treat them, the nurse must have a basic knowledge of normal sleep physiology and its development. The normal 24-hour cycle of sleep is known to have a restorative function for our bodies and perhaps also our minds. Differences among individuals exist in the amount of sleep required, but the time spent asleep decreases with age, from an average of 16 hours per day at 1 week old, to 8 hours for an adult. Two biological clocks control sleeping and waking. A circadian clock controls the 24-hour sleep–wake rhythm and an ultradian homoeostatic system controls the rhythm of two distinct types of sleep: rapid eye movement (REM) and non-rapid eye movement (non-REM) sleep. Both the circadian and ultradian rhythms mature during early development, as the child's 'clocks' become coordinated with regularly occurring external signals such as the light–dark cycle, recurring changes in atmosphere or noise level, and regular periods of social interaction, together with internal signals, such as hunger, core temperature, pain and hormone secretion. Initially there is no distinction between night and day, the newborn sleeping and waking throughout the 24-hour period and not being asleep for more than 3 or 4 hours at a time. By 6 months, there is a definite pattern of night-time sleep and day-time wakefulness. The child will require about 14 hours' sleep in 24 hours and most of this will be at night, with just two 1–2-hour naps during the day. Gradually, the amount of sleep needed in 24 hours slowly decreases and night-time sleep becomes consolidated. By the age of 2, children require only one day-time nap, and in the pre-school years, depending on social expectations, most give up all day-time sleep. By the time the child has reached pre-adolescence, he/she will require only 10 hours' sleep. By 14 years, many teenagers are sleeping for only 7 or 8 hours a night during the week, but often complain of tiredness and, when left to wake naturally at weekends, tend to sleep longer. It seems likely that during puberty more sleep is actually required and that 7–8 hours is perhaps culturally imposed rather than truly adequate (Ferber, 1986; Anders, 1994).

The ultradian rhythm, consisting of REM and non-REM sleep, also begins in infancy and continues to mature through to adolescence. During REM sleep, the body is profoundly relaxed with poor muscle tone, the heart and breathing rate become irregular, blood flow to the brain increases and there are striking rapid eye movements. The brain is active and this is the stage of sleep when dreams and nightmares occur. It is possible that REM sleep has a psychological function, allowing us to process the day's emotional experiences and transfer recent memories into longer-term strorage. The other important characteristic of REM sleep is that we can be woken easily if the outside stimulus is sufficiently important. For example, an alarm clock may not wake us, but a baby crying or someone shouting 'fire' will. When woken from a state of REM sleep, we feel alert and ready for action. There is also a tendency to wake automatically during REM sleep, after an episode of dreaming, but return to sleep is almost immediate and there is usually no recollection of this waking. Some evolutionists believe that REM sleep has an important protective function, providing an intermediate stage between non-REM and waking, when the mind is 'woken' before the body, enabling a speedy escape from predators once fully awake and allowing an animal to check its environment whilst sleeping.

Non-REM sleep is characterised by tonic muscle activity, slow, regular heart and respiratory rates, and no rapid eye movements. It is during non-REM sleep that repair and revival of the body occurs. This stage can be divided into four stages, each representing a deeper level of consciousness. On hearing your name called, you will probably rouse easily from stage II, but be oblivious in stage IV. However, in emergency situations, it is possible to be woken from stage IV sleep, but you are likely to feel confused and disoriented. A period of REM sleep alternates with a period of non-REM sleep to form a 'sleep cycle'; an 8-hour sleep episode in an adult will contain about five sleep cycles (Ferber, 1986; Clore and Hibel, 1993).

The proportion of time spent in REM sleep decreases from about 50% in a neonate to 20% in an adult. Adults enter REM sleep approximately 90 minutes after falling asleep, whereas infants frequently enter REM sleep immediately. By about 3 months, a baby will enter non-REM sleep before REM sleep. A young child progresses rapidly through the stages of non-REM sleep and may be soundly asleep in as little as 10 minutes. In the early stages of the night, non-REM sleep in a youngster is an extremely deep sleep and it is virtually impossible to rouse the child. For example, if a child falls asleep in the car, it may be possible to carry them into the house, change them into their pyjamas and put them into bed, with only the slightest arousal. After about 1 hour of deep stage IV sleep, the child will have a brief partial wakening and then descend quickly back into stage IV again. After 50–60 minutes, another partial wakening will occur, which will probably be followed by the first REM sleep. During this and subsequent periods of REM sleep, the child will experience brief wakenings. The child's sleep cycle continues to recur every 50–60 minutes, unlike in the adult, where it recurs every 90 minutes. After 3 months, although the total amount of REM and non-REM sleep remains the same, the proportion in each sleep cycle begins to shift. In children, non-REM sleep predominates in early night cycles and REM predominates the later cycles. The natural wakenings that occur through the night are significant for many sleeping problems. During partial wakenings in non-REM sleep, parasomnias, such as night terrors and sleep walking or talking, may occur, and during the brief wakenings in REM sleep children may experience difficulties in returning to sleep (Figure 8.1).

Problems with sleeping are likely to have multiple contributing factors and research has produced considerable contradictory evidence. Possible aetiological factors include:

◆ Biological predisposition affecting the body's biological rhythms

◆ Slower neurological maturation

◆ Temperament

◆ Perinatal problems

◆ Maternal attachment experiences

◆ Maternal anxiety or depression

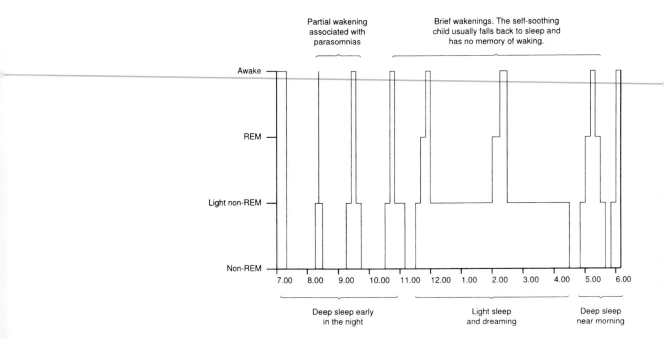

Figure 8.1 Typical progression of sleep stages.

◆ First-born child

◆ Parental management of sleep

◆ Present attachment between caregiver and child

◆ Stressful life events

◆ Poor sleep habits in adolescence

As sleeping problems are common in healthy young children and maturation may be an important factor in developing an ability to sleep well, the reader may question their relevance in a book about mental health problems. However, emotional and behavioural factors do appear to be relevant in their aetiology, and psychological treatment has proved to be effective.

One of the obstacles to research has been subjective reporting of sleep problems. For example, some parents may not consider getting up to their child once in the night a problem, whereas others will. Nevertheless, after taking into account the developmental stage of the child, professionals should base their decision regarding intervention on the level of parental concern. In other words, if the parents are experiencing it as a problem, then they need help. This chapter is concerned with difficulties falling asleep at night, frequent waking during the night, nightmares and parasomnias (episodes or unwanted events that occur during sleep). The most common parasomnias that occur in childhood include night terrors (pavor nocturnus), sleep-walking (somnambulism) and sleep-talking (somniloquy).

ASSESSMENT

MEDICAL ASSESSMENT

Some research suggests a correlation between perinatal problems and later night waking, whereas other studies have found no correlation (Kerr and Jowett, 1994). Perhaps perinatal problems alter parents' behaviour, which in turn contributes to the development of sleeping problems. A birth history may reveal the emergence of such behaviour. Parents of a child who has required medical treatment after birth are likely to be more anxious than other parents and may be quicker to respond to their child when she/he cries (see below – *Parental management of bedtime and sleeping disturbances*).

Any acute illness, especially one with a fever, teething pains or colic, is likely to disrupt a baby's normal sleeping pattern. A health visitor should be able to offer advice to parents on how to ease their child's discomfort. Sleeping will generally improve without any specific intervention, but sometimes can persist because the child has adopted poor sleeping habits. For example, if the baby has been rocked to sleep, he or she may have become accustomed to this, which can lead to problems (see below – *Parental management*). A discussion with parents about the general well-being of the child may highlight the trigger of current difficulties. Sometimes the persistence of sleeping problems may have a biological basis. During a fever, stages II and IV of non-REM sleep are suppressed. Afterwards, there is a rebound increase in these stages, which can predispose to parasomnias.

A chronic medical condition may contribute to sleep problems. For example, asthma can result in the child having difficulty breathing, which may be particularly frightening at night; eczema can result in annoying itchy skin; scoliosis may require the child to wear an uncomfortable brace, and so on. Certain medication may also disrupt sleep, such as the stimulant methylphenidate, used to treat attention deficit disorder or the sedative phenobarbitone, used in epilepsy (Ferber, 1986).

Parents will generally be aware of any medical conditions affecting their child's sleep, but occasionally a physical problem will first be recognised when sleeping disturbances are reported. Parents are certainly likely to be worried that something is wrong with their child and medical problems must be excluded. For example, middle ear disease, which causes a build-up of fluid in the middle ear, can become infected and result in severe pain, but can also disrupt sleep even when not infected and the child is not complaining of any discomfort during the day. The doctor should enquire about any previous ear infections and examine the child's ears for signs of fluid behind the eardrum. It is not known how middle ear disease disrupts sleep, but possibly drainage from the middle ear cavity is worse when the child is lying down and pressure builds up, causing discomfort (Ferber, 1986). Sleep-disordered breathing is a common, yet often unrecognised, cause of chronic sleep disruption in children. Despite large tonsils and adenoids in these children, most breathe normally while awake but, once asleep, decreased muscle tone further reduces the size of the airway, leading to intermittent obstruction. Another, but more rare, example of a medical condition causing sleep problems is the occurrence of temporal lobe seizures. These can mimic parasomnias, but electroencephalograhpy and sleep studies can rule this possibility out (Clore and Hibel, 1993).

Although a medical condition may contribute to a sleeping problem, this is not always the case. Therefore, it seems likely that, in many cases, it is not the illness alone that is disrupting sleep, but a number of factors. For example, the child's emotional status, the parent–child relationship and the coping mechanism used by the parents may all play a significant role (Tirosh et al, 1993).

INTERVIEWING THE PARENTS

Description of the problem and gathering sleep-related information

A thorough interview with the parents should start by gathering basic details concerning the nature and frequency of the problem and sleep-related information. A description of the problem, including duration, frequency and any changes that occur at weekends or in response to other environmental factors, such as stress, should be obtained. It is also important to ascertain the child's usual sleep–wake pattern, bedtime routine, behaviour during the night, morning routine and any symptoms of sleepiness during the day. More detailed information will be obtained as the interview proceeds and once the parents have kept a diary (see below – *Sleep diaries*). The description of the child's behaviour will obviously go hand in hand with the parents' account of how they manage their child's bedtime and their attempts to overcome the problem (see below – *Parental management*).

When parasomnias are the presenting problem, the following information should be ascertained (Ferber, 1988; Clore and Hibel, 1993):

✦ *Behaviour during episode* During sleep-walking, the child is likely to have an affectless expression and engage in clumsy, purposeless activities, but, as the episode proceeds, the activity may become more purposeful and coordinated. In contrast, a child who is having a night terror is likely to be confused, agitated or in a state of panic. The episode may begin with the child moaning, sobbing, crying out or screaming. The child may thrash and roll about, with eyes open, and have a peculiar expression on their face. Changes to the autonomic nervous system occur, including tachycardia, tachypnoea, dilated pupils and sweating. Sleep-walking may accompany a night terror. Sleep-talking is a relatively benign occurrence, when the child mumbles or speaks incoherently during their sleep. It does not generally pose a problem, although may sometimes awaken the child.

✦ *Time length of episode* If the child is uninterrupted, a sleep-walking episode can last up to 40 minutes. If the child is guided back to bed before they are ready, they are likely to get up again. A night terror usually lasts less than 10 minutes, but can continue for half an hour.

✦ *Can the child recall the episode?* It is important for the nurse to differentiate between night terrors and nightmares. A child will recall a nightmare, but not a night terror.

Age of onset and duration of problem

The nurse's history should establish when the sleeping problem started and how long it has persisted. Often the problem has existed since birth, but sometimes a settled sleep pattern may be disrupted by illness, separation and so on (see below – *Major life events*).

Some research has suggested that neurological maturation is a significant contributory factor in the development of sleeping problems. However, this theory is incongruous with the findings of a study by Wolke et al (1995), which demonstrated no difference between the night waking patterns of pre-term and full-term babies; in fact, pre-term babies tend to wake less often. However, sleeping patterns do go through a developmental process and so it is important to establish whether the parental expectations are realistic. For example, it is probably unreasonable to expect a baby of less than 6 months to sleep through the night. Parasomnias also follow a developmental pattern. Infants as young as 6 months may have partial wakenings, when they cry and cannot be calmed, but more defined and complex parasomnias occur as children get older.

Family history

There is often a family history of parasomnias. This may suggest a biological origin, and indeed families that have high amounts of non-REM sleep are those that tend to present with parasomnias, but these findings could, of course, also be linked to family patterns of communication or life events (Dahl, 1992). A family history of day-time sleepiness may be significant in identifying certain sleep disorders, such as narcolepsy, and in making a differential diagnosis.

Major life events or stressful situations at time of onset

A significant relationship exists between environmental stress and sleeping problems. Social stressors, such as financial difficulties in the family, poor housing conditions, family illness or an accident, and maternal depression, are more common in families of children who sleep poorly (Kerr and Jowett, 1994). Current stressors may also trigger parasomnias. Experts differ in their opinion as to whether emotional factors trigger the partial wakening or affect the child's response to partial waking, but, in either case, the child's mental state seems important.

General day-time behaviour and mood

Older children who exhibit parasomnias are typically well behaved and find it difficult to express difficult or painful feelings, such as jealousy and anger. During a partial wakening, their 'guard' is let down. A general enquiry about the child's day-time mood and behaviour may also highlight current stressors in the child's life that may have significance for any type of sleeping problem.

Parental management of bedtime and sleeping disturbances

It is important to ask parents whether their child has a bedtime routine, and, if so, what this involves, and to ascertain what measures the parents have tried to overcome the presenting problem. Patterns of parental interaction with the child have been linked with good and poor sleeping behaviour. Johnson (1991) found that infants whose parents soothed them to sleep, by rocking or comforting them in some way, were more likely to wake at night than infants who were left to fall asleep alone. Some 80% of those who fell asleep alone were sleeping through the night, compared with less than a third of those whose parents were present while they fell asleep. All children briefly wake between one and three times a night, but some will soothe themselves back to sleep, while others signal distress. Anders (1994) suggests that it is inaccurate to describe children as 'sleeping through the night' or as 'night-wakers', but more accurate to talk about 'self-soothers' and 'signallers'.

Anders and co-workers (1992) identified a significant developmental pattern in the emergence of self-soothing behaviour and in the increasing use of a sleep aid. In the first month, 95% of infant arousals were accompanied by crying (signalling) and required a parental response before returning to sleep, but by 8 months 60–70% were able to self-soothe and return to sleep on their own. The use of a sleep aid, such as a teddy bear or blanket, was associated with children who were self-soothers and the emergence of an ability to use a sleep aid was associated with children who were left to sleep alone. Parents may reinforce signalling behaviour, perhaps by giving drinks, cuddles or taking the baby into the parental bed. They may also inhibit the development of self-soothing behaviour, by soothing the child to sleep themselves and attending to them the moment they start crying, so denying the child space to develop their own coping skills (Atkinson et al, 1995; Wolke et al, 1995).

Sleeping problems are common in children with severe learning difficulties. Quine (1992) suggests that this may in part be due to maternal responsiveness. Mothers of children with learning difficulties are more likely to attend to their child immediately when they wake at night, offering cuddles, drinks and attention, and less likely to play music or read with their child at bedtime, to help settle them.

Some studies have suggested that first-born children are more prone to sleep problems, and this may also be the result of increased parental responsiveness (Pollock, 1992).

It can be very disturbing for parents to be woken by their child in the midst of a night terror and extremely worrying that the child may come to harm if sleep-walking. However, attempts to waken or comfort the child are likely to be unsuccessful and may even aggravate the child's behaviour. The nurse must establish what safety precautions the parents have taken and whether they have tried to intervene in the child's parasomnia and, if so, the consequence of their intervention.

Mental health of caregivers

Mothers of children with sleeping problems are reported to have a higher incidence of nervousness, depression, alcohol problems and marital difficulties (Kerr and Jowett, 1994). In a study by Atkinson and colleagues (1995), a mother described how the death of her mother coincided with the start of chronic sleeping problems in her toddler. Feelings will be picked up by the child and parenting behaviour is likely to be affected by ill-health. Enquiring about the mental and physical health of parents is therefore an important component of the assessment. Ask questions such as, 'How are you feeling in yourself?', and to mothers, 'It can take a long time to recover from the birth of a baby. To what extent do you feel that you have recovered from your child's birth?'

Child's temperament

A child's temperamental style seems to be an important contributory factor in sleeping problems. Children who are 'easy', that is adaptable, rhythmic, mild in intensity and positive in mood, tend to sleep better (Atkinson et al, 1995). A child with an 'easy' temperament is perhaps more able to tolerate changes in their environment, such as a wet nappy, changes in temperature or light intensity. Asking about the child's temperament may give some insight into sleeping difficulties, and the knowledge that temperament is significant can give some relief to parents who feel totally to blame for their child's problem. Ask questions such as, 'How would you describe your child's temperament', 'How does your child behave in new situations?', 'Has your child's behaviour fallen into a daily routine?' and 'How would you generally describe your child's mood?'. Children who are reluctant to adopt self-soothing techniques are also more likely to be poor sleepers and so it may be helpful to ask, 'Are you aware of your child being able to comfort him/herself? Does he/she use a comforter of some kind or is he/she dependent on you for soothing, such as cuddles?'.

Nutrition and feeding

The relationship between feeding and night waking remains controversial. Many mothers report that a good feed before bedtime helps to ensure a good night's sleep. However, Wright and co-workers (1983) found that the sleep–wake pattern of infants fed on an enriched diet did not differ from that of those fed on a regular diet. Kahn et al (1989) identified cow's milk allergy in a group of infants with persistent night waking who failed to respond to behavioural interventions. Methods and styles of feeding have also been studied (breast vs. bottle and demand vs. schedule), but results have been inconsistent. Perhaps, it is the parent–child interaction rather than the feeding itself that is important.

Sleep diaries

Asking parents to complete a sleep diary (Figure 8.2) will provide a clear record of the child's sleep–wake pattern and parental behaviour, and avoids distorted memories. It also checks the parents' level of motivation to correct the sleeping problem; parents who fail to complete a diary are unlikely to comply with treatment intervention (Douglas, 1989).

OBSERVATION OF PARENT–CHILD RELATIONSHIP

Infant–caregiver attachment

The attachment relationship serves a developmental function, ideally promoting curiosity and exploration, together with security and comfort. Patterns of parent–child interaction will lead to distinctive characteristics of the attachment relationship. Four categories of attachment can be recognised cross-culturally: secure, avoidant, anxious and disorganised. Sensitive and consistent patterns of caregiver responsiveness lead to secure attachment; inconsistent and/or intrusive interactions lead to anxious attachment; distant, uninvolved parenting leads to avoidant attachment; and more serious early childhood trauma, such as abuse or the death of a parent, seems to result in disorganised attachment (Anders, 1994).

Sleeping disturbances have been associated with parent–child relationship problems in young children. Mothers who respond sensitively to their child's pleas for attention, while

DAY AND DATE	MONDAY 30/12/96	TUESDAY 31/12/96	WEDNESDAY 1/1/96	THURSDAY 2/1/96	FRIDAY 3/1/96	SATURDAY 4/1/96	SUNDAY 5/1/96
TIME WOKE IN MORNING							
TIME AND DURATION OF DAYTIME NAPS							
TIME WENT TO BED							
TIME WENT TO SLEEP							
TIME WOKE IN THE NIGHT, WHAT YOU DID AND TIME WENT BACK TO SLEEP							
TIME YOU WENT TO BED							

Figure 8.2 Format for a sleep diary.

encouraging self-soothing, independence and exploration of the environment during the day-time, tend to have children who sleep better. It seems that these children are more able to comfort themselves and tolerate distance from their mothers. This would suggest that lack of a secure infant attachment relationship plays a significant role in infant sleeping problems.

Recent research also suggests that a mother's own attachment history may contribute to the development of good or poor sleeping patterns in her child. Mothers of young children with sleep problems are less likely to have secure attachment than mothers of children with normal sleeping patterns. Mothers with an insecure attachment history may be less emotionally available, less empathic or less flexible in interacting with their infant, and consequently may be unpredictable and inconsistent in the management of their child's bedtime or chronically rejecting (Benoit et al, 1992).

As well as using her/his observational skills during history-taking, the nurse should attempt to observe the parent–child interaction in a variety of settings, such as during feeding, at bedtime, and so on. This will ensure that a more accurate picture of the overall relationship is obtained. The nurse should note the style of interaction, that is whether it is age-appropriate, chaotic, inconsistent, intrusive or detached, and the affective tone of the interaction – whether it is hostile, anxious, balanced or dependent (Anders, 1994).

TALKING WITH THE CHILD

An older child may be able to describe their own sleeping problems. Some children may feel frightened at night. During the day-time, it is easier for children to keep worries under control; they are usually busy and there is less time available to brood over problems. At night, while waiting to fall asleep, the child can do little except think, and fantasies may run free. As she or he becomes sleepy, the child has less control over their thoughts and feelings. For some children, their worries may take the form of monsters or ghosts, and children may stall going to bed for fear of their 'appearance'.

Nightmares are frightening dreams that cause us to wake, feeling anxious and afraid. If dreams reveal the content of our unconscious, as psychoanalytical theory suggests, nightmares must reflect psychological distress and conflict. At each stage of development, all children are faced with new and sometimes frightening experiences and feelings, which may cause nightmares. For example, temporary separation from a caregiver may arouse feelings of fear and anger, a new sibling may lead to jealousy and the awakening of sexual impulses may result in feelings of confusion and anxiety. All children will have nightmares at one time or another, but some will have persistent, terrifying nightmares which may be a sign of more serious distress. These children may be referred for professional help as a direct result of nightmares. Alternatively, the occurrence of nightmares may become apparent during the assessment of another problem, such as fear or anxiety. Children may be able to describe their nightmare or find it easier to draw a picture. The nurse should look at the context in which nightmares are occurring, asking the child and parents about current life events. For example, the child may have experienced the death of a grandparent or a change of school. It may be enlightening to record the day's events to see whether these correlate in any way with the occurrence of nightmares. For example, a child who has been abused may be more prone to experience a nightmare after contact with the perpetrator.

ASSESSMENT BY A PSYCHOANALYTICAL PSYCHOTHERAPIST

Children presenting with sleeping problems *per se* are unlikely to require a psychotherapy assessment, but if the sleeping problems are associated with other mental health problems, an assessment by a psychotherapist may be appropriate. A psychotherapist, together with the child, may be able to shed some light on the meaning of dreams and nightmares, which can then be utilised in other areas of treatment intervention, as well as in ongoing psychotherapy.

FAMILY ASSESSMENT

The family assessment may be a part of the general history-taking and assessment, rather than a specific family meeting with a view to family therapy, and so may be conducted by a nurse. If it becomes apparent that family dynamics are significant in the cause of the child's sleeping difficulties, family or marital therapy may be prescribed as part of the treatment intervention. For example, a child wakeful at night may provide a convenient diversion for parents with marital problems, allowing them to avoid closeness and intimacy (Quine, 1994). Conversely, a child with sleeping problems will impact on the family. The causal links are likely to be complex, but during assessment some working hypotheses may be formulated.

NURSING/MULTI-DISCIPLINARY INTERVENTION

Most sleeping problems can be dealt with on an outpatient basis, although some children admitted to general paediatric or psychiatric wards for other problems may also have a sleeping problem and so benefit from appropriate intervention. In the community, the health visitor will be one of the key professionals involved, working alongside a clinical psychologist.

BEHAVIOURAL THERAPY

Behavioural approaches are recognised as the most effective method of dealing with difficulties in settling and night waking. A review of research by Leeson et al (1994) suggests an 80–90% success rate. This is based on the premise that, although a number of factors contribute to the development of a sleeping problem, parental management of bedtime and night waking can reduce or exacerbate sleeplessness.

Sleep programmes are more likely to be effective if tailor-made for the individual child and parents. This can be achieved after a thorough assessment and by planning the programme with parents. It is important to ask parents to clarify the exact nature of the problem, which may involve amending statements such as 'my child takes ages to settle and wakes throughout the night' to 'my child settles at around 11pm and then wakes two or three times during the night'. Initially, it is probably better to establish a single goal of treatment, rather than several. For example, parents of a child who is taking a long time to settle and wakes during the night should decide which area of concern they wish to tackle first. Often, when a difficulty in settling is overcome, night waking ceases (Mindell and Durand, 1993). This phenomenon can be explained by a change in the child's behaviour and/or by a change in the parents' approach. The child, having learnt how to fall asleep on their own at bedtime, can then automatically return to sleep after waking at night; the parents, having adopted a behavioural approach at bedtime, are less likely to respond immediately to the child the moment they start crying in the night, which, in turn, allows the child time to fall asleep unaided.

Behavioural therapy may take a number of approaches.

Shaping behaviour or graduated extinction

Extinction refers to the complete removal of problem reinforcers, such as drinks, cuddles, being taken into the parental bed, and so on. Shaping or graduated extinction refers to a more gradual and kinder approach. The ultimate goal of the programme is broken down into small intermediate goals, the first of which is not too far removed from the present situation, and reinforcers of the problem are slowly withdrawn. For example, if a child is used to being held and rocked to sleep, the ultimate goal is for the child to fall asleep alone. However, the first target of the programme may be that the child falls asleep with a parent sitting by the cot, gently stroking their back. Similarly, the child who cries the moment parents leave the room may be expected to go for increasing lengths of time, before the parents return to offer some comfort. The aims of such programmes are to increase self-soothing in the child and correct unhelpful sleep associations. We all associate a certain set of conditions with falling sleep; for example, we may prefer a certain side of the bed, always read before turning out the light, need darkness to fall asleep, and so on. When we wake in the night, the conditions have not changed and we generally fall asleep again and do not even remember waking. If we have difficulty returning to sleep automatically, we may use our usual sleep associations to help us, such as reading. Children who have not learnt to self-soothe but have become accustomed to an adult helping them to fall asleep, such as being held and rocked or fed at the breast, will find it difficult to return to sleep after waking at night without these conditions being reinstated.

It is not possible to teach a child a new set of sleep associations without listening to some crying. Once the parents have settled the child (see below – *Restructuring bedtime routines*), they must leave the child to fall asleep alone. The literature varies in the amount of time recommended between returning to the child to offer brief reassurance, and the author suggests that this is one area that needs to be tailored to the individual child and parents. Ferber (1986) recommends that, on the first night of the programme, parents return to their child 5 minutes after settling him or her, then after 10 minutes if the child is still crying and subsequently every 15 minutes until the child is asleep. On the following night, parents increase each time interval by 5 minutes and likewise on subsequent nights. Leeson et al (1994) adopt shorter time intervals of 2, 4, 6 and 8 minutes, and thereafter 10 minutes. Leaving a child to cry for even short periods is a controversial issue, some believing that it can affect the child's long-term feeling of security. However, the rapid improvement in sleep that is seen after using such a programme would be unlikely if anxiety or lack of parental attention were causing the sleeping problem (Richman et al, 1985). If anything, babies appear more secure and contented once they have learnt to sleep unaided and parents, who are less exhausted, are more able to give positive attention during the day (Leeson et al, 1994). Parents will differ in the amount of time they are able to leave their child crying and the nature of the crying/distress will vary between children. Similarly, parents must decide on the type of brief reassurance that they will give the child on their return. This may involve patting their back and/or talking quietly to them or picking them up briefly, although this is not generally recommended. The most important thing is that the parents find out what works for them and their child (Figure 8.3).

Night waking can be tackled in a similar way to settling the child. On being woken, parents go to their child and offer brief reassurance, once they have satisfied themselves that the child has come to no harm. They should then leave the room regardless of whether the child is still crying. The parents return to their child after waiting for a planned length of time and continue in a similar fashion, increasing the time interval between going to the child, until the child has fallen asleep again. To carry through this programme, parents must be satisfied their child does not require night feeding. As a general rule, most babies of 6 months can sleep a 6–8-hour stretch without needing a feed (Leeson et al, 1994), and Ferber (1989) suggests that babies aged over 3 months do not require a bedtime feed or feeding during the night. Certainly, if the child has previously managed to sleep through the night, this would indicate that they can manage without feeding. The nurse must help the parents to decide what they believe their child's feeding requirements are. Leeson et al (1994) suggests that a late feed, at about 10pm, is sufficient to see the child through the night, and advocates that this is given with minimal waking of the child, to enable him/her to resume sleeping quickly.

Sleeping problems can be linked to feeding if the child has learnt to associate feeding with falling asleep or the quantity of fluid and calories consumed at night is directly disrupting sleep. Stimulating the digestive system and creating wet sodden nappies, which leave the child feeling cold and uncomfortable, can cause wakefulness (Ferber, 1989). The nurse's assessment will involve identifying whether there is a problem of association or an excess of fluid and/or calories is being consumed. If the child is drinking less than about 8 ounces in total (at bedtime and during the night), the problem is more likely to be one of association. However, other inappropriate sleep associations should be considered, as many children have a bedtime feed and have no difficulties sleeping through the night. Falling asleep at the breast or on the bottle is likely to lead to problems, and consuming more than 8 ounces at bedtime is probably inadvisable. Figure 8.4 shows an example of a sleep programme to reduce night feeding. When the mother is breast feeding, it is particularly helpful for the father or someone other than the mother, to go to the child during the night, as the baby's crying will stimulate the let-down reflex and the sight of the mother and smell of milk will further distress the child.

Sufficient time should be allowed to plan the programme thoroughly with parents, giving them the opportunity to problem-solve any foreseeable obstacles. The child may share a bedroom with a sibling, and so parents might decide to move the brother or sister into another room temporarily, to avoid unnecessary disturbance of their sleep; parents will need to agree on how they will share the responsibility for the programme and support each other, and so on. It is

JAMES' SLEEP PROGRAMME

1/ Settle James at bedtime with his usual routine i.e. a bath with time to play before putting him into his pyjamas, a drink of warm milk (4ozs) sitting on your lap, followed by a look at a book together. Wind up his music box, and sing softly along with the tune, placing James into his cot as the music is finishing. Put teddy next to James, kiss him, say goodnight and leave the room, regardless of whether he is crying or stands up.

2/ Return to James after 2 minutes if he is still crying. Lie him down if he is standing. Stroke his head and kiss him, explaining to him that it is time to go to sleep. Talk gently but firmly. Leave the room regardless of whether he is crying. Remember that you have gone into him to reassure him and yourself, that he is O.K; not to help him fall asleep. The goal of the programme is to help him learn how to self-soothe and fall asleep on his own. In the long run he will feel more secure when he has to be on his own, and benefit from a good night's sleep.

3/ Repeat this action after 4 minutes, then after 6, 8 and 10 minutes, all the time that James is still crying.

4/ Continue this action every 10 minutes, until James is asleep.

N.B. Take it in turns to go into James and turn off the baby intercom between checking on him. It will feel even harder if you wait listening to him cry at full volume. Support each other. If one of you decides that you want to go to James before the agreed interval in the programme — discuss it before making a joint decision. If you both decide to abandon the programme one night, discuss the incident at your next appointment.

Figure 8.3 Example of a programme to help a one-year-old child fall asleep with appropriate associations.

also important to decide when the programme should start. For example, it is unlikely to be successful if there are concerns that the child may be in pain, perhaps because of teething. Parents must feel that it is all right to leave their child crying, because any hesitancy about this will probably lead to inconsistency in the programme. It is also inadvisable to begin a programme at a time when one or other parent can ill afford to lose sleep, such as whilst sitting exams or attending interviews for a new job.

SUSAN'S SLEEP PROGRAMME

1/ At bedtime, on the first night, feed Susan for 9 minutes, instead of the usual 10. Place her in the cot, even if she's not yet asleep or crying. Rub her back, say goodnight and leave the room.

2/ If Susan wakes in less than 2½ hours, Peter should go to her, checking that she is not unwell and reassuring her. He will need to leave the room in about 2 minutes, despite her probably still crying. Jenny must not feed Susan before 2½ hours is up. and so Peter may need to check on Susan 2-3 times. After 2½ hours Susan should be fed for 9 minutes. Continue offering feeds every 2½ hours.

3/ On the second night of the programme offer 8 minutes of feed every 3 hours if it is required.

4/ Continue reducing the amount of time spent feeding and increase the time interval between feeds on successive nights.

DAY	MINUTES AT THE BREAST	MINIMUM NUMBER OF HOURS BETWEEN FEEDS
1	9	2.5
2	8	3.0
3	7	3.5
4	6	4.0
5	5	4.5
6	4	5.0
7	3	5.5
8	2	6.0
9	1	6.5
10	NO FEED AT BEDTIME OR DURING THE NIGHT	

N.B. You may decide to stop feeds altogether sooner once feeds have reduced substantially you may find that a very small feed is more distressing for Susan than no feed at all.

Figure 8.4 Example of a programme to help eliminate night feeding in an eight-month-old baby.

Restructuring bedtime routines

Adopting a bedtime routine can help to prompt sleep and foster self-soothing. The routine might involve having a bath, getting into night clothes, looking at a picture book or having a story read, and so on. Encouraging the child to adopt a soft toy, blanket or other article, as a comforter, will enable them to cope better when parents have left them to sleep and when they wake alone at night. Parents need to agree on a specific bedtime for the child and decide roughly how long the bedtime routine will take. This will ensure that parents are consistent.

Swaddling a young baby has been found to shorten the initial crying period (Leeson et al, 1994), perhaps because it simulates the feeling of being held tightly and/or the security of the womb. However, care must be taken not to overheat the child because overheating has been associated with cot death. Swaddling in a sheet, rather than a blanket, is probably advisable.

Positively reinforcing appropriate bedtime behaviour

Older children may be encouraged to behave appropriately at bedtime by parents' positive reinforcement. Praise, privileges and incentive charts can be a helpful adjunct to shaping and adopting bedtime routines. Incentive charts should be individualised and rewards given immediately after the appropriate behaviour has occurred (see Chapter 7 – *Points to remember when using incentive charts and rewards*).

Adolescents, who commonly complain of sleepiness during the day or whose parents identify a problem, may be helped by a strict behavioural contract between them and their parents. This should specify the number of hours to be spent in bed, including at weekends, and could also target contributory factors, such as frequent late-night activities, caffeine intake, erratic napping, and so on (Dahl, 1992).

Day-time routines

If babies become overtired they do not sleep well at night. A fairly regular pattern of day-time naps will facilitate any night-time behavioural programme, and a similar approach to settling the child should be taken during the day. If inappropriate sleep associations have been identified, it will be important that these are not allowed to occur before day-time naps, such as the child falling asleep at the breast.

COGNITIVE–BEHAVIOURAL THERAPY

Cognitive–behavioural treatment may be helpful for older children who have night-time fears. Verbal self-instructional training is probably the most frequently used procedure. This is based on the premiss that irrational self-talk is one cause of emotional distress. Ollendick et al (1991) described a programme, consisting of verbal self-instruction, self-induced relaxation and self-monitoring, to treat children with night-time separation anxiety.

Mary, a 10-year-old girl, expressed excessive worries about her mother's well-being and reported night-time fears related to burglars, monsters and being afraid of the dark. Mary requested to sleep in her mother's bed, refusing to sleep alone or with friends. She explained that she had lost her father (her parents had recently divorced) and her brother (who had gone to college) and was now afraid of losing her mother.

During the initial **monitoring phase** of treatment, Mary was asked to record:

◆ Whether she went to bed within 15 minutes of being told.

◆ Went to bed without complaining, arguing or crying.

◆ Slept in her own bed with lights and noise turned off.

◆ Slept in her own bed throughout the night.

◆ Whether she had any anxious thoughts and how she behaved in response to these.

◆ How her mother responded to her night-time problems.

Mary's mother was asked to record:

◆ The amount of time between telling Mary to go to bed and this happening.

◆ Avoidant behaviours used by Mary.

◆ Whether Mary slept in her own bed throughout the night.

During the **self-control phase**, Mary was encouraged to problem-solve and evaluate her own progress using four questions: 'What's my problem?' (problem definition), 'What can I do about it?' (focused attention), 'How is my plan working?' (self-evaluation and error correction) and 'How did I do?' (self-reinforcement). The therapist modelled self-instruction, by talking through the process out aloud, demonstrating how the questions could serve as prompts to engage in deep breathing relaxation and positive self-statements. The latter include statements such as, 'I am brave', 'I can take care of myself in the dark', and so on. Examples of relaxation exercises can be found in Chapter 4 (*Individual work, Relaxation*). In verbal self-instructional training, the child initially talks through the process out aloud, then in a whisper and finally to themselves. Reinforcement, in the form of praise, is given by the therapist at each stage of the problem-solving process.

In the final **self-control plus reinforcement phase,** role-play and didactic instruction are used to train mothers to firmly instruct their child to go to bed; to ignore whining, crying or similar behaviour; to ignore their child if he/she insists on getting into bed with the parents; and to reward appropriate behaviour in the morning. Reinforcement involves using praise and treats, such as being given a pair of earrings, having a 'special time' with one or other parent, or being allowed to hire a video.

> Mary completed 2 weeks of monitoring, six weekly sessions of 50 minutes of self-control training (SCT) and 12 30–50-minute weekly sessions of SCT plus reinforcement. Mary made steady progress and, by the end of treatment, was able to sleep in her own bed, spend time away from home with friends and generally became less 'clingy' (Ollendick et al , 1991).

As well as learning relaxation techniques and skills in positive self-talk, children and adolescents may be taught to adopt other methods of self-help. For example, if a child has always had a story read to them at bedtime, they may be able to listen to a tape of a story in the night, rather than waking their parents.

GROUP WORK

Meeting with groups of parents who have children with sleeping problems facilitates the mutual support of parents and makes efficient use of health resources. There are several examples in the literature of groups being successfully run by a psychologist and health visitor. Carpenter (1990) reported an improvement in the sleeping of 73% of children whose parents joined a group in Glasgow. The group approach described by Reeve and Miers (1994) is relaxed and informal. Parents are offered tea on their arrival and arrangements are made for children to be cared for in an adjacent room. The group process involves parents recalling their own experiences and brainstorming ideas on how to solve their problems, with the group analysing each option that is suggested. The main emphasis of the group is on building the parents' confidence. Balfour (1988) describes an alternative, more structured, format:

Meeting 1

◆ An 'ice-breaker' name-game to introduce group members.

◆ A discussion of the aims of the group and group rules, such as confidentiality.

◆ Completion of a problem identification sheet, including rating how severe and upsetting their child's problem is.

◆ Discussion of problems in the group, using the sheets completed earlier as a prompt.

◆ A brief presentation by the facilitators of problem-solving, using a flip chart.

◆ Parents volunteer to work on a problem using the framework that has been described.

◆ 'Homework' tasks are set by the parents themselves, who volunteer, and these are recorded on the flip chart. Small goals are encouraged and parents are asked to pre-empt anything that might sabotage successful completion, to prevent failure.

Meetings 2–6

◆ Each group begins with coffee and a review of homework tasks.

◆ The original homework is revised or new tasks set.

◆ Other parents are encouraged to work through problems in the group.

◆ Homework agreements are made.

One of the difficulties experienced by Balfour (1988) was maintaining the boundaries of the group. Parents may start to bring other problems that they are experiencing with their children and/or marital and emotional problems. It is important for group facilitators to deal sensitively with these issues, explaining that they are best talked about in an alternative setting and ensuring that provision is made for this.

FAMILY THERAPY

Perhaps not surprisingly, Mindell and Durand (1993) have demonstrated that successful behavioural treatment of a child's sleeping problem can significantly improve parental mood and marital satisfaction. However, occasionally family therapy is warranted, either because the sleeping problem is creating unbearable tension in the family or because parents and/or professionals believe that family factors are significant in creating the problem. This does not mean that contributing factors need necessarily be dealt with directly; on the contrary, this may not be helpful. Focusing on the present problem and utilising the natural abilities of the family to find a solution can be successful in treating the presenting problem and may have a snowballing effect which will touch other underlying problems.

Prest and Keene Carruthers (1991) described the use of Michael White's 'externalising technique' (see Chapter 7 – *Encopresis, Assessment, Interviewing the parents*), to treat an 11-year-old boy who had difficulties separating from his parents at night and going to sleep. 'Rather than focusing on the individual and pressuring him/her to change, externalising the problem allows the family to work together on solutions to a common problem' (p. 67). This case example illustrates how this technique enabled a change to occur within the inter-personal patterns of behaviour in the family, which were helping to maintain the problem.

During the evening Jon would become sad and anxious, and at bedtime it would often take the parents an hour to settle him in his room. Jon would cry when left, pace the hall and knock on his parent's door, insisting that one of them be by his bedside. Although the parents had been creative and resourceful in ensuring that Jon had a bedtime routine, a 'special time' to talk to one or other parent and a story, they were unable to limit the length of time spent with Jon at night because of his distress. Mr Peters had requested family therapy because he felt that Jon's difficulties originated from his mother's death 2 years ago and was now confounded by step-family issues (Mr Peters had recently remarried and his new wife also thought that Jon's behaviour was problematic). Because the family, in particular Mr Peters, had identified the 'origin' of the problem, the therapist reframed Jon's behaviours as helpful, as they reminded the family of the unresolved grief process. After instigating various strategies to facilitate the grieving process, which produced moderate, but not lasting, success with Jon's difficulties, the therapist decided to 'externalize the problem' and the theme of a 'sneaky sleep thief' arose. Externalising the problem seemed to alleviate the conflict between the step-mother (who was increasingly casting Jon as the villain) and father (who maintained a neutral view of his son), and enabled the parents to start working together to solve the problem. The idea evolved of the 'sneaky sleep thief' sneaking up on Jon and then on Mrs Peters and then Mr Peters. The idea of Jon needing to 'fight off' the 'sneaky sleep thief' was congruent with the step-mother's belief that Jon needed to take more responsibility for himself and Mr Peter's view that Jon was a 'victim'. The siblings, who until now had not been engaged in therapy, formed the 'sibling swat team' whose job was to be alert for the appearance of the 'sneaky sleep thief' and to rescue Jon by diverting his attention, for example using play, music or chores. Mr Peters was to be alert to the sneaky sleep thief sneaking up on his wife, so that he could rescue her, taking her out to dinner or into their bedroom for some time alone.

White (1989) also described a specific intervention to help children overcome fears, in particular those that occur at night. He suggested that, in many instances, the family's response to the child's fears is actually perpetuating them. Parents' eagerness to protect their child from the fear, such as sitting with the child until he or she falls asleep, can result in the child losing the confidence to overcome the fear, and so it intensifies. White encourages the family to confront the fear together and so disrupt the system that is allowing it to survive. The child is encouraged to draw pictures of their fear. It may take the form of monsters, but even if less specific, the child is asked to 'put a face' to their fear. White then goes on to explain to the child his strategy for 'taming monsters' and checks whether the child already knows the 'fourth rule of monsters'. This states that monsters grow more fearsome with night-time practice and more funny with day-time practice. Therefore, if children want a funny time, they need to stop their monster from having night-time practice. The parents are asked to provide a box large enough to contain their child's drawings and a piece of rope. Before bedtime the child is instructed, with parental assistance, to place the drawings in the box, tie the box up with one end of the rope and use the other end to secure the box outside, hanging it from either the branch of a tree or a washing line (it is explained that monsters are less tiresome if their feet cannot touch the ground and, if put outside, will cause less disturbance to the household). The child is told to keep some shoes by their bed, so that if the monsters escape in the night they can be returned to the box. In the morning the child lets the monsters out for day-time practice. Each evening the parents are instructed to reflect on the monster-taming progress and discuss any attempts the monsters have made to provoke them into facilitating their survival. The parents also take photographs of the proceedings, which are taken to the next family meeting.

Tiredness confounds the stress these families are under. Sleep deprivation makes people tired, irritable, depressed and less able to carry out sleep programmes. Parents can easily end up resenting each other, believing that the other should do more to help or be able to manage the child better. Whether the family of a child with a sleep problem has family therapy or not, the nurse must be aware of the effects that the problem is having on the family. These may not only be detrimental to the family but may also become part of a vicious circle that maintains the sleeping problem.

INDIVIDUAL WORK

Individual work with the nurse might include cognitive–behavioural treatment for sleeping difficulties (see above), supporting behavioural programmes for older children (see above) or treatment that is generated from family work.

Sometimes children can be taught to gain control over their nightmares by writing a description of them or drawing a picture, as soon as they wake up, and having a 'special' time to talk about them. It may be possible for the child to create a fantasy superhero, whom they can call on at bedtime to fight off the scary characters in their nightmare (see Chapter 5 – *Individual work, Problem-solving work* on using visual imagery to fight against the symptom). Individual sessions could use role-play to reduce the scary nature of monsters, the key nurse helping the child to see

Paul, aged 11, had recurring nightmares of monsters and witches. He had been admitted to the psychiatric unit because of behavioural problems, which were partly a manifestation of complex partial seizures. His older sister, who was diagnosed with atypical Kleine–Levin syndrome, had severe behavioural problems, which included aggressive outbursts. During family work, the ideas of White (1989) were adopted (see above – Family therapy). Paul drew four pictures of his monsters and witches (e.g. Figure 8.5) in individual work. Whilst on weekend leave, his parents helped him to secure the drawings in a box and tie them outside and during the week, while on the unit, his key nurse assisted him in the ritual. Eventually, once the nightmares ceased, Paul requested that his mother take the pictures to 'the dump' for disposal (Figure 8.5 is a photocopy of the original).

the funny side of them. If two nurses work together, one could act as the monster and the other help the child to frighten the monster off or make friends with 'this rather pathetic creature'.

INDIVIDUAL PSYCHOANALYTICAL PSYCHOTHERAPY

Psychoanalytical psychotherapy may be indicated where the sleep problem is considered to be a symptom of psychological disturbance.

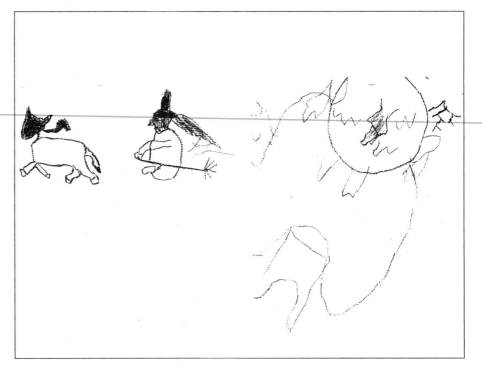

Figure 8.5 Paul, aged 11, drew pictures of his recurring nightmare. Reproduced with permission from the artist.

> Paul's nightmares (first mentioned above) seemed to represent his frightening feelings of being out of control, both of his own seizures and of his sister's aggressive outbursts. Some monsters trod on him, flattening him; others ate him up. Psychotherapy helped Paul to gain some understanding of why they occurred and consequently reduced their scary nature. It also enabled the parents and multi-disciplinary team to have a greater understanding of Paul's behaviour.

MEDICATION

Although sedatives are widely prescribed for sleeping problems, research suggests that they are of extremely limited use in wakeful children (Richman, 1985). Medication may result in short-term improvement in sleeplessness, but there is little long-term benefit. Intolerance to the drug and withdrawal effects may occur. In addition, children who cannot self-soothe are likely to fight against sleep despite sedation, which may result in a paradoxical response, the child becoming extremely 'wired' (Dahl, 1992).

TREATMENT OF PARASOMNIAS

Parasomnias tend to occur more in childhood because the depth and amount of non-REM sleep is greater. Added to this, greater amounts of deep non-REM sleep tend to run in families. However, the amount of deep sleep and, hence, parasomnias can be reduced if measures are taken to reduce excessive tiredness, such as not going to bed very late. Research suggests that changes in sleep schedules, such as giving up a day-time nap, increased stress and heightened activity during the day, and during 'recovery' nights, following sleep loss, night terrors and partial night wakings are more common (Dahl, 1992). Treatment of parasomnias should therefore address the adequacy of the child's sleep.

Treatment must also address any worries, fears and psychological conflicts that may be contributing to parasomnias. Individual work with the nurse, including cognitive–behavioural treatment, psychoanalytical psychotherapy and/or family therapy may be indicated. There is some evidence that helping children to express feelings during the day can reduce the frequency of night terrors (Dahl, 1992).

Kohen and colleagues (1992) described the role of self-hypnosis in the management of night terrors. As children typically cannot recall night terrors and only learn about the night's events from parents in the morning, it is not uncommon for them to express doubts, and also confusion, worry and feelings of guilt. Self-hypnosis gives the child the opportunity to take control. Kohen et al describe the brain to the child, as being like a computer, and the night terror behaviour as an 'accidental bad habit', which can be undone or reduced by 'reprogramming' the computer. This is achieved by training the child in relaxation and mental imagery (self-hypnosis), so that each night before the child goes to sleep, they remind themselves, in a deeply relaxed state, that they will have 'a peaceful, restful, quiet night's sleep in their own bed, and wake up in the morning happy and proud'. Kohen et al used this approach with children aged 8–12 years, who had frequent, prolonged or dangerous night arousals, but no known significant psychological problems. After a 2–3-year follow-up, all children remained asymptomatic, and so it would appear that self-hypnosis is highly successful in treating parasomnias. However, it should be noted that a professional who is trained in hypnosis, usually a clinical psychologist, should always be involved in this intervention.

Perhaps the most important intervention is to educate parents about parasomnias. They can be extremely frightening for the family and are likely to leave parents feeling helpless and concerned for the psychological well-being of their child. The facts that they tend to run in families, are more common in childhood because of the nature of sleep cycles, and that psychopathology is not normally present in young children may be a comfort to parents. Parents should be advised to take all possible measures to ensure the safety of their child during a night terror and, if they are woken themselves, to stay close to their child to avert injury, but not to attempt to wake or comfort them, as this may agitate the child further (a child who is having a nightmare can be woken and comforted). However, waking the child 10–15 minutes before the usual time of the night terror has been shown to be a successful treatment. After 1 week of this intervention by parents, Lask (1988) reported a 100% cessation of night terrors. After 7 weeks, night terrors returned in 3 of the 19 children, but the problem was resolved by reinstating waking for a further week.

MEDICAL TREATMENT

If, during the assessment, it has become apparent that there is a physical cause for the sleep disturbance, medical treatment may alleviate the problem. For example, it is obviously important to address the source of airway obstruction where there is sleep-disordered breathing.

CONCLUSION

The stress caused by sleeping problems should not be underestimated. In extreme cases, it may contribute to child abuse. Health visitors are probably in one of the best positions to identify problems and initiate help.

A thorough assessment of the problem is essential to plan an effective sleep programme. The programme must be tailored to the family. It must obviously address the specific problem, but must also have the parents' support. Unless parents believe that the approach suggested is right for their child and themselves, it is unlikely to succeed.

Where family tensions run high, it may be useful to externalise the problem. This process can take the pressure off the identified child and cause a change in family dynamics, which may have been contributing to the maintenance of the problem.

With imagination and creativity, the nurse can help the young person who is having nightmares to gain a sense of control. Drawing, role-play and imagery can all be used. More straightforward practical measures can be taken to reduce the incidence of parasomnias, although teaching the child self-hypnosis can be particularly effective.

REFERENCES

Anders T, Halpern L and Hua J (1992) Sleeping through the night: a developmental perspective. *Pediatrics* **90**: 554–560.

Anders TF (1994) Infant sleep, nighttime relationships and attachment. *Psychiatry* **57(1)**: 11–21.

Atkinson E, Vetere A and Grayson K (1995) Sleep disruption in young children. The influence of temperament on sleep patterns of pre-school children. *Child: Care, Health and Development* **21(4)**: 233–246.

Balfour AM (1988) A group for parents who have children with sleeping problems. *Health Visitor* **61**: 316–318.

Bartlett L, Johnson C and McGrigor V (1992) Five years experience of a clinic for children's sleep problems. *Association of Child Psychology and Psychiatry Newsletter* **14**: 67–71.

Benoit D, Zeanah CH, Boucher C and Minde KK (1992) Sleep disorders in early childhood: association with insecure maternal attachment. *Journal of the American Academy of Child and Adolescent Psychiatry* **31(1)**: 86–93.

Carpenter A (1990) Sleep problems: a group approach. *Health Visitor* **63(9)**: 305–307.

Chavin W and Tinson S (1980) Children with sleep difficulties. *Health Visitor* **53**: 477–480.

Clore ER and Hibel J (1993) The parasomnias of childhood. *Journal of Pediatric Health Care* **7(1)**: 12–16.

Dahl RE (1992) The pharmacologic treatment of sleep disorders. *Psychiatric Clinics of North America* **15(1)**: 161–178.

Douglas J (1989) Bedtime and sleeping problems. In *Behaviour Problems in Young Children*, pp 116–134. London: Tavistock/ Routledge.

Errante J (1985) Sleep deprivation or postpartum blues? *Topics in Clinical Nursing* **6**: 9–18.

Ferber R (1986a) What we know about sleep. In *Solve Your Child's Sleep Problems,* pp 22–34. London: Dorling Kindersley.

Ferber R (1986b) What your child associates with falling asleep. In *Solve Your Child's Sleep Problems,* pp 53–77. London: Dorling Kindersley.

Ferber R (1986c) Feedings during the night – another major cause of trouble. In *Solve Your Child's Sleep Problems,* pp 78–85. London: Dorling Kindersley.

Ferber R (1986d) Colic and other medical causes of poor sleep. In *Solve Your Child's Sleep Problems,* pp 86–94. London: Dorling Kindersley.

Ferber R (1986e) Sleeptalking, sleepwalking, thrashing and terrors – a spectrum of sudden partial wakings. In *Solve Your Child's Sleep Problems,* pp 127–153. London: Dorling Kindersley.

Johnson M (1991) Infant and toddler sleep: a telephone survey of parents in one community. *Journal of Developmental and Behavioral Pediatrics* **12**: 108–114.

Kahn A, Mozin MJ, Rebuffat E, Sottiaux M and Muller MF (1989) Milk intolerance in children with persistent sleeplessness: a prospective double-blind crossover evaluation. *Pediatrics* **84**: 595–603.

Kerr S and Jowett S (1994) Sleep problems in pre-school children: a review of the literature. *Child: Care, Health and Development* **20(6)**: 379–391.

Kohen DP, Mahowald MW and Rosen GM (1992) Sleep-terror disorder in children: the role of self-hypnosis in management. *American Journal of Clinical Hypnosis* **34(4)**: 233–244.

Lask B (1988) Novel and non-toxic treatment of night terrors. *British Medical Journal* **297**: 592.

Leeson R, Barbour J, Romaniuk D and Warr R (1994) Management of infant sleep problems in a residential unit. *Child: Care, Health and Development* **20(2)**: 89–100.

Mindell JA and Durand VM (1993) Treatment of childhood sleep disorders: generalization across disorders and effects on family members. *Journal of Pediatric Psychology* **18(6)**: 731–750.

Morrison DN, McGee R and Stanton WR (1992) Sleep problems in adolescence. *Journal of the American Academy of Adolescent Psychiatry* **31(1)**: 94–99.

Ollendick TH, Hagopian LP and Huntzinger RM (1991) Cognitive–behavior therapy with nighttime fearful children. *Journal of Behavior Therapy and Experimental Psychiatry* **22(2)**: 113–121.

Pollock JL (1992) Predictors and long-term associations of reported sleeping difficulties in infancy. *Journal of Reproductive and Infant Psychology* **10(3)**: 151–168.

Prest LA and Keene Carruthers W (1991) The case of the sneaky sleep thief – White's externalizing technique within a broad strategic frame. *Journal of Strategic and Systemic Therapies* **10(3–4)**: 66–75.

Quine L (1992) Severity of sleep problems in children with severe learning difficulties: description and correlates. *Journal of Community and Applied Social Psychology* **2(4)**: 247–268.

Reeve A and Miers S (1994) Managing sleep problems in children with special needs. *Health Visitor* **67(7)**: 230–231.

Richman N (1985) A double-blind drug trial in young children with waking problems. *Journal of Child Psychology and Psychiatry* **26**: 591–598.

Richman N, Douglas J, Hunt H, Lansdown R and Levere R (1985) Behavioural methods in the treatment of sleep disorders – a pilot study. *Journal of Child Psychology and Psychiatry* **26**: 581–590.

Tirosh E, Scher A, Sadeh A, Jaffe M, Rubin A, and Lavie P (1993) The effects of illness on sleep behaviour in infants. *European Journal of Pediatrics* **152**: 15–17.

White M (1989) Fear busting and monster taming: an approach to the fears of young children. Selected papers. *Dulwich Centre Review* 107–113.

Wolke D, Meyer R, Ohrt B and Riegel K (1995) The incidence of sleeping problems in preterm and fullterm infants discharged from neonatal special care units: an epidemiological longitudinal study. *Journal of Child Psychology and Psychiatry* **36(2)**: 202–223.

Wright P, Macleod H and Cooper M (1983) Waking at night: the effect of early feeding. *Child: Care, Health and Development* **9**: 309–319.

9 DISTURBED OR UNUSUAL THINKING, ALTERED PERCEPTIONS AND COMMUNICATION DIFFICULTIES

INTRODUCTION

This chapter is concerned with young people who think and perceive the world differently from most others and have difficulties communicating. Some of these children represent the group of patients that are most readily associated with mental illness and are themselves the victims of other's misconceptions. The social isolation that these children may suffer is not only the product of their own difficulties. Essentially this chapter is concerned with two groups of children: those who are psychotic and those with pervasive developmental disorders.

The term 'psychosis' actually means no more than a condition of the mind, although clinically it is accepted as meaning a condition in which there are disturbances of thinking, perception and mood (Steinberg, 1985). Disturbances of thinking include delusions (firmly held beliefs that are not true); a pressure of ideas (the person's mind being bombarded with thoughts); thought block (when the mind becomes blank); disorganised thinking, leading to disorientation and confusion; concrete thinking (a lack of abstract and intuitive thought); and a preoccupation with one's own thoughts, leading to social withdrawal. Disturbances of perception refer to hallucinations (false perceptions), which are most commonly auditory, visual and somatic, and disturbances of mood include manic–depressive swings of mood (although this is rare in childhood) and depression (Wilkinson, 1983).

Children and adolescents may be psychotic as result of a serious psychiatric illness, such as schizophrenia, a neurological disorder or neurological damage, or as a result of contamination with toxic substances. The prevalence of psychotic disorders in adolescence is about 1% (Steinberg, 1985). They are thought to occur less often in infancy and early childhood. However, there is some controversy surrounding the existence of schizophrenia in early childhood and, because a positive diagnosis depends largely on the child's ability to describe symptoms and so convey the presence of thought disturbance, it is quite probable that early childhood schizophrenia is often missed. This view is strongly held by Cantor (1984), who describes 'pre-schizophrenic' signs in early infancy.

Pervasive developmental disorders, such as autism and Asperger's syndrome, have certain features in common with psychoses, such as concrete thinking, an inability to understand other people and a preoccupation with one's own thoughts, together with a lack of awareness of conventions of social interaction. Childhood autism used to be regarded as a form of childhood psychosis, but it is now recognised that autism has more in common with other developmental disorders. The prevalence of autism is 2–4 per 10 000 population, although the rate rises to 20 in

10 000 if severely learning impaired children, who have some autistic features, are included (Rutter, 1985).

Reviewing the literature on schizophrenia and autism in young people, it is easy to see how these disorders were once placed in the same diagnostic category. They present with some remarkably similar problems. It can be confusing to read the scope of opinion regarding the aetiology, diagnosis and treatment of these disorders. Perhaps all that is clear, is that there are still enormous gaps in our knowledge concerning the way that the mind works and what influences it.

To summarise, the nurse will come across children and adolescents who have disturbed thoughts, or at least think differently from most others, who perceive the world differently and who have difficulties communicating. Some will be given a diagnosis but, regardless of this, the nurse must identify the problems the child is experiencing and subsequently plan effective intervention. In addition, whatever the diagnosis may be, the aetiology is most likely to involve a number of factors. Possible contributing factors include:

✦   Genetic predisposition

✦   Perinatal trauma producing neurological damage

✦   Other trauma producing neurological damage

✦   Neoplasms resulting in neurological damage

✦   Poisoning or drug intoxication

✦   Neurological infection

✦   Stress

✦   Sensory overload

✦   Family patterns of communication

ASSESSMENT

MEDICAL/PSYCHIATRIC ASSESSMENT

Medical/psychiatric assessment will include a thorough history of the family, the child's birth and developmental progress, and a description of the parent's concerns. The psychiatrist will assess the child's mental state and initiate a thorough physical assessment, which may involve other medical colleagues. The onset of symptoms may have been precipitated by organic factors which are amenable to medical treatment.

The history is likely to help in the process of differential diagnosis. For example, in certain disorders, such as schizophrenia and affective disorders (mood disorders), genetic factors have a clear contribution to aetiology. Therefore, a family history of such disorders would alert the doctor to the possibility of the child's symptoms being a manifestation of a similar problem. Certain developmental trends may suggest a particular diagnosis, although some similarities may occur across diagnoses, such as schizophrenia and autism. Gordon (1992) actually suggests that young children with autistic features may well go on to develop either autism or schizophrenia.

INDIVIDUAL ASSESSMENT

Interviewing the child

Care should be taken that the doctor's mental state examination is not duplicated. The important thing is that certain information is obtained by the multi-disciplinary team. A mental state examination consists of six components: appearance and behaviour, speech, thought content and flow, mood and affect, perceptions, and cognitive capacity. It is important that a psychiatrist is involved in assessing the child's mental state, but it may be that a nurse will continue pursuing certain areas. What is vital is that there is good team communication, so that the child is not bombarded with questions.

It is particularly important to meet the child in a quiet place free from distractions. The child who has disordered thinking is likely to feel threatened by questioning and so it is paramount that the assessment is approached with sensitivity, and care is taken to gain the child's trust. It may be helpful to meet the child with one of the parents. Wilkinson (1983) usefully points out that the psychotic child may not perceive the nurse's personality and behaviour as it is intended or expected, and indeed those with autism or Asperger's syndrome are unlikely to perceive nurse's demeanour accurately.

One approach might be to start with simple, general, life questions, such as what the child enjoys doing, where they go to school, who is in the family, leading on to what the child's understanding is of why their parents have brought them to the hospital/clinic. Sometimes it will be immediately apparent that the child does not understand, is confused or has more outrageous thought disturbances. At other times the nurse may simply believe that the child is somehow 'different' from other children.

Some children may be unable to differentiate themselves from the outside world. The child may report that objects or people are inside them or that things happening in the environment are also happening to them. This phenomenon is often referred to as the **blurring of ego boundaries** and is a feature of psychosis. It is important that the nurse not only enquires about the content of these experiences, but also asks how the young person feels about them. The child may be equally frightened or comforted by them (Barker, 1985).

The blurring of ego boundaries may extend to a belief that the child's actions are being controlled from some outside force. The child may describe thoughts being drained from him/her and this may be demonstrated by **thought blocking**, when the child suddenly appears to stop thinking. Alternatively, **thought broadcasting** may be described, when the child believes that others can 'tune in' to their thoughts. This loss of personal control is often thought to be indicative of schizophrenia.

Dissociation of affect refers to a blunting of feelings. It is not uncommon for people who are under stress to experience this phenomenon, for example following a bereavement. The person feels as though they are outside the situation, looking in, feeling calm and detached. One can see how useful this may be as a defence against overwhelming emotion. However, if this experience occurs in a variety of settings, without the evidence of stress, it may suggest a serious emotional disturbance.

Asking a child what sort of things they like doing may help the nurse to start forming an idea of what the child values and believes in. It can also highlight any obsessive interests and lead to a question concerning whether the child likes to be alone and has a tendency to be introspective, or enjoys mixing with others. Extreme beliefs or convictions and obsessive interests can become a problem if they influence daily life significantly. The nurse's questioning should therefore attempt to discover their effect on the child's and the family's life, as well as their content.

Delusions must be assessed with the child's developmental age in mind and in the context of the child's family and culture. Deciding whether someone's belief is false or true is highly subjective, and so the nurse must take care to view the child's belief in context. It is also important to discover how much these thoughts dominate the child's mind and whether they interfere with everyday living. Delusions can take many forms, including 'persecution' (the young person believing that others are against them),'jealousy' (for example, believing that a parent loves a sibling more than them), 'grandeur' (the young person believing that they have abilities that are far superior to reality), 'ill-health' (believing that they are seriously ill) and 'guilt' (the young person having extreme feelings of reproach for some act they have perpetrated).

Hallucinations or false perceptions can also take many forms. They should be distinguished from illusions, which are distortions of reality, and are a common occurrence. Illusions make us question reality, whereas hallucinations are experienced as reality. It is helpful to establish whether voices are heard inside or outside the child's head. We all experience 'voices inside our head' (when we talk to ourselves in our head or simply have thoughts), but voices outside are indicative of an hallucination.

Whilst meeting with child, the nurse should make a note of the child's appearance and behaviour during the interview:

◆ *Describe the child's general appearance* What was the young person's racial background, was he/she thin or overweight, tall or short, and so on. Was the child clean and reasonably well dressed or was there evidence that they were not caring for themselves? It is likely that this child will need help, or at least supervision, to care adequately for him/herself.

◆ *Describe the child's posture and any strange mannerisms or movements* Various anomalies in posture, difficulties in fine and gross motor function, and odd mannerisms and movements have been associated with schizophrenia, autism and Asperger's syndrome. For example, hypotonia is associated with schizophrenia, clumsiness with Asperger's syndrome and odd movements, such as arm flapping, with autism. Those already on anti-psychotic medication may also exhibit extra-pyramidal motor effects, such as facial tics, a shuffling walk, muscle rigidity and tremors.

◆ *Assess speech for its style, rate, volume and quantity* Did the child have to be coaxed to talk or did he/she talk spontaneously? Did the child demonstrate any control over what was being said, or did he/she seem to say whatever came into his/her mind? Did the child speak loudly or softly, and was there variation in tone? Did the child demonstrate any unusual speech characteristics, such as repeating words said to him/her (echolalia) or using made-up words (neologisms)? Speech anomalies are characteristic of both schizophrenia and autism.

◆ *Describe the child's social interaction* For example, did the young person use eye contact? Did they place themselves at a comfortable distance from you or inappropriately close? Did they appear to have an understanding of social norms in communication and behaviour?

◆ *Evaluate the child's mood* This should be done subjectively, asking the child how they feel, and objectively, the nurse making her/his own observation based on the child's appearance and behaviour.

Catherine, aged 14 years, was admitted to the psychiatric unit for assessment. Her individual assessment is summarised:

Catherine presented as a tall, thin, white girl, standing with a stooped posture and pacing up and down the room restlessly. When asked to sit, she did so, but continued to move her legs compulsively. Some paucity of movement would be in keeping with her medication, chlorpromazine. Catherine's speech was fast, with a flat intonation, and she giggled at inappropriate moments in our conversation. At times she appeared distracted, as if listening to something else. She seemed to have some insight into her problems. However, she may simply have been repeating what she has heard her parents talk about. They talk openly in front of Catherine about her being mentally ill. Catherine talked about peers at school picking on her and conveyed a belief that they were trying to kill her. She explained that that is why she has stopped going to school. She also talked about a famous boxer who she believes is controlling her. She conveyed feeling comforted and reassured by this person. Her father is very keen on boxing, often going to watch live fights, as well as watching boxing on television. It is not unusual for him to have a number of friends at the house to watch the sport with him. Catherine has a very close relationship with her father and spends much time with him.

Observation of play

Atlas (1990) describes using play to assist in the differential diagnosis of schizophrenia and autism. In his research study, children were shown ten play articles, which were arranged in a circle (black and white baby dolls, a truck with movable human figures, a dump truck, aeroplane, hand puppet, telephone, teddy bear, teaset, bottle and a cradle with a blanket). The 'evaluator' named the objects, told the child that they could play with them and withdrew to the corner of the room. The evaluator or a second person then recorded the spontaneous behaviour of the child every 15 seconds. The child's play was rated as 'symbolic' (pretend play, using the toys symbolically), 'stereotyped' (symbolic, but repetitive and lacking purpose or goals) or 'not symbolic'. Schizophrenic children played symbolically, whereas autistic children showed no symbolic play. Stereotyped play was a characteristic of children who presented with a condition somewhere in between autism and schizophrenia.

In reality, the characteristics of play are not so clearcut according to the child's disorder; for example, some autistic children will play symbolically to a limited extent and may demonstrate stereotyped play. However, observation of a child's play will certainly give some indication as to the nature of the problem and may also highlight possible areas of internal conflict for the child. Play not only serves a developmental function, enabling the child to practise social and creative skills, but is also a medium through which the child can process thoughts and feelings. The nurse should simply record what she/he observes, rather than making interpretations or diagnoses, so that these observations can be used along with other aspects of the assessment to establish a holistic view of the child. The description of play might usefully include:

◆ *The type of play* Symbolic, not symbolic and/or stereotyped.

◆ *A description of the content of play*

◆ *A description of the feelings evoked in the nurse by play* This may give some indication as to the feelings the child was re-enacting through play.

◆ *The child's interaction with the nurse* Did the child involve you in play (unlike in the research study mentioned, the author would suggest being available to the child and not withdrawing to observe) or play in isolation.

◆ *The apparent mood of the child*

◆ *A description of the child's use of language* Was language delay apparent and/or speech anomalies?

◆ *Any evidence of unusual posture, movements or mannerisms*

◆ *Any evidence of altered perceptions* Did the child's behaviour suggest altered perceptions, such as hallucinations or delusions? Perhaps the child seemed to be suddenly distracted, as if hearing another's voice, or the content of play appeared indicative of some delusion. Obviously, a healthy imagination could be misconstrued as delusional thinking, and so, again, it is paramount that the nurse's observations are seen in the context of the whole assessment.

INDIVIDUAL PSYCHOTHERAPY ASSESSMENT

The psychoanalytical understanding of psychosis is that it represents a defence mechanism. The outside world is experienced as unbearable and so the person withdraws to a more tolerable fantasy world, denying reality. Whether the primary cause of the child's problems are psychological or not, there will certainly be emotional sequelae. Therefore, assessment by a child psychotherapist may usefully begin to highlight some of the internal conflicts the child is experiencing.

At one time, many psychoanalysts believed that 'autism' (a Greek word meaning a preoccupation with internal stimuli) was a part of natural development and that the disorder, similarly named, represented either a failure in development or a regression to this state. The mother–child relationship was seen as fundamental in determining successful development. Today, most psychoanalysts accept the evidence that there is probably an important physical basis to autism, but that, as in any disorder that disrupts life, there will be emotional consequences and these in turn may cause 'secondary handicap' (C. Hughes, 1994).

FAMILY ASSESSMENT

The family is likely to be frightened of the diagnosis that their child may be given, worried as to what lies behind his/her problems and anxious for the future to look brighter. The family assessment should attempt to establish the family's understanding of the child's problems and how the family is coping. The child's behaviour may have changed suddenly or the family may have been struggling with a 'difficult' child for a long time. Equally, the family may have ideas regarding the cause of the child's problems or may be baffled and confused.

Research suggests that certain characteristics of communication in the family, high 'expressed emotion' (EE) and 'communication deviance' (CD), are associated with the onset and maintenance of schizophrenic symptoms (Rund et al, 1995). Expressed emotion is a measure of the extent to which a relative expresses highly critical, hostile and/or over-involved attitudes towards the patient. Communication deviance is a measure of the degree to which an individual is unable to establish and maintain a shared focus of attention with a listener during verbal transactions. It is a measure of egocentricity and an inability to take the perspective of others. During the family assessment, the therapist should attempt to gain some understanding of how the family members interact. It has been suggested that high EE develops in response to the patient's behaviour. Frustration, distress and concern can sometimes lead to intrusive and/or critical interactions between the patient and his/her relatives. Such negative experiences precipitate a relapse in psychotic symptoms and so a vicious circle of harmful communication evolves (Kavanagh, 1992).

Earnshaw (1994) describes how family management of autistic children may confound their lack of a sense of self.

When visiting one particular family and asking how the 8-year-old autistic child slept, the 15-year-old brother explained:
' "Well, I take her up to bed at 8 o'clock – that's her bedtime, and she comes into bed with me for a cuddle and we watch T.V. When she goes to sleep, I go downstairs and do my homework. When I'm ready for bed I go up and lift her across into her own bed (in the same room), and I go to sleep myself in my bed". Mother carried on: "She always wakes up in between me and her dad every morning, she gets in quietly some time in the night" '. When Earnshaw 'asked if the family thought that all this could be confusing for her, mother said "That's what I've always said", but brother said, "But it's so nice!" Father said absolutely nothing' (p. 89).

The families of autistic children that Earnshaw met appeared unable to set limits and tended, instead, to go along with their child's wishes and preferences. She conjectures that the autistic child, with a lack of a sense of self, is not recognised as a unique individual, but comes to represent someone else unconsciously by the parents. This other person is someone in the family who has died and for whom the family has not successfully grieved. Family deaths through generations have been a recurring theme in Earnshaw's work with families of autistic children. Whether or not an autistic child becomes a focus of unresolved family feelings, family management of the child will influence his/her developmental progress.

HOME VISIT

See Appendix A – *Home visit*. Visiting the family in their own home environment will enable the nurse to gain further insight into family dynamics and coping skills, and provides an opportunity to offer the family support. Parents are likely to be more relaxed and able to ask questions away from the hospital or clinic setting. Concerns about mental illness and psychiatry should be brought out into the open and any myths dispelled. A common misconception regarding schizophrenia is that it is a disorder in which the personality is split. 'Schizophrenia' is a Greek word meaning 'split mind', but actually refers to the split or incongruency that occurs between emotions and thoughts, for example laughing whilst describing a tragic event.

SCHOOL VISIT

Visiting the child's school and talking to his/her teacher will provide further information concerning the child's development and behaviour (see Appendix B – *School visit)*. Particular areas of discussion should include:

◆ *The child's intellectual capacity and language development*

◆ *Ability to understand abstract concepts*

◆ *Characteristics of play* Does the child use symbolic play; are there signs of stereotypy; and does the child play alone, with peers, or in parallel?

◆ *Social skills* Does the child mix easily with peers? The schizophrenic and, indeed, autistic child is likely to be apart from his/her peers, either behaving as though others do not exist or trying to control and boss other children around, unable to hear their point of view. How does the child relate to adults?

◆ *Particular interests* Does the child have a tendency to perseverate over things or have a particular interest from which they cannot easily be distracted?

◆ *Anxiety or depression* Does the child appear more anxious than most or is he/she consistently sad or upset?

◆ *Motor development* Is the child well coordinated or clumsy; able to perform fine motor skills; have any unusual movements or mannerisms.

◆ *Evidence of hallucinations or delusions*

MILIEU ASSESSMENT

The milieu assessment will provide a valuable opportunity to record further information along the lines already mentioned, but in a less formal environment and over a period of time. The nurse can observe whether the child behaves differently under different circumstances, for example whether certain stimuli seem to make the child anxious or provoke hallucinations.

EARLY DETECTION OF PROBLEMS

Early detection of serious psychiatric illness is very important. Delays in receiving treatment for schizophrenia are associated with a slower and less complete recovery (Edwards et al, 1994). During this period, the normal development of the young person is put on hold, and family and social relationships are strained. Werry and co-workers (1991) identified a 15% mortality rate amongst adolescents with schizophrenia, which was attributed to suicide and delusional driven accidents.

Similarly, children with pervasive developmental disorders, such as autism, will benefit from early diagnosis. It can only be to the benefit of the child to receive appropriate education and management as soon as possible, and for the family to receive much needed support.

NURSING/MULTI-DISCIPLINARY INTERVENTION

The initial concern must be whether the child is best treated as an outpatient or admitted to a child or adolescent psychiatric unit. A decision will be made based on:

✦ The impact that the child's difficulties are having on the family and their ability to cope.

✦ Whether the child is likely to come to any harm or to harm others.

✦ The perceived need, or otherwise, of assessment and treatment in an alternative environment from home, where skilled nursing staff can observe the child around the clock and a therapeutic milieu is considered necessary to achieve therapeutic goals.

Some children will, of course, be on general paediatric wards, either because they require treatment for a seemingly unrelated problem or because disturbed thoughts and/or altered perceptions are primarily the result of organic pathology or a toxic reaction. Paediatric nurses should liaise with psychiatric services, including a child psychiatric clinical nurse specialist or nurses working within child psychiatry, to facilitate the provision of truly holistic care.

Most children that the nurse will come across who have disturbed or unusual thinking, altered perceptions and communication difficulties cannot be 'cured', but nursing/multi-disciplinary intervention can go a long way to help the child and family to function optimally with the disabilities they have. It is therefore important that the nurse sets realistic, achievable goals, so that all involved do not become disillusioned and demoralised.

FAMILY THERAPY AND PARENTAL COUNSELLING/EDUCATION

There is considerable evidence that family-based psycho-education, which focuses on communication skills, support and problem-solving, can help in the management of schizophrenia, reducing cognitive symptoms in the patient and enabling the family to cope (Zastowny et al, 1992).

Psycho-education might begin by teaching the family about the prevalence, aetiology, symptomatology and course of the child's disorder, dispelling myths and reassuring the family that they have not caused the illness. Sessions could then move on to problem-solving and enhancing family communication.

Early relapse of psychotic symptoms is three to four times more likely in high expressed emotion (EE) than low EE households (Parker and Hadzi-Pavlovic, 1990; Kavanagh, 1992). Therefore, in families where high EE has been identified, the family therapist should aim to facilitate change. Strategies for intervention to reduce EE might include:

◆ Enhancing the family's listening skills.

◆ Teaching the family to speak concretely and concisely.

◆ Teaching parents calmly to set clear, firm limits of behaviour with their children.

◆ Promoting the individual growth of each family member to reduce enmeshment.

Teaching parents problem solving skills and getting them to practise these in family meetings will help to empower them, improving their self-esteem and ability to cope. An example of problem-solving would be for the parents to find a way of spending time alone together. The strategies that they could come up with include: asking another relative to 'baby-sit'; booking a table at a restaurant; preparing the relative for all feared eventualities; agreeing to telephone home once, on their arrival at the restaurant; agreeing to support each other whilst out, not allowing discussion to veer towards talking about their child. This particular example of problem-solving also tackles parental over-involvement, which is a component of high EE.

McFarlane et al (1995) have demonstrated that meeting with groups of families, rather than meeting with individual families, is more effective in the treatment of schizophrenia. Intervening processes that might account for this include:

◆ Enabling families to meet together expands their network for support.

◆ Multiple-family groups absorb more of the anxiety and stress generated by psychotic symptoms than single-family treatment sessions.

◆ Problem-solving capacities are expanded with an increase in the number of participants.

◆ Over-involved families tend to become less so, once they start to develop relationships outside the family.

◆ Multiple-family groups tend to have a more positive emotional tone, with greater warmth and humour than in single-family meetings.

Similar approaches to family work are likely to be helpful where the child has autism or Asperger's syndrome. The case example cited from Earnshaw (1994) demonstrates how families may inadvertently confound the child's problems, by colluding with their child's preferences and probable underlying anxieties.

INDIVIDUAL WORK

Coursey and colleagues (1995) undertook a piece of research looking at the value of individual psychotherapy for those with serious mental illness. Some 72% of patients found individual therapy to be helpful and thought that it had brought a positive change to their lives. In relation to medication, only 16% considered that medication alone was most useful, 25% found talking therapy was most useful and 60% believed that a combination of the two was most effective. Of those with schizophrenia, 84% preferred brief, less frequent, reality-oriented therapy over longer, more frequent, insight-oriented therapy. Reality-oriented therapy addressed current, often practical, problems that the patient wanted to overcome. Persons who felt empowered by therapy spent less time in hospital, expected a shorter time in therapy and were better informed about their problems. Although this research involved adults with serious mental illness, it probably also has some relevance for children and adolescents. In the author's experience, it seems particularly useful to have concrete goals in individual work. This is also the case when working with children with autism or Asperger's syndrome. Obviously, the extent and type of individual work that can be done will depend entirely on the individual child and the present state of their condition.

Ideas for individual work include:

◆ *Play a game* Care must be taken to choose a game that the child can manage and which will not heighten their anxiety. For example, many children with autism and Asperger's syndrome seem to enjoy activities involving numbers, counting and construction. They are perhaps less likely to enjoy games that require abstract thought or imagination.

◆ *Play particular games to enhance specific skills* For example, 'Face games' by Nes Arnold promotes the ability to recognise, perform and comprehend a variety of facial expressions. Alternatively, make up your own game (Figure 9.1).

◆ *Read a story* Similarly, care must be taken in choosing the story. Children who have a tendency to think concretely or who cannot distinguish reality from fantasy may be easily frightened. It may also be important to point out each time that you read a story, that it is just that.

David, an 8-year-old boy with Asperger's syndrome, had a pet rabbit about which he thought a great deal and spent hours taking care of, when he was at home. His key worker chose a children's country tale to read to David in the evening. Unfortunately, soon into the story, a rabbit was cooked for tea. David was distraught and ran about the room screaming.

◆ *Simple cognitive work to address delusions* See Chapter 4 – *Individual work, Cognitive therapies*. It may be possible to challenge or reality-test certain delusions, such as those of persecution.

◆ *Teach a social skill* See Chapter 3 – *Targeting the behavioural problem* for the case vignette of David.

◆ *Teach relaxation skills* See Chapter 4 – *Individual work, Relaxation*.

◆ *Make a life book* This may help the young person in their struggle to find a sense of self (see Chapter 2 – *Individual work, Improving self-esteem*).

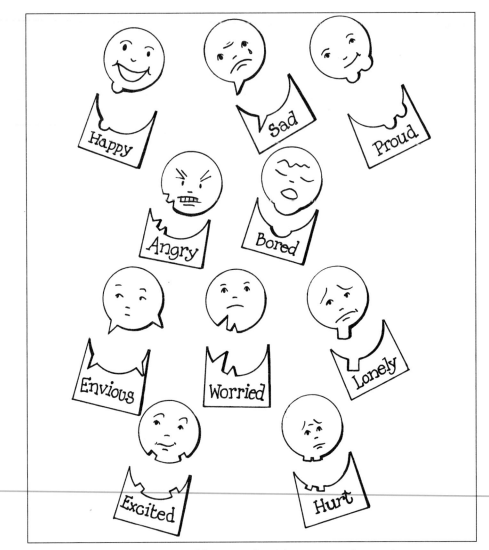

Figure 9.1 A game of faces: cardboard cut-outs to fit together.

◆ *Teach the young person about their disorder and the positive steps that can be taken to gain some control.*

◆ *Activities to raise self-esteem* See Chapter 2 – *Individual work, Improving self-esteem.*

◆ *Growing up work* Entering puberty can be particularly frightening for the schizophrenic child, who may view the menarche or the occurrence of nocturnal emissions as the loss of his/her own ability to control bodily secretions. Preparation and continuing reassurance and support are therefore paramount. Some will regress and need firm behavioural intervention to enable them to learn how to care for themselves, such as during the menstrual cycle. The young person entering puberty is likely to become increasingly preoccupied with their body and may be prone to bodily delusions. Awakening sexuality may evoke confusion, fear and/or disgust, and the teenager may masturbate inappropriately, in public, or insert objects into their body, so putting themselves at risk of harm (see Chapter 10 – *Individual work, Growing up work*).

Catherine (mentioned above) became noticeably agitated during her menstrual cycle and would leave soiled sanitary towels around the unit. She would giggle inappropriately when asked to put them in the sanitary bin and run about the unit exposing herself. During group activities or whilst watching television with other children, she would masturbate. On one occasion, Catherine had been found alone in her bedroom, trying to insert a pencil into her vagina. As well as firm limit-setting and practical help, Catherine appeared to benefit from simple growing up sessions.

Cantor (1984) described a 14-year-old boy who appeared to respond to his increased muscle mass by developing the delusion that he was the 'incredible hulk'.

Obviously there are likely to be other factors, besides puberty, that will contribute to such extreme reactions and determine the type of reaction. Catherine was known to have been sexually abused and the boy who Cantor described, was thought to be unable to verbalise his rage with his alcoholic father.

Another finding of the research conducted by Coursey et al (1995) was that friendliness was the most desired quality in the therapist. As the child is likely to suffer social isolation, he/she may want the nurse to be their friend. There is a fine line between being friendly and being a friend, and so the nurse will need to establish clear boundaries sensitively.

INDIVIDUAL PSYCHOANALYTICAL PSYCHOTHERAPY

Although the author has stressed the importance of practical reality-based individual work, it is not her intention to negate the value of psychoanalytical psychotherapy. As mentioned in the assessment, whether important psychological factors have contributed to the aetiology of the child's problems or not, there will certainly be emotional sequelae and possibly 'secondary handicap'. As well as giving the child space to vent feelings and attempting to make sense of these, the psychotherapist can play an important role in enabling the young person to develop a sense of self.

Hughes stresses the importance of using counter-transference in trying to understand Dean and of commenting on 'what' his experience was, rather than 'why.' After 18 months in therapy, Dean started to play symbolically, talk about his thoughts and feelings, ask pertinent questions and grapple with complex emotional ideas. Outside therapy, he started to become more involved in the life of his foster family, would play with other children and became more aware of social norms of behaviour.

Carol Hughes (1994) describes her therapy sessions with a 9-year-old autistic boy called Dean. His mother had suffered prenatal and postnatal depression, the parents had separated when he was 18 months old, and he was taken 'into care' after his mother declared she could no longer cope.

'Looking past me – anywhere but into my eyes – he insistently asked innumerable questions about my car. What colour was it? What year? Did it have electric windows or central locking? I found it difficult to think and felt coerced into mindlessly answering his questions… I·tried to get him to tell me why he was interested … His response to my refusal to answer his obsessive questioning was to deteriorate into a flap. He lay on the floor flapping his arms, kicking his legs up rhythmically and spinning the wheels of the toy car from time to time. He screamed 'Pack your bags!' almost continuously for the rest of the session. It lasted many months … He conveyed in a most powerful way his experience of mindlessness. In the countertransference I would be unable to think. I felt baffled, bewildered and at times quite violent … Dean conveyed to me a powerful sense of panic – that he was literally in a flap … I found myself on the floor with him stroking his back, murmuring gently, 'Calm down, calm down'. I do not think that he heard my words for many sessions but felt the physical presence and the tone of reassurance and calm. Gradually over time he would quieten enough to allow me to talk in a general way about the fear, the panic, the flap' (pp 46–48, 50–51).

SOCIAL SKILLS TRAINING

Research suggests that social skills training can improve social skills, including assertiveness, in those with schizophrenia and can increase the discharge rate from hospital and delay relapse (Stirling, 1994).

Any child who has extreme difficulties interacting socially should be entitled to the opportunity of some social skills training. Programmes should aim to improve verbal and non-verbal skills, and enhance more accurate social perception. Sessions might start by addressing basic communication skills and progress on to assertiveness. Direct instruction, communication games, role modelling (live and video), direct feedback, practice in sessions and homework tasks are some of the training methods that can be used (Edwards et al, 1994; Dobson et al, 1995).

The young person may also need help in learning more concrete, practical, social skills, such as washing, dressing, shopping, using a telephone, and so on. Where a child has a particular skill, such as memorising train timetables, the nurse should make use of it in training, to enhance self-esteem. This child may easily become frustrated and demoralised if social skills training does nothing but reinforce their inadequacies.

MUSIC, ART, DRAMA AND DANCE THERAPY

Music therapy has been used successfully to improve social skills in both individuals with autism and schizophrenia. Tang et al (1994) demonstrated how music therapy could improve the ability of those with schizophrenia to converse with others, reduce their social isolation and increase their level of interest in external events. Therapy involved listening to music, talking about the content, style and imagery of the music, singing along to music, singing in rounds and playing with instruments. This therapeutic use of music could easily be facilitated by nurses with some musical skill.

Other forms of expressive therapy, such as dance, drama and art, can help to reduce social isolation if used in a group setting, and provide a means of communicating feelings that cannot easily be expressed verbally. Children and adolescents with language difficulties and thought disorder will find it particularly difficult to talk coherently about their thoughts and feelings.

MILIEU THERAPY

An environment of low expressed emotion

For children with schizophrenia, it has been shown that a climate of low expressed emotion is most helpful. This is probably true for most children, and particularly for those with autism and Asperger's syndrome. Staff should approach the management of children in a matter-of-fact style, not becoming too 'heated' or emotional themselves. Limits should be set firmly, but kindly, and clear concise language used.

Structure and close supervision

The child must be given every opportunity to develop to his/her optimum potential. Children with cognitive difficulties or disturbed thoughts will benefit from a structured timetable, similar to that described for the overactive child (see Chapter 3 – *Milieu therapy, Structure and individual attention*). A high level of individual supervision and attention is necessary both to keep the child involved in an activity and to prevent perseveration. The young person's development will be enhanced if they are 'kept on track'. However, in the case of the child with schizophrenia, care must be taken not to swamp the child and become intrusive, as this is likely to exacerbate their psychotic symptoms.

Social integration

The daily timetable should include socialising, such as joining others at mealtimes and for group activities. Dobson et al (1995) have demonstrated the positive effect of social activity groups in the treatment of schizophrenia. Autistic individuals generally avoid interaction with others and therefore need gentle coercion. It may also be helpful to consider rewarding interaction in some way. However, social goals must be manageable for the child. If the young person believes that they have 'lost contact' with the group, they are likely to become distressed and disruptive. An example of an appropriate goal for a child who finds group activities particularly difficult might be to spend a limited time in groups, followed by time with their key nurse. If the nurse is to help raise this child's self-esteem, the child must not be set up, albeit inadvertently, to fail.

Utilising the child's strengths

A child's special interest may be used constructively to help raise their self-esteem. Obviously, it is not helpful to allow the child to perseverate on one aspect of their interest but, with creative management, it may be possible to expand and develop their interest, and subsequently gain the child much admiration from others.

> David, a 10-year-old boy with Asperger's syndrome (first described in Chapter 3), was fanatical about the London Underground map, and knew it off by heart. While on the psychiatric unit, David was encouraged to complete a project on the Tube system in London. This included writing a questionnaire to take to the nearby station to find out the role of different employees, such as the ticket collector; taking a trip on the Docklands light railway with his key nurse; and visiting the London Transport Museum.

Firm limit-setting

The shaky ego of the young person is revealed by an inability to comprehend social norms (the ego is the part of the psyche that regulates behaviour, listening to basic internal drives and wishes, and modifying behaviour according to learnt social expectations). The child may have difficulty in understanding the need for privacy of those around them. He/she is likely to stare, interrupt conversations, approach others uncomfortably closely, and talk loudly or laugh at inappropriate moments. Any attempt to explain socially acceptable behaviour is likely to be met with a perplexed look and/or an increase in anxiety and disruptive behaviour. However, it is important to help the young person to learn about appropriate behaviour, and so firm limits should be set. The child needs to be put in touch with reality, rather than allowed just to respond to internal drives and wishes.

Protect the child from bullying

A lack of awareness of social norms, particularly sexual disinhibition, may lay the young person open to ridicule and scapegoating. Other teenagers, who are having to deal with their own insecurities during puberty, may encourage the child to expose themselves. The unit or ward must have a policy for dealing with bullying in order to protect children, safeguarding their self-esteem and teaching the need for self-respect. The unit philosophy should not tolerate bullying and there must be sanctions for such behaviour.

Challenging hallucinations

The child who is hallucinating will need reassurance that what is seen or heard is not actually happening. The nurse must acknowledge that the experience feels very real, but can gently point out that the 'pictures' or 'voices' are in fact inside the child's head, 'a bit like a dream'. Some children may not be able to talk about their hallucinations, but if the child is behaving in such a way as to suggest hallucination, the nurse should attempt to intervene. For example, if the child is talking into space, the nurse could ask who they are talking to. If the child describes a person, the nurse can explain that this picture of a person is actually only inside their head and that really there is no-one there.

Challenging delusions

Helping the child to feel safe with reality is one approach for managing delusions. For example, the boy who over-identifies with a tomato could be gently, but repeatedly, told that 'boys are much nicer than tomatoes', and the girl who has delusions of grandeur and says that she can swim miles, when she cannot in fact swim at all, might be reminded that 'it is OK not being able to swim, because you can easily learn' (Cantor, 1984).

Maintaining the child's safety

The child's safety must be maintained at all times. The young person, frightened by their symptoms and/or depressed, may attempt to self-harm or to harm others. The unit environment must be kept as safe as possible and supervision of the child increased when considered appropriate. Occasionally nurses may need to restrain the young person in order to ensure their safety (see Chapter 3 – *Milieu therapy, Safety*).

The child who is socially disinhibited is also vulnerable to abuse. Personal safety issues may be addressed in social skills training, but this should be consolidated on in the milieu. Firm limit-setting and simple explanations are required.

Facilitating language development

Children who have difficulty articulating their thoughts need encouragement to do so, whereas those who have a tendency to allow all their thoughts to spill out need to be taught to gain some control. The nurse will need to use all her/his listening skills to try to understand what the young person is trying to communicate. Where there is 'poverty of speech' and the child replys to questions with brief phrases or even monosyllables, the nurse will need to ask many questions and reflect what she/he believes is being said, in order to gain any understanding. The nurse may also need to decipher language anomalies, such as 'word salad', when a numbers of words are spoken but sentences are not formed.

Preventive nursing management

Finally, in relation to the milieu, it is worth noting the role that the nurse can take in preventing certain psychoses in general paediatrics. For example, it is recognised that patients in intensive care units (ICUs) can develop delirium with psychotic-like symptoms, including auditory or visual hallucinations and distortions of reality, involving time, place and person. Sleep deprivation, sensory monotony and stress are thought to be important contributory factors. Julie Hughes (1994) described a case of ICU psychosis in an 18-month-old girl following cardiac surgery. The nurse in the paediatric ICU can play a significant role in reducing the likelihood of a child developing this condition. Pre-hospital admission preparation, family-centred care, enabling children to use play to overcome fear and gain a sense of control, and ensuring adequate sleep are some of the ways that the nurse can reduce the trauma of hospitalisation and subsequent risk of ICU psychoses.

MEDICAL TREATMENT

Early identification of psychosis resulting from drug toxicity can ensure speedy treatment and subsequent recovery. For example, anticholinergic toxicity can be treated with drug discontinuation, sedation and hydration, together with small doses of neuroleptic drugs to treat the psychotic symptoms. Similarly, psychoses resulting primarily from organic pathology may be amenable to treatment.

MEDICATION

Little is known about the response of childhood schizophrenia to neuroleptic medications (i.e. drugs that affect the nervous system), although limited research suggests that the response is similar to that of adults (McClellan and Werry, 1992; Campbell et al, 1993) .

Overt psychotic symptoms, that is hallucinations and delusions, are often responsive to neuroleptic medication, such as chlorpromazine and haloperidol. However, a minority of patients show little or no response and, because the individual rate of response also varies, it is necessary to wait 4–6 weeks before realising the full therapeutic effect. These are powerful drugs with unpleasant side-effects and so dosage should be kept to a minimum. For those with chronic psychotic disorders, following an acute psychotic episode, dosage is either lowered to a maintenance level or a 'targeted approach' is taken, whereby prodromal signs of a psychotic episode are identified and medication is administered at these times.

The nurse must be aware and observant of the side-effects of neuroleptic drugs. These include:

✦ *Dystonias* Acute and often painful involuntary movements, commonly seen in the neck or trunk muscles and in the extraocular muscles, leading to opisthotonos and oculogyric crisis respectively. If dystonias are observed, the prescribed antidote must be given immediately and medical staff informed.

✦ *Parkinsonism* Tremor, rigidity, akinesia (absence of movement) and bradykinesia (decrease in movement).

✦ *Akathisia* – A subjective sensation with or without objective restlessness. The young person may complain of feeling that they are 'crawling out of their skin' and/or the nurse may observe shuffling of the feet or an inability to sit in one place. Akathisia is difficult to identify because similar signs are indicative of psychosis itself or anxiety.

✦ *Tardive dyskinesia* Involuntary choreoathetoid movements, most commonly lip smacking, tongue oscillations and hand/finger clenching.

✦ *Seizures*

◆ *Neuroleptic malignant syndrome* This is a life-threatening condition with a mortality rate of 4–22%. The most common medical problems are respiratory and renal. The nurse may become aware that the young person's mental state has changed, that they are very hot and are showing signs of extra-pyramidal symptoms. Immediate medical treatment is necessary.

◆ *Non-neuroleptic side-effects* Skin flushing, dry mouth, urinary retention and sexual dysfunction, allergic skin reactions and hypersensitivity to the sun, and weight gain may occur. The nurse should ensure that the child wears sunblock when out in the sun. Cholestatic jaundice and agranulocytosis are more serious non-neuroleptic side-effects.

FUTURE PLANNING

An important part of the nursing/multi-disciplinary team intervention will be planning for the child's future together with the parents and community services. With appropriate schooling, family support and therapeutic input, these young people can be given the chance to reach their own individual potential. However, sadly, it must be recognised that, at present, some young people will have a very difficult time ahead. For example, the outcome of adolescent schizophrenia is currently very poor. Cawthron et al (1994) found that 78% of adolescents with schizophrenia are continuously ill and socially handicapped.

SUPPORT GROUPS

National support groups can offer parents and young people the opportunity to share experiences and information. Some useful addresses include:

National Autistic Society
276 Willesden Lane
London NW2 5RB
Tel: 0181-451 1114

Young Minds
22a Boston Place
London NW1 6ER
Tel: 0171-724 7262

National Schizophrenic Fellowship
28 Castle Street
Kingston-upon-Thames
Surrey KT1 1SS
Tel: 0181-547 3937

CONCLUSION

The child who has disturbed or unusual thinking, altered perceptions and/or communication difficulties essentially needs structure, clarity, encouragement to socialise and the opportunity to build on his or her own strengths.

A structured daily timetable of activities with a high level of supervision will help to focus the child's attention and, because he or she is likely to avoid socialisation, gentle coercion to join group activities will probably be necessary. Giving clear expectations of behaviour and limit-setting will contribute to the child's sense of security and facilitate social integration. Often this group of children will have a particular interest, which is so all-consuming that it contributes to their problems. Channelling this energy into positive pursuits related to their particular interest will help to raise their self-esteem and distract them from repetitive purposeless behaviour.

Children on neuroleptic medication must be observed closely for side-effects and to monitor the effectiveness of the drug. Obviously, the aim must be to reduce the level of medication to the minimal therapeutic dose.

Family work will be an important component of treatment. The parents will need tremendous support, along with advice on how best to help their child and manage his or her behaviour.

REFERENCES

Atlas JA (1990) Play assessment and intervention in the childhood psychoses. *Child Psychiatry and Human Development* **21(2)**: 119–133.

Barker PJ (1985) On the edge of experience: the patient with a psychotic disorder. In *Patient Assessment in Psychiatric Nursing*, pp 268–302. London: Croom Helm.

Campbell M, Gonzalez NM, Ernst M, Silva RR and Werry JS (1993) Antipsychotics (neuroleptics). In *Practitioner's Guide to Psychoactive Drugs in Children and Adolescents*, pp 269–296. New York: Plenum Press.

Cantor S (1988) *Childhood Schizophrenia.* New York, Guildord.

Cawthron P, James A, Dell J and Seagroatt V (1994) Adolescent onset pychosis: a clinical and outcome study. *Journal of Child Psychology and Psychiatry* **35(7)**: 1321–1332.

Coursey RD, Keller AB and Farrell EW (1995) Individual psychotherapy and persons with serious mental illness: the client's perspective. *Schizophrenia Bulletin* **21(2)**: 283–301.

Dobson DJG, McDougall G, Busheikin J and Aldous J (1995) Effects of social skills training and social milieu treatment on symptoms of schizophrenia. *Psychiatric Services* **46(4)**: 376–380.

Earnshaw A (1994) Autism: a family affair? *Journal of Child Psychotherapy* **20(1)**: 85–101.

Edwards J, Francey SM, McGorry PD and Jackson HJ (1994) Early psychosis prevention and intervention: evolution of a community-based specialist service. *Behaviour Change* **11(4)**: 223–233.

Gordon CT (1992) Childhood-onset schizophrenia. *New Directions for Mental Health Services* **54**: 71–75.

Hughes C (1994) From confusional entanglement to sense of self: etiology, thinking and process in work with an autistic boy. *Journal of Child Psychotherapy* **20(1)**: 43–55.

Hughes J (1994) Hallucinations following cardiac surgery in a paediatric intensive care unit. *Intensive and Critical Care Nursing* **10**: 209–211.

Kavanagh D (1992) Recent developments in expressed emotion and schizophrenia. *British Journal of Psychiatry* **160**: 601–620.

McClellan JM and Werry JS (1992) Schizophrenia. *Psychiatric Clinics of North America* **15**: 131–148.

McFarlane WR, Lukens E, Link B et al (1995) Multiple-family groups and psychoeducation in the treatment of schizophrenia. *Archives of General Psychiatry* **52(8)**: 679–687.

Parker G and Hadzi-Pavlovic D (1990) Expressed emotion as a predictor of schizophrenic relapse. *Archives of General Psychiatry* **45**: 806–813.

Rund BR, Oie M, Borchgrevink TS and Fjell A (1995) Expressed emotion, communication deviance and schizophrenia. *Psychopathology* **28**: 220–228.

Rutter M (1985) Infantile autism and other pervasive

developmental disorders. In Rutter M and Hersov L (eds) *Child and Adolescent Psychiatry – Modern Approaches,* pp 545–561. London: Blackwell Scientific Publications.

Steinberg D (1985) Psychotic and other severe disorders in adolescence. In Rutter M and Hersov L (eds) *Child and Adolescent Psychiatry – Modern Approaches,* pp 567–583. London: Blackwell Scientific Publications.

Stirling J (1994) Schizophrenia and expressed emotion. *Perspectives in Psychiatric Care* **30(2)**: 20–25.

Tang W, Yao X and Zheng Z (1994) Rehabilitative effect of music therapy for residual schizophrenia – a one-month randomised controlled trial in Shanghai. *British Journal of Psychiatry* **165(supplement 24)**: 38–44.

Werry J, McClellan J and Chard L (1991) Childhood and adolescent schizophrenia, bipolar and schizoaffective disorders: a clinical and outcome study. *Journal of the American Academy of Child and Adolescent Psychiatry* **30**: 457–465.

Wilkinson TR (1983) Psychotic symptoms. In *Child and Adolescent Psychiatric Nursing,* pp 133–154. London: Blackwell Scientific Publications.

Zastowny TR, Lehman AF, Cole RE and Kane C (1992) Family management of schizophrenia: a comparison of behavioral and supportive family treatment. *Psychiatric Quarterly* **63(2)**: 159–186.

10 PROBLEMS RELATING TO SEXUALITY

INTRODUCTION

Sexuality is a part of one's personality or self-concept. It does not just involve sexual drives and behaviour, but is an integral part of who we are and determines how we function. Sexuality includes gender identity, that is, our self-awareness and expression of being male or female, and gender role, the behaviour reflecting our gender identity. It determines one's ability to establish and maintain intimate relationships and, ultimately, affects our self-esteem.

The development of sexuality begins in infancy or possibly even before birth. Certainly from a biological viewpoint, automatic genital activation probably starts in the womb. At birth penile erection is observed in all boys during rapid eye movement (REM) sleep, spontaneously when awake and from manual stimulation, and research suggests that early arousal also occurs in girls (Langfeldt, 1993). During infancy the child experiences their first relationships with other people. Touch and eye contact are thought to be important factors contributing to the child's feeling of security and bonding. The infant will also experience other new sensations, such as the taste and smell of milk and feeling of satiation. They are beginning to learn about their inter-action with the world and how they can influence what happens to them. Positive interactions are thought to contribute to an ability to trust others and the development of a healthy social and sexual life (Nelson, 1995). For example, a caregiver who is consistently responsive to the child's physical and emotional needs will be teaching the infant to trust others, and a positive loving relationship between parents will model a positive attitude towards intimacy.

Gender identity starts to develop the moment the child is born when parents ask, 'Is it a boy or girl?'. Personal and cultural attitudes, and expectations, affect the way parents and others behave towards the child. The tone of voice, how the child is dressed, the toys provided and the approach to play will all influence the child's developing self-concept. Even today in a climate of sexual equality, boys are generally played with boisterously, whereas girls are often dressed in pretty clothes and handled more gently. This process of socialisation is actually important to establish a clear gender identity, which is achieved by about the age of 2, when the boy or girl starts to take on their gender role (Smith, 1993).

During the toddler stage of development, the child starts to take more interest in their body and begins to develop more self-control, such as learning to be toilet trained. They discover that touching their genitals creates a pleasurable sensation, and a parent's reaction to this behaviour may contribute to healthy sexual development, or otherwise. A parent giving a negative response, such as scolding the child, will convey the message that such pleasurable feelings are bad, whereas a parent who is supportive will encourage the child to feel positive about their body and sexuality. During the toddler years, the child learns more about their interaction with the world, what is acceptable and unacceptable behaviour and, as cognitive and language skills grow, their ability to communicate increases. The child learns the names of the parts of the body and Smith (1993) suggests that this is probably a good time for parents to teach the child that the genitals are a special part of the body that feel good to touch, but are private, and best not touched in public.

The pre-school years are a time of great curiosity and questioning. Questions about the difference between boys and girls, and where babies come from, are common. Simple, but true, answers, appropriate for the child's level of comprehension, will satisfy rather than frustrate the child, and convey a message that sexuality is a good thing, instead of something that is bad or embarrassing, and should not be talked about. The pre-school years are also a time when the child may develop competitive feelings with the parent of the same sex, for the affection of the parent of the opposite sex. Freud referred to this as the oedipal phase. The child may say that they want to marry the parent of the opposite sex. It is important for both parents to continue to show love and affection towards the child, explaining sensitively why marriage is not possible. An adult role model of the same sex is also important during these years. This does not mean that children need to observe stereotypically 'masculine' or 'feminine' behaviour, but that they will benefit from being able to enjoy an activity with an adult of the same sex. This helps to reinforce the child's gender identity and appropriate behaviour. During the pre-school years the child is continuing to learn more about their sexual role; what sort of things they should say and do, so that by the time they reach school they have a fair idea of expectations for boys and girls (Smith, 1993; Nelson, 1995).

During the early and pre-adolescent school years, children are believed to have a reduced sexual interest. Freud referred to this stage of development as the latency phase. The child is more concerned with what is happening in the world around them and tends to choose friends of the same sex, considering those of the opposite sex to be repulsive (Smith, 1993). However, contrary to Freud's theory of latency, sexual play, particularly involving others of the same sex, is common amongst schoolchildren. Modesty becomes important during these years and disclosing sexual activity is embarrassing for most children, having dramatic negative effects on the adult sexual life of some. It is therefore important for parents and other adults to respect a child's privacy and act discreetly (Langfeldt, 1993).

Adolescence is a time of rapid physical growth, sexual maturity, and emotional, intellectual and social development. Girls have a growth spurt after about their 11th birthday and boys about 2 years later. Girls begin to menstruate between 10–13 years and boys have nocturnal emissions between 13 and 15 years. Secondary sexual characteristics develop and the young person's adult body shape begins to emerge. In the Western world, there is a tremendous cultural emphasis on the 'perfect body' and children very quickly pick this up. The adolescent experiences an awakening of sexual feelings and sexual orientation emerges, although homosexuality is believed to be established early in childhood (Coleman and Remafedi, 1989). Some teenagers may experience homosexual feelings and develop a close sexual relationship with a friend of the same sex, but later go on to establish heterosexual relationships. This is different from the emerging gay or lesbian teenager but, nevertheless, a part of healthy adolescent sexual exploration and experimentation. Peer relationships become very important as adolescents struggle together to find their own identity and autonomy. However, parents and other significant adults will play an important role in providing information, guidance, support and limit-setting. In Kenya, the disappearance of the extended family, and its influence on adolescents' developing sexual knowledge, attitudes and behaviour, is thought to have contributed to the high incidence of pregnancy amongst teenage girls (Ojwang and Maggwa, 1991).

Obstacles that may hinder the development of healthy sexuality include:

◆   Disability

◆   Illness

◆   Abuse

◆   Parental attitudes and behaviour

◆   Cultural influences

Problems relating to sexuality in children and adolescents include:

◆   Sexual acting out or promiscuity and vulnerability to sexual abuse

◆   Prostitution

◆   Teenage pregancy

◆   Acquired immune deficiency syndrome (AIDS)

◆   Other sexually transmitted diseases

◆   Inability to form close or intimate relationships

◆   Dissociative or somatic symptoms

◆   Self-injury

◆   Sexual aggression

◆   Sexual dysfunction

ASSESSMENT

Some problems are obviously related to sexuality, whereas others may at first seem unrelated. The child who shows overtly sexualized behaviour will immediately alert parents and professionals to instigate an assessment, including exploration of the child's sexuality, and the child who is cutting her or himself will cause the initiation of a general psychiatric assessment, but any problems relating to sexuality may not be apparent initially. Therefore, sexuality must form part of any nursing assessment, but the direction and distance that exploration should take will vary, depending on circumstances. For example, in a school health check, discussion with an adolescent about sexual orientation may reveal anxieties that need to be explored further; a child on an inpatient psychiatric unit disclosing sexual abuse will need the opportunity to talk about her or his abusive experiences; the toddler who is found by parents engaged in sexual play may simply require observation, to ensure that it is a part of normal healthy development and not an indicator of abuse.

The nurse will need to draw on other chapters in this book to plan a comprehensive assessment. For example, the child who has been sexually abused may present with self-harming behaviour and physical symptoms that cannot be medically diagnosed (see Chapters 2 and 5).

INDIVIDUAL ASSESSMENT

As with many other chapters in this book, it is difficult to separate assessment from intervention; there will be considerable overlap. Problems are likely to unfold slowly as intervention proceeds.

Routine history-taking

As part of a nursing history, sexuality should be included for all adolescents. Sexuality is often a forgotten area of health care, particularly in relation to those who are chronically sick or disabled. Society tends to ignore or discourage the expression of sexuality amongst disabled people, assuming that sexual drives, self-image and the forming of intimate relationships are unimportant. Williams and Wilson (1989) found that, although 92% of paediatric nurses working in oncology thought that sexuality should be an important component of care, less than half actually discussed sexuality with adolescent patients. Professionals seem uncomfortable in initiating such discussions, which may in part be due to society's view that sex and sexuality is a taboo subject and partly the result of inadequate training. Nurses are in an ideal position to help children and adolescents, with or without disabilities, to develop a healthy sexuality.

Being non-judgemental and showing a genuine interest and concern about the young person's sexual health is paramount. The teenager is likely to find the subject embarrassing and so starting with general statements and broad questions, moving on to more specific, may be perceived as less threatening, for example talking about teenagers in general and then moving on to the individual's personal experience. It is also important to use simple and unambiguous words and terms, such as 'sexual intercourse' rather than 'sleeping with' or 'making love'. Throughout the discussion, the nurse must clarify that the young person understands what is being talked about. For example, it seems that many teenagers believe that they are not 'sexually active' if they have not had intercourse in the past week or two, even if they are actually having regular sex (Smith, 1993).

Areas to cover in a history include the following:

Sexual development

Discussion about puberty may take place in conjunction with a physical examination by a doctor. Teenagers need reassurance that their body changes are normal and healthy. For example, it is quite usual for girls to have one breast bigger than the other, for boys to have one testicle lower than the other and to have uncontrolled erections. Cultural background plays an important part in determining attitudes towards puberty. Most cultures have a negative attitude towards menstruation. Trans-culturally, menarche has been described as dirty, debilitating and evil in myths and folklore. The silence and concealment that has surrounded the menstrual cycle for generations has enabled these attitudes to pass from mother to daughter unchecked. Some research suggests that Afro-American females have a more negative attitude than white Americans, although this has been refuted by Dashiff and Buchanan (1995). Negative attitudes are linked with inadequate preparation for the menarche and black females do menstruate at an earlier age than girls from other ethnic groups, and so require earlier preparation. Discussing menstruation with the teenager enables the nurse to allay fears, correct any faulty beliefs and encourage a more positive attitude. Menarche can generate a more positive self-image, pride of entering womanhood, a sense of maturity and femininity. Adequate preparation of menarche has also been linked with decreased symptom experience and pain.

Body image

Although the teenager has little choice regarding the final shape of their emerging adult body, Western culture cruelly defines what their body should look like. It is important to identify any unhealthy dieting or exercising practices and help to educate the teenager about respecting and looking after their body.

Sexual orientation

It is not unusual for teenagers to have homosexual feelings. It is reassuring to compare body changes with someone of the same sex, and sexual experimentation is not uncommon. However, a proportion of teenagers will be homosexual and so facile reassurance or labelling should be avoided. Most teenagers, gay and straight, are likely to have misconceptions regarding homosexuality and gay lifestyles. 'Myths surrounding homosexuality abound and continue to have a powerful influence on both popular and professional thought' (Bidwell, 1988). These can lead to reduced self-esteem only in the young person who is sure they are gay. The nurse must explain that sexual orientation is not a choice, nor is it contagious or the product of pathological upbringing, or some flaw in the personality of the individual. Rather it is a natural and valid human experience. It is important that the nurse identifies any serious concerns that a teenager may have concerning sexual orientation. Possible hostility and rejection from family or peers mean that the gay teenager is particularly vulnerable to psychosocial problems. Running away from home, prostitution, sexual victimization and attempted suicide have been reported (Coleman and Remafedi, 1989).

Sexual intercourse

A large percentage of teenagers will have had sexual intercourse, and the rebellious nature of adolescence means that risk-taking is likely to be high. It is important to ascertain the number of partners, sex of partner(s), sexual practices and use of condoms, and to ask whether the young person has noticed any symptoms associated with sexually transmitted disease. Whether or not the teenager has sexual experience, this discussion is a good opportunity for the nurse to talk about safe sex and sexually transmitted diseases.

Relationships

As mentioned in the introduction to this chapter, sexuality is more than just about sexual practices. The ability to form relationships comes into sharp focus during adolescence. Awkwardness and shyness can cause the young person great distress, shatter self-confidence and result in feelings of loneliness. There may be peer pressure to behave in a certain way: engage in sexual intercourse, take drugs, smoke cigarettes, and so on. Talking about this phenomenom in general terms, and mentioning that other teenagers have talked to you about such pressures, may be a helpful approach to this sensitive subject.

Facilitating disclosure of abuse

A specific area of assessment relating to sexuality, which warrants special consideration, is that of sexual abuse. Sadly, we are constantly reminded in the media of the enormity of this problem.

The social services department acting for the local authority and the police child protection team have a responsibility for investigating suspected child abuse. Therefore, it is imperative for the social worker in the multi-disciplinary team to inform social services of cases of suspected abuse. Depending on the degree of suspicion and the current safety of the child, a decision will be made regarding investigation. For example, a low-level suspicion of abuse by one parent of a child who is currently on a 7-day inpatient psychiatric unit can be dealt with very differently to a high level of suspicion in the community. The advantage of the inpatient psychiatric setting is that the child can feel safe, build a therapeutic relationship with staff and, in their own time, find a way of communicating their experiences. It is in these situations that the nurse is most likely to be involved in facilitating disclosure.

The child is likely to be fearful of the consequences of disclosure. On hearing an emotionally disturbed child accuse a respectable adult of perverse behaviour, most adults will fault the child. 'Disbelief and rejection by potential adult caretakers increase the helplessness, hopelessness, isolation and self-blame that make up the most damaging aspects of child sexual victimization. Victims looking back are usually more embittered toward those who rejected their pleas than toward the one who initiated the sexual experiences' (Summit, 1983 p. 178).

The multi-disciplinary team, in conjunction with social services, must decide who is most appropriate to help the child to talk about their abuse. The number of 'interviewers' should be kept to a minimum to reduce the risk of secondary trauma to the child (Kienberger Jaudes and Martone, 1992) and the person(s) to be involved should be guided by the child's behaviour. For example, the child may first drop hints about their trauma to a particular staff member with whom they feel comfortable. Ultimately, the child will decide who they wish to confide in and so it is important to be responsive to their wishes. Although it is essential to have policies and written procedures for dealing with abuse, it is also important to remember the particular individual involved and not to be so rigid in procedure that the child feels betrayed by those who she or he thought could be depended on for sensitivity. It is imperative that any staff member facilitating disclosure has clinical supervision from someone experienced in handling child sexual abuse.

In working with children who have been sexually abused, it is helpful to remember that there are five typical reactions which most children have to their victimization (the child sexual abuse accommodation syndrome). These include (Summit, 1983):

✦ *Secrecy* Abuse by a known adult is three times more common than abuse by a stranger. The child, who is totally unprepared for abuse by a trusted adult, will have to rely on that adult for an understanding of the experience. The most likely things that they will be told is that it must be kept a secret and the consequences of telling anyone. These might include the parent killing the child, him or herself, the other parent, the family breaking up, and so on. Therefore, to disclose abuse, the child must feel safe and able to trust adults to react sensitively, believing what they are told and ensuring the whole situation is handled carefully, for example ensuring the safety of other family members.

✦ *Helplessness* Children may be told to avoid strangers, but they are expected to obey trusted adults. Therefore, in the abusive situation they are helpless. Adults may find it hard to understand why the child does not disclose the abuse and may even believe that they are somehow consenting because they fail to disclose. However, it is important to remember that children and adults are not equal in their power to say no to a parental figure.

✦ *Entrapment and accommodation* Sexual abuse is not generally a one-off occurrence. A compulsive, additive pattern emerges and the child learns to accommodate and develop their own survival skills. It feels too unsafe to conceptualise a parent as bad; this would be equivalent to abandonment, and so the child conceptualises her or himself as bad. It feels safer to direct their anger inwards and believe that they have provoked the abuse and must learn to be good. The abusing parent reinforces this notion, perhaps promising rewards if the child is 'good' and meets their sexual demands, and threatening punishment if the child complains. The parent may talk about going to a younger sibling or warn the child that if they tell anyone it would break up the family. The child is given the responsibility of keeping the family together and must therefore search for some sanctuary from this burden. They may turn to an imaginary friend or develop dissociative symptoms, which enable them to escape reality. Non-epiletic fits are often associated with sexual abuse (Alper et al, 1993). If such measures fail, the child's rage must find another outlet, which for girls often means self-mutilation, promiscuous or suicidal behaviour, and running away, and for boys, outward aggressive and antisocial behaviour. Accommodation mechanisms can be overcome only if the child is placed in an environment that can provide consistent, non-contingent caring and acceptance. Working individually with these children the nurse is likely to be tested and provoked.

◆ *Delayed, conflicted and unconvincing disclosure* Most sexual abuse is never disclosed: cases that are identified, investigated and treated are exceptional. Most adults confronted with an angry and disturbed child or adolescent are unlikely to believe their fantastic story. Very few mothers, to whom the child has disclosed abuse by the father, seek professional help. Therefore it is perhaps not surprising that children delay disclosure and give conflicting and unconvincing accounts.

◆ *Retraction* Fear of the consequences of disclosure, feelings of guilt and a sense of responsibility to keep the family together will make retraction of the child's accusation likely. The nurse must be prepared for this and continue to stand by the child, not alienating them, as so many will.

When interviewing a child for suspected sexual abuse, it is important to have an open mind and not to enter the interview with preconceived ideas. The child should be interviewed alone if possible, because one of the parents or a close family friend may be the perpetrator. The setting should obviously be child oriented and the nurse should use body language and posture that reflects the child's developmental age. For example, it may be appropriate to sit on the floor with a very young child. It is vital not to pressure the child – to go at their pace and, when appropriate, to ask simple, direct questions in the child's language. It is helpful to know, for example, what the child calls the genitalia.

Some examples of questions to facilitate disclosure might include:

◆ Can you tell me what happened?

◆ Has anyone touched you in places or in a way you didn't like?

◆ Has anyone made you touch them in a way that you didn't like?

◆ Has anyone made you take your clothes off when you didn't want to?

◆ Can you remember when it first started?

It is important to acknowledge that it is difficult for the child to talk about what has happened, but that they are showing great courage. Abused children often believe that they are alone in their experiences and so it may be helpful to explain that you have talked with other children who have had similar things happen to them. The child will need reassurance that you believe what they are telling you and that what has happened is not their fault. The nurse must also remember not to make any promises that cannot be upheld, such as making sure that the family stay together (Rappley and Speare, 1993).

Children or adolescents may find it easier to communicate their abusive experiences by using a medium other than talking face to face. Talking through puppets, dolls, a telephone, or perhaps drawing or writing, are just some of the possibilities to be considered.

> Stewart, aged 15 years, had been sexually abused by a young man who befriended him. He was angry, felt ashamed and had concerns that he must be homosexual. Initially, the only way he was able to communicate about his abuse was to tape record himself talking about it in private and then listen to it with his key worker. Eventually he was able to talk directly to his key worker with a policewoman present.

Wolbert Burgess et al (1995) suggest that a child's memory is four-dimensional: somatic, behavioural, verbal and visual. The ability to retrieve a memory verbally may not be possible for some children who have been abused, owing to developmental parameters and/or repression of the traumatic experience. However, the memory may manifest itself in behavioural, visual or somatic terms. Visual memory can be conveyed through drawings.

Peterson et al (1995) warn of the dangers of relying solely on qualitative analysis or 'inter-pretration' of human figure drawings. Instead, they have identified seven quantifiable indicators of abuse, which have been proven to be statistically significant in differentiating sexually abused from non-sexually abused children. These are referred to as the 'serious seven' and include:

- *Explicit drawings of genitals* Penis, vagina, pubic hair or breasts displayed.
- *Concealment of genitals* Drawn objects placed over genitals or breasts.
- *Omissions of genitalia* Body mid-section, genitals and/or breast deleted.
- *Omissions of central part of figure* Absence of head or torso.
- *Encapsulation of drawing* Figure partially or completely enclosed by lines.
- *Fruit trees added* Fruit trees spontaneously added and designated.
- *Opposite sex drawn* Figure of the sex opposite to that of the child drawn.

Kinetic family drawings, where the child is asked to draw their family 'doing something', have been shown to differeniate homes characterised by abuse, divorce and juvenile delinquency. The Peterson–Hardin kinetic family drawing screening inventory includes both qualitative and quantitative analysis:

- *The quality of the drawing is noted* – the feeling or emotion that it invokes and the extent of order or disorder in the drawing.

◆ *The child's perceptions of the family are evaluated* – the size, shape and distortion of family members and their relationship to each other on the paper.

◆ *The absence or presence of quantifiable components is scored* – actions with negative aspects (aggression, the presence of weapons, blood, fearful expressions, and so on), treatment of figures (rubbing out, slanting and so forth), and styles (encapsulation, barriers, compartmentalisation, and so on) are noted.

Figure 10.1 is a drawing by Christy, an 8-year-old girl, described by Peterson et al (1995). Christy's father had recently lost his job and Christy talked about him being unhappy. Her mother was enduring violence from her father. Father's sadness (sad faces on buttons) and aggressive arms are clearly shown. The line between the parents represents a barrier or compartmentalisation. Christy depicts her angry mouth and later revealed that she was also being physically abused.

A child's drawings should not be viewed in isolation, but used as part of a holistic assessment. Qualitative and quantitative evaluation should reduce the risk of misinterpretation, together with

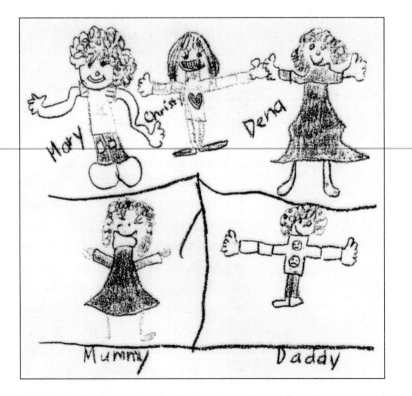

Figure 10.1 Kinetic family drawing by Christy. Reproduced from Peterson et al. (1995) The use of children's drawings in the evaluation of child sexual, emotional and physical abuse. Archives of Family Medicine 4, 445–452, with permission from the American Medical Association.

ensuring that the child's developmental age and cultural background is recognised. For example, drawings of genitalia in Western culture are a strong indication of sexual abuse, even when nudity is commonplace in the home. However, children within the Tellensi in the Gold Coast of the Northern Territories in Australia are known to draw explicit genitalia normally (Peterson et al 1995).

Accurate and detailed report-writing is paramount to enable any legal steps to be taken. Such action may be necessary to ensure the child's safety as well as enabling prosecution of the perpetrator. It is important not to ask any leading questions that could jeopardise prosecution and perhaps cause further trauma to the child, and to check that you have understood what the child has been communicating. Anatomical dolls may help to clarify the abuse and provide the child with an alternative to having to describe their painful experience. However, they cannot be relied on alone to assess child sexual abuse accurately (Realmuto and Wescoe, 1992) and, for some children, using these rather strange dolls may cause further trauma.

Unless the safety of the child is likely to be jeopardised, the parents must be informed that abuse is suspected. Many parents will have thought already about this possibility and will be concerned that professionals may think that they are the perpetrators. It is far better to have an open discussion about the feasibility of abuse having occurred (see below – *Family assessment*). Finally, it is important to acknowledge that, on hearing about child sexual abuse, the nurse is likely to experience her/his own strong feelings, such as anger, disgust or denial. These feelings are natural and should be shared with the multi-disciplinary team, in order to gain professional support and reduce the likelihood of such feelings having a detrimental effect on work with the child.

FAMILY ASSESSMENT

A family assessment is likely to be initiated after referral for emotional or behavioural disturbance, rather than a specific problem relating to sexuality. However, just as an individual assessment should consider sexuality, so should a family assessment. The development of sexuality can be fraught with anxiety and confusion. Having the support and guidance of parents is therefore very important. Meeting with a family where there is an adolescent should therefore include discussion about the child who is 'growing up'. How does the family feel about having an adolescent? What changes have occurred in the family? Who does the teenager go to for support? Perhaps the parents have denied that their child is emerging into adulthood and the young person has looked outside for support or resisted growing up themselves. It seems very important for children to have a parent as a confidant, to buffer the effects of stressful events (Aro et al, 1989), and this must be especially true for the adolescent who is experiencing so many changes, particularly relating to sexuality.

Family assessment where sexual abuse is suspected

When a child or adolescent shows signs of having been abused, saying that they have a secret that cannot be talked about and/or presenting with a psychiatric disturbance, sexualised behaviour and/or physical signs of trauma, discussion about the possibility of abuse must be raised with the family. Some families may actually be relieved that the subject has been brought into the open, as they may have had their own concerns. Where there is a low level of suspicion, it can be put to parents that, 'Some children who have similar problems to…have been hurt or touched inappropriately by someone. Is this anything that you have ever worried about?' Observing the parents' reaction and listening to what they have to say will lead to further areas for discussion.

It must be recognised that a large proportion of child sexual abuse does occur within the family and is representative of a currently dysfunctional system. Family sexual abuse has no socio-economic, religious, ethnic or geographical boundaries. Family behavioural patterns that characterise many families where there is sexual abuse or those where there is a high risk of abuse include (Rappley and Speare, 1993; Stern et al, 1995):

◆ Social isolation

◆ Extreme mistrust of outsiders

◆ Dysfunctional communication patterns

◆ Imbalance of parental power, usually with the father being authoritative

◆ Role reversal, so that children take care of adult needs

◆ Enmeshment

◆ Shame-based family, where mistakes represent catastrophes

◆ Drug or alcohol dependency

◆ Unemployment

◆ Poor mental health of mother

◆ Other forms of violence within family relationships

◆ Marital breakdown, including sexual dysfunction

◆ Previous incidents of sexual abuse

However, although it may be helpful to be aware of some of the characteristics that have been identified in abusive families, care must be taken to avoid making swift judgements. For example, in some ethnic groups, the patriarchal structure should be recognised as culturally appropriate, rather than an imbalance of parental power contributing to abuse (Heras, 1992). Conversely, a family tradition of silence among women and children may severely inhibit disclosure. Furthermore, research identifying the characteristics of abusive families has concentrated mainly on father–daughter incest, not considering abuse by another family member or a close family friend.

HOME AND SCHOOL VISIT

A home and school visit can shed further light on the child's life at home and in school (see Appendices A and B). In terms of sexuality, the nurse is concerned with the child's ability to form relationships, and their sexual knowledge and behaviour (if appropriate to the referral). Establishing what sex education the young person has had at school may be relevant, if this is an area identified for nursing intervention.

GENERAL OBSERVATION

A child's behaviour may give clues of problems related to sexuality, for example difficulties in forming relationships, withdrawal and isolation, or overt sexualised behaviour without an awareness of safety.

Observations that suggest sexual abuse

If the child's verbal memory is fragmented or irretrievable (see above – *Facilatating disclosure of abuse*), behavioural patterns, play characteristics and somatic symptoms may be important indicators of abuse (Wolbert Burgess et al, 1995). Possible indicators of sexual abuse include (Rappley and Speare, 1993):

✦ *Overcompliance* The child, lacking a sense of self, looks to others for acceptance and approval, and does and says what she/he believes others would like.

✦ *Acting-out behaviour* Some children will behave in the reverse, being uncooperative and socially inappropriate in their behaviour.

✦ *Pseudo-maturity* The child looks, talks and acts as if older than their chronological age. They may take on adult responsibilities, such as looking after young siblings, and, although they may appear confident outwardly, inside they are likely to be frightened, lonely and unhappy, and have a low self-esteem.

✦ *Sexualised behaviour* The sexually abused child may exhibit highly sexualised behaviour, including open masturbation, excessive sexual curiosity and exposure of the genitals. They may rub or poke themselves in their genital or anal areas with toys or other play materials and, whilst playing alone or with others, may assume the role of aggressor or victim during sexual play.

✦ *Frightened, agitated, hypervigilant* The terrified child may appear to be constantly scanning their environment for potential danger, frequently tearful for no apparent reason, very 'clingy' or develop excessive fears.

✦ *Withdrawal* The child may withdraw from social situations, have poor peer relationships and become socially isolated.

✦ *Regression* The child may regress to an earlier stage of development, perhaps talking in a babyish voice, developing enuresis, returning to thumb-sucking, and so on.

✦ *Self-destructive behaviour* The child may stop looking after themselves, perhaps not eating, or may actively try to hurt themselves, cutting their arms, burning themselves, attempting suicide.

✦ *Development of somatic symptoms* It is not unusual for children who have been abused to somatize their distress.

✦ *Sleeping problems* Children may develop difficulties sleeping, nightmares, refuse to go to their bedroom, go to sleep.

✦ *Mood swings* The young person may experience excessive mood swings, with depression reaching suicidal depths.

MEDICAL ASSESSMENT

As mentioned previously, routine medical examination of adolescents should include an assessment of puberty, and provides the doctor and nurse with an opportunity to ask about sexual development and the young person's adjustment. The nurse may then be made aware of areas that require individual work.

Medical assessment where sexual abuse is suspected

When abuse is suspected or has been disclosed, medical examination of the genital area may clarify suspicions, enable prosecution and, perhaps most importantly, allay the young person's fear of irreparable damage. However, it is myth that physical examination alone can determine whether a child has been sexually abused. Most kinds of abusive touching leave no signs of trauma, and even vaginal and anal penetration are not necessarily discernible. The hymen is elastic and can stretch to allow penetration without injury, and the anus is also expandable. Furthermore, when injury does occur, healing in the genital and anal area is fast (Adams, 1992).

Physical indicators of abuse include (Child Protection Policy and Procedures, Great Ormond Street Hospital, 1995):

◆ *High index of suspicion*

Semen in the vagina, anus or on the external genitalia.

Pregnancy in a minor where the identity of the father is unknown.

Laceration or scarring of the hymen, attenuation of the hymen with loss of hymeneal tissue, in the absence of another credible explanation.

Laceration or scarring of the anal mucosa extending beyond the anal verge into the perineal skin, also in the absence of another credible explanation.

Bruises, scratches or other injuries to the genital or anal areas, or other 'sexual' areas, such as lips and breasts. Such damage may be minor but inconsistent with accidental injury.

Signs of sexually transmitted disease.

◆ *Medium suspicion*

Perineal itching, soreness, discharge, pain on micturition.

Anal warts.

◆ *Low suspicion*

Recurrent urinary tract infections.

Recurrent abdominal pain, headaches or other symptoms of somatisation.

A medical examination should include a top-to-toe assessment, both to exclude injury and to reduce the trauma to the young person of immediately focusing on the anogenital area. To give the child some control over the examination, the doctor and/or nurse could ask: 'Which part of your body shall we look at next?'. The nurse has the important role of distracting the child's attention when necessary, providing reassurance and sometimes asking the doctor questions, for the sake of the child, such as, 'Is there any damage that cannot heal?'.

NURSING/MULTI-DISCIPLINARY INTERVENTION

Because sexuality is influenced by physical, emotional, intellectual, social and cultural factors, a holistic, multi-disciplinary approach to treatment is most likely to be successful. The nurse will need to consult other chapters of this book for the management of problems that are not concerned directly with sexuality; for example, the child who has been sexually abused may behave aggressively, be frightened, and so on.

MILIEU THERAPY

Encouraging healthy sexuality

It is important to provide children and adolescents with an environment that can foster social and sexual development. This is particularly important for young people with disabilities or a chronic illness. Children can become socially isolated due to lack of mobility, communication difficulties and by over-protective parents and other providers of care (Nelson, 1995). Organising group activites and facilitating communication can help to overcome some of these difficulties.

Adolescence is a time of increasing independence. For the child with a chronic illness or disability, who has relied on others for their everyday care, this will be a particularly difficult time. Lack of experience in self-care and over-protection by parents can lead to a degree of 'learned helplessness'. The nurse can play an important role in helping the young person to become more independent, encouraging them to participate in self-care and to join in social activities. The child who has been sexually abused may also lack confidence in their ability to be independent and self-caring or, alternatively, may be pseudo-mature, assuming an adult role. The young person needs encouragement to behave age-appropriately, which may involve the nurse positively reinforcing acts of independence and assertiveness but discouraging the child from taking on adult responsibilities.

Children and teenagers, particularly those with a disturbed body image, are likely to benefit from positive role models of the same sex. Boys who have been abused by men frequently experience confusion about their sexuality and need the opportunity to relate to a healthy group of males.

Managing sexual acting-out

Sexual acting-out may be a symptom of sexual abuse, delinquent behaviour or age-appropriate exploration of sexuality. Such behaviour may evoke feelings of anger, fear and helplessness amongst nursing staff. Carrey and Adams (1992) found that an educational approach was the most helpful intervention for dealing with this behaviour. Children expressed relief at being able to discuss sex openly. Education on sexuality occurred in a group setting and in individual sessions (see below – *Individual work* and *Group work*). Behavioural measures can also help to modify behaviour and may be necessary to safeguard other children (see Chapter 3 – *Targeting the behavioural problem*).

Stewart (mentioned previously) expressed his rage at having been abused through sexualised verbal aggression, which he directed towards staff. He would also entice other children to join in the barrage of insults thrown at staff. As well as supportive individual work, which included sex education, Stewart received daily points for positive involvement with peers, such as initiating games, and was separated from the group for a morning or afternoon for inappropriate provocation. During this time away from positive reinforcement, Stewart made some reparation for his behaviour, perhaps writing a letter of apology to the assaulted staff member, which was followed by an individual activity with a member of staff. Having the opportunity to let off steam, by playing football in the local park, was also important in reducing his aggressive behaviour.

When there are concerns about sexualised behaviour, nursing staff must be vigilant to ensure the safety of other children. Those who have been abused may attempt to abuse others in order to gain some control over their own experience and/or through ignorance regarding appropriate sexual behaviour. Clear boundaries to behaviour are essential and an appropriate level of nursing supervision should be organised.

INDIVIDUAL WORK

'Growing up work'

From an early age, parents influence their child's sexual knowledge, attitudes and behaviour. During the pre-school years the child receives not only factual information from parents, but also their sexual values (Lober Aquilino and Ely, 1985). The inquisitive child will ask questions about mummy's breasts and daddy's penis, observe characteristics of the parental relationship and have their own expression of sexuality encouraged or repressed. Intimacy, gentleness, a belief in equality or otherwise will be learnt.

During adolescence, parents are in an ideal position to increase their child's knowledge of sex-related issues and play an important role in shaping their sexual attitudes and behaviour. However, research suggests that information from parents is often vague and young adolescents do not hear or retain what parents believe they are communicating (Newcomer and Udry, 1985; Tucker, 1990). When adolescents are asked where and from whom do they learn about sex, most cite the media and peers, and place parents among the least important sources of information. Sex education at school is rarely mentioned (Campbell and Campbell, 1990). The problem with these sources of information is that peers are often misinformed themselves and the media tend to portray a distorted picture of reality. Adolescents who rely on television for information are likely to have a narrow concept of female beauty, believe that extra-marital sex with multiple partners is acceptable, that the use of contraceptives is unimportant (they are rarely seen or mentioned in sex scenes), and so on. Sex is rarely seen in the context of a loving relationship, but is generally associated with power struggles and violence. Research suggests that television can increase young people's acceptance of promiscuity and sexual infidelity, increase sexual callousness towards women, encourage rape to be trivialised, and lead to comparison of sexual satisfaction with television images (Brown et al, 1990).

Nurses can help to improve children's knowledge of sex and sexuality, and promote healthy sexual behaviour. Health visitors can discuss the development of sexuality with the parents of young children, perhaps helping them to decide how they will answer their child's probing questions; school nurses can promote effective sex education, and so on. However, sometimes sex education will need to be reactive, responding to a problem related to sexuality. It will then not only have a preventive function, but also a healing purpose. Individual sessions can provide a space for this work, which I will refer to as 'growing up work'.

Although I refer to 'growing up work' as individual work, I believe that parental involvement is generally essential. However, there may be occasions when the child will not benefit from their parents' presence, for example where a girl's mother does not believe that her daughter has been abused. Many parents feel inadequate to teach their children about sex, perhaps because they think that they need to be totally knowledgeable or because they still feel confused about their own sexuality. These issues need to be addressed before growing up sessions with the teenager begin. Having a discussion with the parent about their thoughts and values is an important starting point for growing up work. It enables the parent to help clarify their own views and wishes for their child and, of particular importance, communicates these to the nurse. Different attitudes and perspectives are likely to occur within different ethnic groups, and must be respected.

One of the possible reasons why school sex education is relatively ineffective in promoting desirable behaviour is the tendency of curricula to reflect the salient concerns of adults, rather than those of adolescents. Adults tend to place more importance on the long-term consequences of behaviour, whereas adolescents are guided by their present emotional state and the short-term consequences of their actions. Adults will concern themselves with abstract issues, and the adolescent will focus more on concrete realities. For example, an adult's concern about a teenage daughter not using contraception is likely to go beyond worrying about pregnancy and sexually transmitted diseases. An adult will also understand that pregnancy can limit educational opportunities, career development and long-term financial independence (Campbell and Campbell, 1990). Therefore, growing up work must focus on adolescent concerns and address questions and topics that the adolescent wishes to discuss, rather than what adults think the adolescent needs to know. If the adolescent feels their concerns are taken seriously, and even given priority, they are more likely to change their attitudes and behaviour. Sex education in schools tends to avoid certain 'sensitive' subjects, yet research indicates, not surprisingly, that these are of interest to teenagers. Homosexuality, abortion and masturbation are among the topics often avoided. During growing-up sessions, the nurse and parent must try to discover the types of questions the teenager has about sex and sexuality and go on to address them. The adults do not need to know all the answers and, indeed, may need to research new areas themselves and be prepared to learn along with the teenager.

Research into sex education suggests that use of multiple channels of communication is more effective than using a single mode, for example using leaflets, books, television, and so forth. Television programmes can be selected to view and then discuss, a sex education book chosen to read together, and magazines looked at to talk about the 'ideal', but generally unrealistic, images of beauty that are portrayed. DuVal Frost (1984) describes how nurses can use rock music to assist adolescents in developing their sexual identity. She describes group discussions (see below – *Group work*), but the principle could be applied to individual work. The parent could bring a recording of one of their best-liked songs from their teenage years, and the adolescent, one of their current favourites. As well as discussing their understanding of the lyrics of each song, the more explicit nature of present-day lyrics could be talked about. This discussion may help to bridge the generational gap, helping the parent and child see each other's perspective on adolescence.

Growing up work with adolescents who are disabled or chronically sick will need to address how their sexual development and function is affected. For example, the adolescent with cancer will need to know that chemotherapy may cause temporary alterations in ovulation or spermatogenesis, but that, if they are sexually active, contraceptives are necessary to prevent pregnancy. Preventing pregnancy during chemotherapy is particularly important, as certain anti-neoplastic agents are known to cause fetal abnormalities. Contraceptive therapy for the adolescent with cancer must be chosen with care; for example, the intrauterine device or sponge may increase menstrual blood loss and cause haemorrhage during periods of thrombocytopenia (Klopovich and Clancy, 1985).

Contractures and spasticity caused by cerebral palsy are likely to cause difficulties for the teenager managing her own menstruation and make birth control a challenge. Sexual intercourse and masturbation may be difficult but, with creative positioning, are both possible (Nelson, 1995). The nurse organising growing up work will need to liaise with other professionals to acquire expert advice and, during sessions, should not be frightened to say to the teenager, 'I don't know the answer to that, but I'll find out'. It may be useful to 'invite' certain outside people to growing up sessions.

Body image is likely to be a damaged area for the teenager who is disabled, or chronically sick and receiving therapy that has undesirable effects on the body. Alopecia resulting from cancer therapy is likely to signify a loss of attractiveness and femininity for the girl and a loss of sex appeal and virility for the boy. Such changes in body image will adversely effect self-esteem and be detrimental to the development of peer relationships. This problem may be exacerbated by the reaction of others, such as being treated as if their condition is contagious. An important aspect of growing up work is to help the young person feel more at ease with their body and develop skills to facilitate forming relationships with peers (see also below – *Improving self-esteem*).

For the young person who has been sexually abused, early blurring of boundaries between trust and coercion, love and sex, may greatly affect future relationships. Sex may be associated with violence, rather than love and affection, and a disturbed sexual self-concept may emerge. Some youngsters may be sexually aggressive towards peers, or choose partners, consciously or unconsciously, who will abuse them further. The child sexual abuse victim is likely to internalise their abuse, so that they expect, and feel that they deserve, to be abused. They may develop promiscuous behaviour or fall into prostitution, and are likely to be more vulnerable to abuse than other children.

The teenager may have specific concerns regarding their sexuality; it is not uncommon for victims to be concerned that they are homosexual, if they have been abused by an adult of the same sex, and many may experience sexual dysfunction. Suppressed sexual desire, flashbacks during moments of sexual intimacy and resistance to any body contact with others may be present (Gillman and Whitlock, 1989). Growing up work can provide the teenager with valuable and comforting information, such as the difference between a true gay person and the victim of abuse by an adult of the same sex, and provide an opportunity for talking about sensitive issues which may be more difficult in a non-directive counselling session.

As well as covering topics that are directly related to sex and sexuality, growing up work can also include other areas, such as growing independence and autonomy. Issues of contention between the parent and child could be discussed and resolutions made, which could be written in a contract (see Chapter 3 – *Targeting the behavioural problem* on Writing a contract with the child).

Plate 8 (which appears in the unfolioed section between p56 and 57) illustrates part of the 'growing up work' done by Clarissa, aged 14 years (first mentioned in Chapter 5), with her key nurse. Clarissa suffered from precocious puberty, starting to develop breasts at the age of 4 years and experiencing the menarche at 6. During individual work, Clarissa drew pictures of herself growing up and wrote down how she had felt at different stages in her life (top of picture). Getting things down on paper helped Clarissa to talk about the painful experiences that she had in relation to puberty. Her key nurse wrote down the more usual experiences of children growing up, in order to show Clarissa that it was not surprising she had found it so difficult and to illustrate that she could now join with her peers.

Improving self-esteem

Sexual identity is an important contributor to our overall self-esteem. Unfortunately, the sensitivity that surrounds sex and sexuality across most cultures means that children often rely on the media for information. As mentioned previously, this can lead to unrealistic expectations of beauty and sexual peformance. These media impressions need to be challenged, perhaps by discussing particular television programmes, films or magazine articles.

A low self-esteem may result in vulnerability to sexual abuse, and work on self-protection may help not only to prevent abuse but also to improve the young person's self-concept. Training in assertiveness skills is a valuable component of the nurse's intervention for promoting sexual health. Role-playing difficult situations, such as the teenager telling their boyfriend or girlfriend that they do not feel ready for sexual intercourse, may enhance the young person's confidence and belief that they have a choice.

Other general exercises for enhancing self-esteem are mentioned in Chapter 2 – *Individual work, Improving self-esteem.*

Providing an opportunity to communicate particular concerns

Children who have been abused need the opportunity to communicate their experiences to a caring adult. This may be a key nurse, psychotherapist, a parent with a nurse or psychotherapist facilitating, or another professional. A decision should be made in the multi-disciplinary team where, when and with whom a special time is organised. Some children may need to talk about their abuse constantly, and will talk indiscriminately to anyone. However, it is generally more constructive to provide boundaries; the child's feelings will be contained and so they are less likely to be overwhelmed by them. The child may communicate by describing their dreams, playing, drawing, talking, and so on. When the child approaches another staff member and starts talking about their abuse, the nurse can sensitively explain that they are aware that horrible things have happened to the child, but that they are private and best talked about with their key nurse. It could be suggested that the child writes down their current thoughts and shows them to their key nurse at their next individual session. Perhaps the written message could be posted into a box so that the child symbolically gets rid of those thoughts for the time being.

Some children relate images that they experience or describe flashbacks. These occurrences have to be dealt with when they arise, but the child can be helped to gain some control over them.

Katherine, aged 13, had been sexually abused by an adult male who was a family friend. She presented with somatic symptoms but, following her elder sister's revelation that she had been abused by this man, Katherine was able to disclose her experiences. At non-specific times in the day, she would see images of a man dressed in a black cloak coming towards her. A nursing plan was set up whereby Katherine would ask for her key nurse when this occurred, and together they would get rid of the cloaked man. Symbolically, they would take the cloaked figure out of the psychiatric unit and lock the door. When Katherine was discharged, her mother helped her to do likewise at home. This simple process enabled Katherine to gain some control over these intrusive, frightening thoughts and images.

Sometimes the child will be able to identify triggers of flashbacks. They may become aware of unconsious associations with the abuser or traumatic experience, such as adults shouting, particular weather characteristics, a specific smell, and so on. Through individual work using drawing, play, sensory work (see Chapter 4 – *Individual work*, *Addressing sensory delays*) and so on, the child may identify associations with trauma. It may then be possible for the child to develop coping strategies and avert the occurrence of frightening flashbacks.

GROUP WORK

Growing up work

Growing up work can be organised in a group setting and, indeed, some adolescents may find this less embarrassing than in one-to-one discussions. Snegroff (1995) describes group work involving pre-adolescents (10–12 years) and their parents. The presenter begins the group work with sharing memories of their own adolescence, including their thoughts, feelings, observations, behaviours, attitudes and values. Topics include physical changes, social behaviour with family and friends, sexual behaviour and feelings, and so on. A film about puberty is then shown, and parents and children are encouraged to ask questions and make comments, which are written down anonymously on index cards. These are then collected by the presenter and each is discussed in turn.

DuVal Frost (1984) describes how nurses used rock music to assist adolescents in the development of their sexual identity. Current rock music was played half an hour before the group session and printed lyrics were made available. This encouraged the teenagers to arrive at sessions on time and to listen to the music, singing along and dancing. The group then used the lyrics for the basis of their discussion on sexuality. For example, *This Night* by Billy Joel deals with the issue of peer pressure and becoming sexually active. Many songs imply that sexual intercourse is the norm between boy and girl friend. Teenagers may find this a frightening prospect and, although they are eager to 'fit in' with their peer group, may not feel ready for sexual intimacy. This song provoked discussions concerning risks for boys and particularly girls, and provided an opportunity to talk about the right for individual choice. Useful songs today might include *You Oughta Know* by Alanis Morissette, which could be used to facilitate a discussion about the anguish of breaking up with a boyfriend, and *Girls and Boys* by Blur, which could initiate a talk about sexual attractiveness, what 'turns different people on', sexual orientation and the risks involved in sexual intercourse.

Drama and social skills training groups can address issues of sexuality. The drama group could write and perform a short play to be performed to other adolescents or parents, and the social skills group could provide an opportunity for adolescents to role-play situations they find difficult, such as asking a girl or boy to go out on a date.

Group therapy for children who have been sexually abused

Research suggests that group treatment has been used successfully in the rehabilitation of abused children (Lindon and Nourse, 1994; Silovsky and Hembree-Kigin, 1994; McGain and McKinzey, 1995). Nursing staff who have the appropriate skills and experience may be involved in facilitating group work, either with each other or with another member of the multi-disciplinary team. Lindon and Nourse (1994) describe a group model they have used with adolescent girls, which contains three essential components: a skills, psychotherapeutic and educational component.

The skills component of the group includes:

✦ *Relaxation through guided imagery* During guided imagery, the adolescent is asked to imagine their own special place of safety and encouraged to use this technique when experiencing flashbacks.

✦ *Problem-solving skills* The girls brainstorm problems arising from their abuse and discuss ways to resolve them. For example, it is common for the young person to feel responsible for the abuse. The group could brainstorm ideas for gaining some control over these feelings, for example using positive self-statements such as, 'it was not my fault'.

✦ *Assertiveness and other social skills* Training in self-protection and general relationship skills is achieved using role-play and video feedback.

The psychotherapeutic component includes:

◆ *Helping the adolescents to become aware of their feelings towards the perpetrator* This process may enable the young person to shed some of the guilt they feel for the abuse. Each young person draws a picture of the perpetrator and places it on an empty chair. They then address the picture as if it were the perpetrator, describing how they felt about the abuse and how they feel now. Another exercise involves the girls writing a letter to the perpetrator. The adolescents are told not to send it, but can do whatever else they choose with it.

◆ *Feedback of group processes* Lindon and Nourse (1994) cite one example where the youngest girl in the group talked about her personal experience of being abused. The others in the group became angry with each other and there was a general feeling of confusion. This was interpreted as the group possibly mirroring the feelings of the girl during her abusive experience and seemed to bring some sense of relief in the group.

The educative component addresses:

◆ *Education about how the body works* This includes the physiological reaction of the body to sexual stimulation. Some victims of abuse may have experienced sexual arousal, which serves only to confound their feelings of guilt.

Silovsky and Hembree-Kigin (1994) highlight the value of incorporating a snack-time into group sessions. It provides an opportunity to demonstrate nurturance and a means of socialisation. Groups for young children might also include a free play time. Group rules must be made explicit, and should include the prohibition of physical abuse towards other group members and respect for the personal boundaries of others. The sex of group facilitators must always be discussed in the team. Girls who have been abused by men may be more at ease with female facilitators; boys who have been abused by men may also want a woman present, but may benefit from the presence of a sensitive male therapist, and so on. It is probably advisable to consider the specific needs of any one group, rather than make blanket rules concerning the sex of therapists. A group for the non-offending parents may usefully run in parallel to the group for victims. Mothers of children who have been abused may experience similar feelings to their children, such as anger, fear and self-blame. The group process is thought to increase their commitment to treatment.

Group therapy can reduce the feelings of isolation that most victims of abuse feel, and overcome the powerful element of secrecy. Self-esteem may be improved, fear and anxiety reduced, and relationships with friends and family improved.

FAMILY WORK

As parents are a child's primary source of sex education, imparting information and conveying their own sexual attitudes, it seems sensible to involve them in addressing problems related to sexuality. Piercy and co-workers (1993) describe using a brief family therapy model to reduce human immunodeficiency virus (HIV) high-risk behaviours among adolescents. Their model includes helping both parents and child to see each other's perspective, establishing appropriate parental influence, interrupting dysfunctional sequences of behaviour (for example, an adolescent sexually acting out following arguments at home), training the adolescent in assertiveness skills so that they can avoid risky behaviour, introducing peers to some therapy sessions and emphasising family resources (that is, drawing on family strengths). The interesting idea of introducing peers into therapy is based on the rationale that it can reduce the possibility of triangulation (for example, the adolescent taking the role of peace-keeper between parents) by strengthening the connections between the adolescent's friends and his/her parents; reduce the adolescent's resistance to therapy by making positive contact with his/her friends; elicit the peer's support for changes occurring in the adolescent; and engage the adolescent and his/her peers in educating the family and therapist about the risks and challenges faced by teenagers.

Families who become aware that an adolescent is homosexual go through their own process of 'coming out' and have to develop a new identity. They are likely to question their parenting skills and their own sexuality, and have concerns about the future health and happiness of their child. The therapist can help the family only if his or her own attitudes toward homosexuality are positive and consistent with the current scientific knowledge that it is a natural expression of sexuality (Coleman and Remafedi, 1989).

Family therapy for sexually abused children

For the child who has been sexually abused, the family may be an important source of strength. For example, Katherine's mother (mentioned previously) played a vital role in helping her to cope with terrifying images that persistently appeared in her mind.

> Through family therapy, Katherine and her sisters were able to talk openly about their abusive experiences for the first time and gain some comfort from each other. Strong emotions of anger and disappointment were directed towards the parents who had 'failed to protect them', as they were unaware of the abuse. The difficult task of the therapist was to allow these feelings to be vented but, at the same time, give strength to the parents, in particular the mother, who needed understanding and to be given the opportunity to provide emotional support to her daughters now. Another important task of therapy was to help each family member to express their rage towards the perpetrator. This was achieved using an empty chair on which the perpetrator was imagined to be sitting.

When an incestuous relationship is discovered, action must obviously be taken to protect the child from further abuse. Most family therapists advocate the removal of the perpetrator from the home, rather than the victim. Contrary to popular myth, most mothers are not aware of their partner's abusive behaviour. The survival of marriage depends on trust. Therefore, on hearing about abuse for the first time, a mother is likely to react with disbelief and protective denial. Rejection and blaming of the child are typical reactions. Individual therapy for the mother will undoubtedly be necessary to enable her to listen to, protect and support her child. Family therapy may have to wait until the mother is strong enough to hear her daughter's story and bear the anger that is likely to be directed towards her, for not preventing the abuse from happening. In situations of father–daughter incest, strengthening of the mother–daughter relationship is often a component of treatment. The long-term aim of therapy may be to re-unite the whole family, if the perpetrator is willing to engage in treatment and every family member wishes to aim for this goal. The non-offending adult must take responsibility for protecting the child from further abuse; the perpetrator must accept full responsibility for the abuse; and an appropriate hierarchy in the family must be established. The marital relationship must be strengthened, and parental roles and age-appropriate roles for the children established. However, the family therapist must work with the family in the context of their culture. For example, in white American culture, the strength of the parental relationship is seen as essential to healthy family functioning, whereas in Asian and Hispanic culture the mother–child relationship is often emphasised. Similarly, communication styles are likely to differ between cultures. In some families it may be appropriate to use more non-verbal means of communicating, and it is therefore inappropriate for the therapist to tell the family that they must express their feelings more openly and directly (Heras, 1992).

Several factors have been identified as poor predictors of outcome in family therapy (Silovsky and Hembree-Kigin, 1994):

◆ Refusal to admit that abuse has occurred by the perpetrator and mother.

◆ Voluntary relinquishment of parental rights.

◆ Refusal to include all family members in family therapy.

◆ Parental psychopathology.

◆ Substance abuse.

◆ Violence in the family.

PSYCHOANALYTICAL PSYCHOTHERAPY

Psychotherapy may be helpful for the teenager who is experiencing difficulties related to sexuality, facilitating the development of a sense of self, including sexual identity. It may also give the young person greater insight into problematic behaviour, such as self-destructive urges in the victim of abuse, where feelings of guilt and self-blame are turned inwards.

CONCLUSION

Sexuality is often a forgotten and neglected area of health care. It is important that the nurse addresses his or her own attitudes and beliefs in clinical supervision. In this way, it will become easier to approach the subject with children and their families, and manage their concerns.

Nurses must be aware of the possible indicators of sexual abuse and relay any concerns that they have regarding a particular child to the multi-disciplinary team. A joint decision will then be taken concerning appropriate action. It is important that professionals do not panic, intervening without foresight and perhaps causing further traumatisation to the child.

Key areas for nursing intervention in relation to sexuality include 'growing up work', assertiveness training and managing sexualised behaviour therapeutically.

REFERENCES

Adams JA (1992) Significance of medical findings in suspected sexual abuse: moving towards consensus. *Journal of Child Sexual Abuse* **1(3)**: 91–99.

Alper K, Devinsky O, Perrine K, Vazquez B and Luciano D (1993) Nonepileptic seizures and childhood sexual and physical abuse. *Neurology* **43**: 1950–1953.

Aro H, Hanninen V and Paronen O (1989) Social support, life events and psychosomatic symptoms among 14–16 year-old adolescents. *Social Science and Medicine* **29(9)**: 1051–1056.

Bidwell RJ (1988) The gay and lesbian teen: a case of denied adolescence. *Journal of Pediatric Health Care* **2(1)**: 2–8.

Brown JD, Walsh Childers K and Waszak CS (1990) Television and adolescent sexuality. *Journal of Adolescent Health Care* **11(1)**: 62–70.

Campbell TA and Campbell DE (1990) Considering the adolescent's point of view: a marketing model for sex education. *Journal of Sex Education and Therapy* **16(3)**: 185–193.

Carrey NJ and Adams L (1992) How to deal with sexual acting-out on the child psychiatric inpatient ward. *Journal of Psychosocial Nursing* **33(5)**: 19–23.

Coleman E and Remafedi G (1989) Gay, lesbian, and bisexual adolescents: a critical challenge to counselors. *Journal of Counseling and Development* **68**: 36–37.

Dashiff CJ and Buchanan LA (1995) Menstrual attitudes among black and white premenarcheal girls. *Journal of Child and Adolescent Psychiatric Nursing* **8(3)**: 5–14.

DuVal Frost A (1984) The use of rock music to assist adolescent sexual identity. *Imprint* **31(4)**: 36–42.

Gillman R and Whitlock K (1989) Sexuality: a neglected component of child sexual abuse education and training. *Child Welfare* **LXVII(3)**: 317–329.

Great Ormond Street Hospital for Children NHS Trust (1995) *Child Protection Policy and Procedures*. London: Great Ormond Street Hospital.

Heras P (1992) Cultural considerations in the assessment and treatment of child sexual abuse. *Journal of Child Sexual Abuse* **1(3)**: 119–123.

Kienberger Jaudes P and Martone M (1992) Interdisciplinary evaluations of alleged sexual abuse cases. *Pediatrics* **89(6)**: 1164–1168.

Klopovich PM and Clancy BJ (1985) Sexuality and the adolescent with cancer. *Seminars in Oncology Nursing* **1(1)**: 42–48.

Langfeldt T (1993) Early childhood and juvenile sexuality, development and problems. *Nordisk Sexologi* **11(2)**: 78–100.

Lindon J and Nourse CA (1994) A multidimensional model of groupwork for adolescent girls who have been sexually abused. *Child Abuse and Neglect* **18(4)**: 341–348.

Lober Aquilino M and Ely J (1985) Parents and the sexuality of preschool children. *Pediatric Nursing* **January–February**: 41–46.

McGain B and McKinzey RK (1995) The efficacy of group treatment in sexually abused girls. *Child Abuse and Neglect* **19(9)**: 1157–1169.

Nelson MR (1995) Sexuality in childhood disability. *Physical Medicine and Rehabilitation* **9(2)**: 451–462.

Newcomer SF and Udry JR (1985) Parent–child communication and adolescent sexual behavior. *Family Planning Perspectives* **17(4)**: 169–174.

Ojwang SBO and Maggwa ABN (1991) Adolescent sexuality in Kenya. *East African Medical Journal* **68(2)**: 74–80.

Peterson LW, Hardin M and Nitsch MJ (1995) The use of children's drawings in the evaluation and treatment of child sexual, emotional, and physical abuse. *Archives of Family Medicine* **4(5)**: 445–452.

Piercy FP, Trepper T and Jurich J (1993) The role of family therapy in decreasing HIV high-risk behaviors among adolescents. *AIDS Education and Prevention* **5(1)**: 71–86.

Rappley M and Speare KH (1993) Initial evaluation and interview techniques for child sexual abuse. *Family Violence and Abusive Relationships* **20(2)**: 329–342.

Realmuto GM and Wescoe S (1992) Agreement among professionals about a child's sexual abuse status: interviews with sexually anatomically correct dolls as indicators of abuse. *Child Abuse and Neglect* **16**: 719–725.

Silovsky JF and Hembree-Kigin TL (1994) Family and group treatment for sexually abused children: a review. *Journal of Child Sexual Abuse* **3(3)**: 1–19.

Smith M (1993) Pediatric sexuality: promoting normal sexual development in children. *Nurse Practitioner* **18(8)**: 37–43.

Snegroff S (1995) Communicating about sexuality: a school/community program for parents and children. *Journal of Health Education* **26(1)**: 49–51.

Stern AE, Lynch DL, Oates RK, O'Toole BI and Cooney G

(1995) Self-esteem, depression, behaviour and family functioning in sexually abused children. *Journal of Child Psychology and Psychiatry* **36(6)**: 1077–1089.

Summit RC (1983) The child sexual abuse accommodation syndrome. *Child Abuse and Neglect* **7**: 177–193.

Tucker SK (1990) Adolescent patterns of communication about the menstrual cycle, sex, and contraception. *Journal of Pediatric Nursing* **5(6)**: 393–400.

Williams HA and Wilson ME (1989) Sexuality in children and adolescents with cancer: pediatric oncology nurses' attitudes and behaviors. *Journal of Pediatric Oncology Nursing* **6(4)**: 127–132.

Wolbert Burgess A, Hartman CR and Baker T (1995) Memory presentations of childhood sexual abuse. *Journal of Psychosocial Nursing* **33(9)**: 9–15.

GLOSSARY

Acting-out Demonstrating internal conflict through behaviours that are socially unacceptable or non-productive without acknowledging the underlying feelings.

Affect A pattern of behaviour that expresses an emotion. Common examples of affect include sadness, anger and elation. In contrast to mood, which refers to a more pervasive and sustained emotional 'climate', affect refers to more fluctuating changes in emotional 'weather'. Disturbances in affect include:

- *Blunted* Significant reduction in the intensity of emotional expression.

- *Flat* Absence or near absence of any signs of emotional expression.

- *Inappropriate* Discordance between affective expression and the content of speech or ideation (ideas or beliefs).

- *Labile* Repeated, rapid and abrupt changes in emotional expression.

Anxiety The apprehensive anticipation of future danger or misfortune accompanied by a feeling of dysphoria or somatic symptoms of tension.

Attachment Dependency needs of children that are focused on adults and are the foundations of relationships.

Behavioural therapy Aims to change behaviour by means of a method of reinforcement.

Boundaries This term may be used in various different contexts in mental health:

- *Ego boundaries* Boundaries that define the limits of an individual's personality. Poor ego boundaries would indicate that the individual has a poor sense of self.

- *Boundaries to behaviour* Limits of acceptable behaviour.

- *Family boundaries* Clear distinction between the roles of different family members, such as parents and children.

Cognitive therapy Aims to change beliefs and thought processes, which are handicapping the patient in some way, through a process of bringing them to the attention of the patient.

Communication deviance A measure of the degree to which an individual is unable to establish and maintain a shared focus of attention with a listener during verbal transactions.

Conversion symptom A loss of, or alteration in, motor or sensory functioning. The symptom cannot be explained fully by a neurological or general medical condition, and psychological factors are thought to be associated with development of the symptom.

Counter-transference The therapist's emotions and behaviour that occur in response to the patient's behaviour and emotions.

Defence mechanism Automatic psychological process that protects the individual against anxiety and from awareness of stressors or dangers. Examples include denial, splitting and projection.

Delusion A false belief that is firmly sustained despite what almost everyone else believes and despite evidence to the contrary. Types of delusion include:

- *Bizarre* A delusion that one's own culture would consider totally implausible.

- *Grandiose* A delusion of inflated worth, power, ability or knowledge, or of a special relationship with a famous person.

- *Persecutory* A belief that one, or someone with whom one is close, is being harassed, attacked or conspired against.

◆ *Somatic* A delusion pertaining to the functioning or appearance of one's body.

◆ *Thought broadcasting* The belief that one's thoughts are being broadcasted.

◆ *Thought insertion* The belief that one's thoughts are not one's own.

Desensitisation Schedule of treatment to replace anxiety with relaxation in the presence of anxiety-provoking stimuli.

Dissociation Cutting off the source of anxiety from conscious thought.

Ego The organised part of the mind; what may be called reason or common sense, in contrast to the id, which contains passions. The ego has been modified by the outside world. An analogy for the ego and id might be a person on horseback: the person (ego) has to hold in check the superior strength of the horse (id).

Enmeshment Lack of clear boundaries between family members which results in a lack of individuality between family members.

Ethnic origin Racial group.

Expressed emotion A measure of the extent to which one expresses highly critical and/or over-involved attitudes towards the identified patient.

Family dynamics Methods of interaction between family members.

Family therapy Treatment of the whole family which focuses on the family system rather than the identified patient.

Family dysfunction Patterns of family interaction that contribute to the development and/or maintenance of mental health problems.

Flashback The recurrence of a memory, feeling or perceptual experience of the past.

Free association Ideas that occur to one spontaneously.

Gender identity A person's inner conviction of being male or female.

Group work In this text, group work refers to the group psychotherapy that may be undertaken by a qualified nurse. This is in contrast to group psychoanalytical psychotherapy or art, drama, dance or music therapy, which require specific training.

Hallucination A sensory perception that has the compelling sense of reality of a true perception but that occurs without external sensory stimulation. Types of hallucination include:

◆ *Auditory* An hallucination involving sound, most commonly voices.

◆ *Visual* An hallucination involving sight, which may include images of people or flashes of light, and so on.

◆ *Somatic* The perception of a physical experience.

◆ *Tactile* The perception of being touched or of something being under one's skin.

◆ *Olfactory* An hallucination involving smell.

Illusion A misperception of an external stimulus.

Individual psychoanalytical psychotherapy Individual psychotherapy which includes psychoanalysis. The key defining concepts of psychoanalysis are free association, interpretation and transference. The patient is instructed and helped to associate freely, to interpret those associations and the obstacles he encounters in trying to do so, and to interpret his/her feelings towards the therapist. The rationale for psychoanalysis is that there is an unconscious part of the mind which the subject is unaware of, but which nevertheless influences his or her behaviour.

Individual work In this text, individual work refers to the individual psychotherapy that may be undertaken by a qualified nurse. This is in contrast to psychoanalytical psychotherapy, which requires specific training.

Internal conflict 'Internal' is frequently used as a synonym for 'psychical' (pertaining to the psyche) or 'mental'. 'Conflict' refers to opposition between incompatible forces. Therefore, internal conflict may occur between instinctual impulses, such as libidinal and aggressive impulses, or between parts, such as the ego and superego.

Internalised representation The mental representation of an object, such as one's mother. This may not represent reality.

Introjection The process by which an internal representaion of external objects, such as parents, is made. Introjection is a defence mechanism, in that it reduces separation anxiety, and a developmental process, in that it renders the person increasingly autonomous.

Key nurse Used in this text to describe an individual nurse designated to oversee the nursing care of an individual child during the course of treatment and to be the identified nurse with whom the child and family can communicate.

Limit-setting Making clear the expectations of acceptable behaviour and facilitating the maintenance of such behaviour by means of identifed strategies.

Milieu therapy The provision of a therapeutic environment, which aims to promote healthy change. Key components include stimulation, positive reinforcement, limit-setting, modelling of appropriate behaviour, and the encouragement of self-appraisal, which includes the nurse identifying transference and counter-transference.

Modelling Demonstrating desirable behaviour.

Mood A sustained emotional state. Examples include:
- *Dysphoric* An unpleasant mood such as sadness, anxiety or irritability.
- *Elevated* An exaggerated feeling of well-being, euphoria or elation.
- *Euthymic* Mood in the 'normal' range, which implies the absence of depression or mania.
- *Irritable* Easily annoyed and provoked to anger.

Nightmare Frightening dream occurring during the rapid eye movement (REM) stages of sleep.

Object As a psychoanalytical term, 'objects' refer to people, parts of people or symbols of either, towards which action or desire is directed.

Organic Concerning the physical structures of the body. Hence an organic disease is one where there is demonstrable physical abnormality of the parts or organs involved.

Parasomnia Events occurring during the non-REM stages of sleep (when there is absence of rapid eye movement), such as sleep-talking (somniloquy), sleep-walking (somnambulism) and sleep terrors (pavor nocturnus).

Phobia A persistent, irrational fear of a specific object, activity or situation that results in a compelling desire to avoid it.

Post-traumatic stress The psychological sequelae following a traumatic event, including flashbacks.

Problem-solving A cognitive technique to help the patient identify strategies to overcome problems.

Projection An unconscious defence mechanism. The individual rejects thoughts and feelings which are unacceptable and relocates them, attributing them to another person or object.

Psyche The mind.

Psychodynamic approach Using the concepts of intrapsychic and interpsychic processes to understand individual and group behaviour.

Psychogenic Of psychological origin.

Psychometric testing Assessment of intellectual capacity.

Psychomotor agitation Excessive motor activity associated with inner tension. The activity is usually non-productive and repetitive. Examples include pacing, fidgeting and wringing of hands.

Psychomotor retardation A slowing of movements and speech.

Psychopathology Pathology concerning the mind.

Psychosexual development Development of the mental aspects of sexual development.

Psychotherapy Any form of 'talking therapy'. It may be individual or group.

Psychotic Profound disorders of thinking, feeling and perception. Some definitions refer to the subject being out of touch with reality and having a lack of insight into the fact that he or she is ill.

Reframing Offering the patient alternative ways of interpreting behaviour, thoughts or feelings.

Sexuality The part of our personality that is concerned with being male or female. Sexuality includes gender identity, sexual orientation, sexual drives and behaviour.

Shaping behaviour A method of reinforcing behaviour which increasingly approximates that which is desired.

Sense of self The sense of who one is and an awareness of the boundaries between oneself and others.

Splitting A defence mechanism that typically aims to reduce the sense of confusion and feeling of unease associated with experiencing opposing emotions towards an object (see Object). These opposing emotions are projected into different objects, usually one being seen as 'good' and the other 'bad'.

Stressor External stimulus that induces stress. A psychosocial stressor would include any life event that could be associated with the onset of mental health problems.

Superego That part of the mind in which self-observation, self-criticism and other self-reflective activities develop, and in which parental introjects are located. It includes unconscious elements. Inhibitions emanating from it may be in conflict with present values (see Internal conflict).

Temperament A person's nature; it influences behaviour.

Transference Attributing one person's qualities to a separate individual and behaving towards that person as to the original.

Glossary definitions were partly informed by the following sources:

American Psychiatric Association (1994) *Diagnostic and Statistical Manual of Mental Disorders*, 4th edn (DSM IV). Washington, DC: American Psychiatric Association.

Ryecroft C (1995) *A Critical Dictionary of Psychoanalytical Terms.* London: Penguin.

Wilkinson TR (1983) *Child and Adolescent Psychiatric Nursing.* London: Blackwell Scientific Publications.

A HOME VISIT

**CHECKLIST FOR
HOME VISITS**

A home visit gives us additional information, from that obtained during meetings with the child and family at the hospital or clinic, about the child, family and their home environment. It can also serve a useful function in helping to prepare the child and family for admission to hospital.

It is preferable to ask all those who live at home to be present during the visit.

Check with other professionals in your team as to whether there are any specific areas that you should cover during your visit.

For safety reasons, always ensure that someone in your team knows the date and time of your visit and your expected time of return. It is advisable to make home visits with another colleague. Visiting in pairs also has the advantage of ensuring a more objective and thorough assessment.

INFORMATION ABOUT THE HOME ENVIRONMENT

◆ Description of the home

    Flat, house, maisonette or other

    Owned, rented or family squatting

    Size and number of bedrooms

    State of repair

    Style of decoration

    Tidy or disorganised

    Garden or back yard

    Does the child have their own bedroom or share with others?

◆ Description of the surrounding area

    Countryside or built up

    Cosmopolitan or essentially one ethnic group

    State of upkeep

    Transport facilities

    Other facilities, such as shops and entertainment

    Proximity to identified child's school

WHO LIVES IN THE HOME

    Parents

    Step-parents

    Siblings

    Step-siblings

    Grandparents

    Lodgers

    Other inhabitants

MEMBERS OF FAMILY PRESENT AT TIME OF VISIT

Who was present?

What was their reception to your visit?

What were they doing at the time of your visit?

Did they join the meeting and, if so, where did they chose to sit in relation to others?

How active a part did they take in the visit?

MEMBERS OF FAMILY ABSENT

Who was absent?

Why were they unable to be present?

CHILD'S UNDERSTANDING OF THE PROBLEM AND TREATMENT

Why does the child think that the parents have asked for help?

Why does the child think that he or she is being admitted to a psychiatric unit/paediatric ward?

What does child believe treatment will entail?

How does the child feel about it; what are their concerns and hopes?

PARENTS' UNDERSTANDING OF THE PROBLEM AND TREATMENT

How do the parents see the problem?

What do they understand about the admission?

What are their feelings about it, in particular in relation to psychiatry?

SIBLINGS' UNDERSTANDING OF THE PROBLEM AND TREATMENT

Why do the siblings think that the parents have asked for help?

Why do they think their brother/sister is being admitted to a psychiatric unit?

What do they believe treatment will entail?

How do they feel about it?

THE UNDERSTANDING OF OTHERS IN RELATION TO THE PROBLEM AND TREATMENT

As above (this might include school friends, others living at home, members of the extended family and so on).

PRACTICAL DIFFICULTIES

Does the family foresee any practical difficulties in relation to treatment, such as travel, time off work for parents, and so on?

What solutions did you all arrive at?

MAIN THEMES OF INTERVIEW

List the main topics covered.

FAMILY INTERACTION

How did individual family members interact with each other?

Did one family member take on the role of spokesperson?

Were there any clear alliances between particular family members?

A checklist of areas to cover in relation to admission may be helpful. For example, what to bring to hospital, giving the child a daily timetable of the unit, discussing unit policies, and so on.

B   SCHOOL VISIT

CHECKLIST FOR SCHOOL VISITS

A school visit gives us extra information to that obtained from telephone conversations and written reports. Furthermore, it is first-hand information.

The visit is important to help build a picture of the child's everyday environment and to help assess the appropriateness of the school for the child.

Parental permission should be obtained before arranging a school visit.

Do not try to obtain information about all of the following areas, but concentrate on those areas most relevant to the child. Before undertaking the visit, check with other professionals in your team and with the parents whether there are any specific areas about which you should enquire or whether there is any information that needs clarification.

FACTUAL INFORMATION ABOUT THE SCHOOL

Age range (primary, secondary, middle school, etc.)

Size, total number of pupils in the school, average class size

Co-educational or single sex

Size of the school site: is it a vast campus, split site (school housed on two different sites), etc.

Comprehensive school, grammar school, grant-maintained school, independent, religious school, special school, etc.

School uniform

Facilities for special educational needs

Facilities for pastoral support

Facilities for medical support

Standards of achievement, pupil expectations: is there an emphasis on academic work, lots of homework, common entrance exam, etc.

INFORMATION ABOUT THE SCHOOL ENVIRONMENT

State of the buildings: are they in good repair, nicely decorated, etc.

Facilities for technology, sports, science, languages, etc.

Aesthetic environment: is work displayed, are there plants, etc.

Sense of order: is there litter, graffiti, noise, children rushing about, etc.

General environment outside the school: is it isolated or close to an industrial estate, is it close to the pupil's home, what is the nature of the pupil's journey, etc.

INFORMATION ABOUT THE CHILD

Does the child attend regularly?

How does the child relate to peers and staff?

Is the child's behaviour manageable in school?

Does the child present illness symptoms in school?

What is the child's academic potential?

Is the child's progress consistent with his or her ability?

What is the child's attitude towards school work, is it completed in class, at home, on time?

Has the child been identified at any stage of the Code of Practice on the Identification and Assessment of Special Educational Needs (Department of Education, 1994)?

Is the school able to meet the child's special educational needs?

Has the school presented any personal or health problems in school?

Has the school tried to help the child; if so, how and with what success?

Does the school have a good working relationship with the child's parents?

NETWORKING INFORMATION

Establish and name a key contact person at the school who will coordinate liaison between the school, the parents and the hospital.

Find out the names and telephone numbers/addresses of relevant teachers and other professionals, for example the special educational needs coordinator (SENCO) at the school, the educational psychologist, the educational welfare officer, the classroom or welfare assistant involved, and the pupil assessment officer for the area.

School Checklist (Tate, 1991, updated 1997, unpublished), reproduced by kind permission of Anna Tate.

INDEX

Note that page numbers in **bold** refer to main discussion, those in *italics* refer to figures and tables